Total Sex

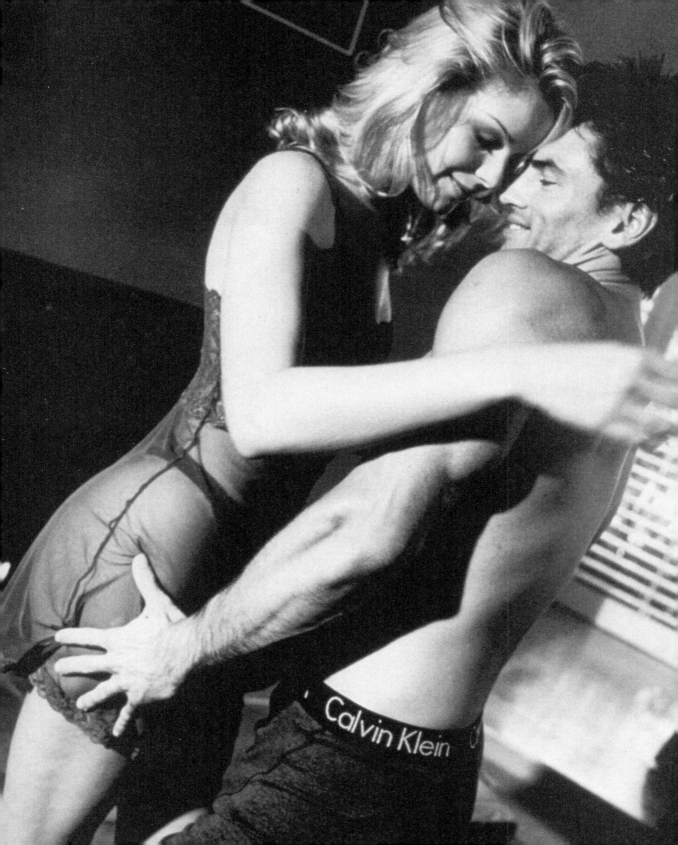

Total Sex

MEN'S FITNESS MAGAZINE'S
Complete Guide to Everything
Men Need to Know and
Want to Know
About Sex

Men's Fitness Magazine
with John and Beth Tomkiw
Produced by The Philip Lief Group, Inc.

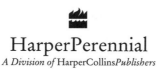

HarperPerennial
A Division of HarperCollinsPublishers

Illustrations page 29, 121, 122, 123, 124,125, 126, 229 by Richard Stodart.

TOTAL SEX. Copyright © 1999 by The Philip Lief Group, Inc. All rights reserved. Printed in the United States of America. No part of this book may be used or reproduced in any manner whatsoever without written permission except in the case of brief quotations embodied in critical articles and reviews. For information address HarperCollins*Publishers*, Inc., 10 East 53rd Street, New York, NY 10022.

HarperCollins books may be purchased for educational, business, or sales promotional use. For information, please write to: Special Markets Department, HarperCollins Publishers, Inc., 10 East 53rd Street, New York, New York 10022.

Designed by Elliott Beard

FIRST EDITION

ISBN 0–06–273629–9

Library of Congress Cataloging-in-Publication Data
     Tomkiw, John.
         Total sex : Men's fitness magazine's complete guide to everything men need to know and want to know about sex / Joe Weider's men's fitness magazine with John and Beth Tomkiw : produced by The Philip Lief Group. — 1st ed.
             p.   cm.
         Includes bibliographical references (p.) and index.
         ISBN 0–06–273629–9
         1. Sex instruction for men.   2. Men—Sexual behavior.   3. Sexual excitement.   4. Sex customs—United States.   I. Tomkiw, Beth.   II. Joe Weider's men's fitness.   III. Philip Lief Group.   IV. Title.
     HQ36.T66 1999   98–31338
         306.7—dc21   CIP

99 00 01 02 03 ❖/RRD 10 9 8 7 6 5 4 3 2 1

Contents

Chapter 6
Sexuality and Aging   180

Chapter 7
Troubleshooting   212

Chapter 8
Relationships or . . . What to Do
with All This Great Information   246

Chapter 9
Hot for the Long Haul   264

Chapter 10
Alternative Nation   280

Acknowledgments

The *Total Sex* team wish to thank the following people, all of whom have helped to make this book what it is:

Cris Bennett of *Men's Fitness* magazine

Dr. Patti Britton

Collin Brown

Paul Cates of the Lesbian and Gay Community Services Center

Celestial Seasonings

Dave, Dawn, and all the Couples Choice members

Cindy DeMarco of House of Whacks

Rose DeSorbo of the New York State Department of Economic Development

Melissa Elsmo

Christa Eskridge

John Gallagher, national correspondent for *The Advocate*

Michael I. Gold, Ph.D.

Nina Hartley

Jacquie Hughett of the Greater Miami Convention and Visitors' Bureau

Stanislaw Kindela

Marilyn Lawrence, Ed.D.

Pfizer

Candida Royalle of Femme Productions

The staff of Adam and Eve, Cupid's Treasures, Erotic Novelties, and Good Vibrations

Norio Sugawara of Sagami, Inc.

Tristan Taormino

Claire Elizabeth Tomkiw

. . . and all of our wonderful, experimental, and forthcoming friends.

This book is dedicated to the memory and work of Mary S. Calderone,
cofounder in 1964 and first president (1964–1982) of SIECUS,
the Sexuality Information and Education Council of the United States.
The mission of SIECUS is "to assure that all people . . . have the
right to affirm that sexuality is a natural and healthy part of life."

Advisory Board

Exercise Physiology

Bryant Stamford, Ph.D. Professor of allied health, School of Medicine, University of Louisville; director, Health Promotion Center, University of Louisville, Louisville, KY; author, *Fitness Without Exercise.*

Dan Wagman, Ph.D. Certified strength and conditioning specialist.

Infectious Diseases

Peter Katona, M.D., F.A.C.P. Director, UCLA Sexually Transmitted Diseases Clinic.

Nutrition

Jerzy Meduski, M.D., Ph.D. Specialist in nutritional biochemistry, president, Nutritional Consultants Group, Inc., Los Angeles.

Pharmacology

Jack M. Rosenberg, Pharm.D., Ph.D. Professor of pharmacology and pharmacy, Schwarz College of Pharmacy, Long Island University, Brooklyn, New York; director, International Drug Information Center.

Psychiatry

Mark Goulston, M.D. Assistant clinical professor of psychiatry, UCLA Neuropsychiatric Institute, Los Angeles; diplomate, American Board of Psychiatry and Neurology.

Andrew Slaby, M.D., Ph.D. Clinical professor of psychiatry, New York University and New York Medical College; specialist in stress management and depression in New York City; author, *60 Ways to Make Stress Work for You.*

Psychotherapy

Sylvia Cary, M.F.C.C. Specialist in addictive behavior; author, *Jolted Sober* and *The Alcoholic Man*; in private practice, Woodland Hills, CA.

Michael Gold, Ph.D., M.F.C.C. Author of *When Someone You Love Is in Therapy*; educator and psychological magic and comedy consultant on *M.A.S.H., St. Elsewhere, Cheers, and Frasier*; 30-year private practice in Beverly Hills.

Contributors

We'd like to gratefully acknowledge and thank all those writers whose articles, which first appeared in *Men's Fitness* magazine, are now used in this book:

James Benning, "The Chemistry of Love," October 1997.

Mark Caldwell, "A Shiver Runs Through It," February 1994; "Fishing off the Company Pier," January 1996.

Sylvia Cary, "Constant Cravings," October 1997.

Michael Castleman, "A Skeptic's Guide to Aphrodisiacs," August 1995; "Lust for Life," December 1996; "Coming Cures," February 1997, "Rock of Ages," March 1996; "Hold Your Fire," September 1996.

Todd Coleman, "Betrayed," October 1996.

Kevin Cook, "Tales from the Crib," November 1996.

Rosemary Daniell, "Is Tough Sexy?" March 1996.

Ginger Darren, "Tough Love," November 1995.

J. Spencer Dreischarf, "Blue Bowling Balls," October 1996.

Sam Dunn, "In-law and Order," June 1996.

Joel Engel, "Terminal Sex," August 1996.

Lee Frank, "Burning Rubber," February 1994.

T. Jesse Goff, "The Rules for Men," March 1997.

Dan Greenberg, "Porn Again," February 1995.

Scott Hays, "Trial of the Century," January 1996.

Paul Karon, "Sexual Healing," February 1997.

Steve Mirsky, "Babe Watch," January 1997.

Steve Mockus, "Sole Mates," January 1998.

Cal Orey, "End Game," August 1997.

Kermit Pattison, "Split Decisions," July 1997.

Joan Price, "The Birds and the Bees," March 1998; "What Is Love? What Is Lust?" March 1998; "A Little Romance," March 1998; "If Women Are from Venus, No Wonder Men Want Satellite Dishes," March 1998.

Ellen Rapp, "Clitoral Translations," February 1995; "A Different Kind of Fitness," February 1996.

Matthew Segal, "Stag Coach," April 1997.

Marc Spiegler, "Meet Market," February 1997.

Michael Szymanski, "Love and Lust and Everything in Between," March 1998.

Beth Tomkiw, "One Woman's Sex Tips," September 1997; "Marathon Men," February 1997; "The Swing Set," June 1997; "Hot for the Long Haul," February 1997.

Louanne Cole Weston, "Talking Bed," September 1997; "Build a Better Orgasm," April 1996.

Foreword

The book you hold in your hands, *Total Sex*, is one of the most unique publications of its kind. The statement may sound hyperbolic, as if it's been dreamed up as some hard sell (pun intended) by yet another marketing whiz. But it's not. Let me explain.

Since attending an international conference of sexologists held in Mexico City in 1979, I've read more books on sexuality than any man should have to read in three lifetimes. It's a chore for most of us to get through one book on sexuality, let alone dozens. However, the intervening years have made something painfully clear: While there have been many excellent tomes published during the last two decades, most are laborious, and often pedantic, and their authors generally assume a ten-foot-pole distance from the subject to give them a sense of clinical authority. That's cool with me, but more often than not these titles don't speak directly to the man in the street, the guy in the real world. *Total Sex* does! Which means that not only do you get crucial, state-of-the-art information, but it's delivered in the language of real people . . . and that includes dirty talk, political incorrectness, euphemism, and ballsy humor to let you know that sex, though serious, must be fun!

While working on my license to become a marriage-family-couples counselor, I inadvertently ended up working with a lot of guys for extended periods of time. This surprised me, since men and therapy generally mate like water and oil. After a lot of soul-searching, I finally came to a couple of conclusions: (1) If you talk to men like men, they'll listen, understand, and integrate the information; and (2) despite the so-called sexual revolution of the sixties and seventies, men (and women) still seek answers and solutions to one of life's most important concerns: What makes great sex?

At *Men's Fitness* magazine, we are broadening the meaning of fitness. Sure, physical fitness is crucial to your sense of well-being, but so are career and financial fitness, and of course, sexual fitness. Since a monthly magazine can rarely cover everything it wants to in depth, this book, *Total Sex*, allows us to bring our energies, talents, and resources to the arena of sex. And I believe we have succeeded. I know you'll agree.

One final note: I wish to thank John and Beth Tomkiw, the husband-and-wife team who authored this book. Bringing together a vast amount of information into a cohesive package while maintaining a sense of real-world language was no easy task, but they carried it off magnificently, managing in the process to sustain the spirit of *Men's Fitness* magazine from first page to last. Thanks guys.

Jerry Kindela
editor in chief
Men's Fitness *magazine*

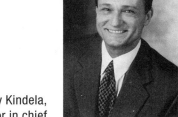

Jerry Kindela,
editor in chief

Total Sex

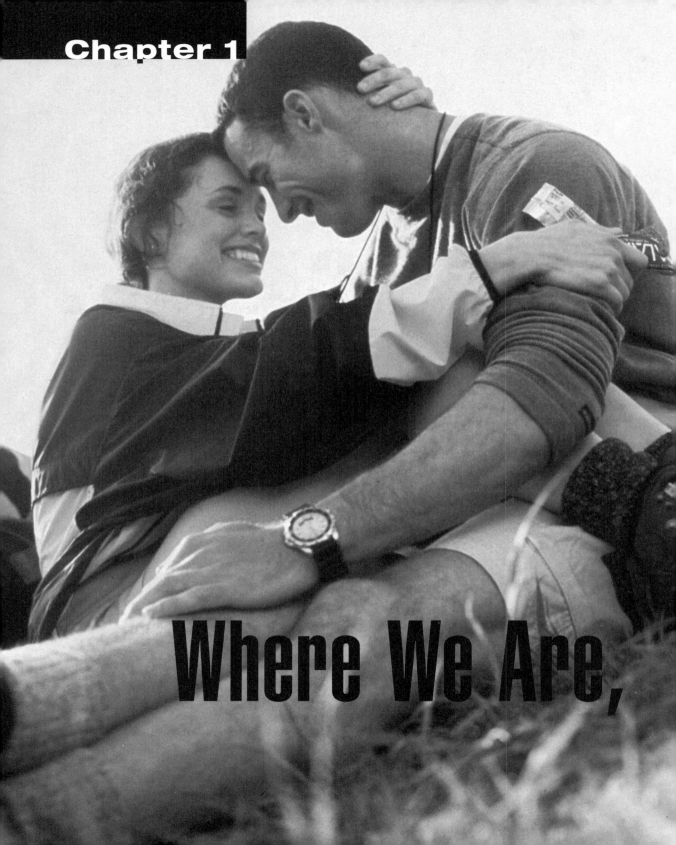

Chapter 1

Where We Are,

The horizontal mambo. Knocking boots. Making the beast with two backs. Bumping uglies. Riding the baloney pony. Taking the skin dolphin to tuna town.

We certainly like our euphemisms for sex. Maybe it's because we, as a nation, aren't all that comfortable talking about it. Sure, we can engage in the typical locker-room banter—"Man! You should've seen this chick go down on me!"—but create a meaningful dialogue about sex? It ain't in our nature. That's why there's a plethora of call-in sex talk shows, on the radio and on television. These shows allow us to remain relatively anonymous—as callers seeking specific information and as just plain listeners, looking for tips or a little entertainment.

Blame it on the birth of a nation. Ours is one steeped in puritanical zeal, based in large part on religious tenets. That's not to say that our founding fathers ignored the demands of the flesh (old Ben Franklin was a notorious ladies' man), or that religion and sex are mutually exclusive (ask the Mormons), just that sex has always been the convenient whipping boy for society's ills in a nation based on "God-fearing" attributes. Up to and including the fifties, good girls didn't —creating the notion that sex was bad or dirty, something you didn't engage in if you cared about your place in the community. In the sixties, however, free love reigned—and the "Establishment" derided those who engaged in it as a threat to national security.

Here's the rationale: *Hippies had sex; and hippies were "Commie pinkos." And since Commies were the antithesis of stolid American virtue, people openly having sex were un-American.*

Okay, so that's a bit of a stretch . . . but not by much. And have matters really changed much since then? Maybe not. Viagra's a perfect example. When *Men's Fitness* magazine queried several members of the clergy, the message was clear: The little blue pill was a Godsend for putting the wood back into the lives of married men, but only for married men. If you're a single guy with erectile problems, well, too bad, because sex outside the conjugal bed is still prohibited by most religions. Who's living in the real world, considering that one billion of those little blue tablets were estimated to have been sold by the end of 1998—in limited international release?

Americans have always been a bit repressed about sex, even after the sixties started changing these attitudes. In the seventies, we could laugh at the "wink-wink" double entendres of *Three's Company,* tittering at the situations set up by a straight Jack Tripper pretending he was gay so he could room with two comely girls. But the laughter was at the expense of gays, who at the time weren't politicized and out. And the jokes were weak attempts by a broadcasting network to tie into a nation's curiosity about sex.

Still, the seventies signaled a sexual revolution of sorts. *Playboy* magazine heralded a new age with an entire philosophy built on sex and hedonism.

Where We're Going

Although the Playboy lifestyle was coveted by many men (as well as a fair share of women), it wasn't until the middle of the decade that the real underpinnings of the "Me decade" took hold—and people became more open sexually. The Pill also accelerated this openness—both men and women felt freer in their sexual pursuits.

Just in time for AIDS.

No other phenomenon has affected our culture so pervasively. And unfortunately, certain religious forces in the early eighties used the disease as a means of accelerating their agenda. Once again, sex was bad—it could kill you—and those engaging in it outside the bounds of marriage were "incurring God's wrath." Luckily, collective cooler heads prevailed, and the misinformation fomented by the Moral Majority and the religious Right was scientifically dismissed. AIDS was not God's wrath, but a disease affecting a variety of populations. Sure, it could be transmitted sexually, but it wasn't designed by a higher being to wipe out a particular group.

If anything, AIDS made a nation aware. And afraid. The hedonism of the seventies and eighties have given way to a more cautious time. And, given the current political climate, when a casual comment may be construed as sexual harassment, it may be difficult for men to feel as confident sexually as in decades past.

That's where this book comes in. *Total Sex* is meant as a calm voice, dispensing clearheaded information and wisdom from a variety of sources—acclaimed counselors and sex therapists, the medical community and real couples. In these pages, you'll find valuable information to assist you in your quest to know everything about sex—everything from general anatomy, physiology, and body chemistry to sexually transmitted diseases, what to expect when you age and the more kinky aspects of the sexual experience. And positions. Lots of positions. What's more, we've provided all this information—and more—in a lighthearted manner, avoiding the clinical tone taken in many books on sexuality. After all, sex should encompass a complete range of emotions. Laughter included.

Percentages, Percentages

Before we can really delve into all things sexual, we need to get a proper perspective on what men are thinking. And for that, we went straight to the source. You.

We at *Men's Fitness* magazine recently commissioned Applied Research-West, Inc. to conduct a sex survey of our readership. Five thousand, four hundred and forty-seven of you red-blooded (or shall we say hot-blooded?) American males responded . . . and the answers to our questions were eye-opening, forthright and—ultimately—an accurate snapshot of our times.

Here's a general makeup of respondents: An overwhelming 71.2 percent of survey participants were 35 years old or younger; 36 percent were 18 to 25, while 35.2 percent were 26 to 35. A little over 18 percent were 36 to 45—then the numbers dropped off considerably, with 7.7 percent aged 46 to 55 and just 2.9 percent aged 56 or older. Now, that's not to say that older gents don't participate in sex surveys—and participate in sex! (Witness the discussion on sexuality and aging in chapter 6.) It's just that the age bracket more closely fits the demographic of *Men's Fitness'* readership.

Forty-four percent of respondents lived in suburban areas, while 36.7 percent lived in what they termed a large city. Only 19.3 percent lived in rural areas.

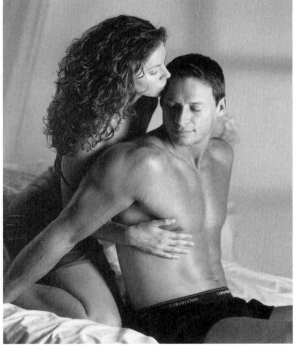

Of the respondents, 36.2 percent said they were married, whereas 32.1 percent said they were single. Monogamy struck a chord with the survey participants, as 20.5 percent mentioned they are in a monogamous relationship. Slightly more than 6 percent were cohabiting (the PC word for shackin' up), while 4.9 percent said they were separated or divorced. Sixty-three percent of respondents had children.

The Goods

Okay, that's the lay of the land, so to speak. Now on to the good stuff. When asked at what age they first have sexual intercourse, 40.8 percent mentioned they were between the ages of 15 and 17—adding credence to the plotlines of all those teen sex-romp movies. Surprisingly, 12.6 percent were 14 or younger. A little over 32 percent were between the ages of 18 and 20 when the Big Event occurred, while 9.9 percent were 21 to 25, and 1.7 percent were between the ages of 26 and 29.

Interestingly, 2.4 percent of the respondents have yet to experience sexual intercourse. There could be a variety of reasons, such as not finding the right partner or the fear of sexually transmitted diseases. In fact, a current fear of such diseases may be what drives another interesting statistic from the survey: 59.2 percent of respondents never would participate in sex with nonmonogamous partners. Apparently, the end of the nineties is about togetherness and longevity, since only 5.6 percent mentioned they frequently have sex with nonmonogamous partners.

While on the subject of "the deed," 38.3 percent of survey participants said they typically have sex two or more times a week. The next highest total: 14.6 percent said they have sex two or more times a month, followed by 14 percent who make the beast with two backs once a week. A sad note: 10.7 percent claim they have sex only a few times a year, while 5.2 percent never have sex. (Here a message to those guys. Read this book. Cover to cover. Chapter by chapter. Then get out there!)

> "... the end of the nineties is about togetherness and longevity, since only 5.6 percent mentioned they frequently have sex with nonmonogamous partners."

When asked about the number of sex partners survey participants have had in their lifetime, quality seems to reign over quantity. In rank order the top selection was two to five partners (29.9 percent), followed by six to ten (a considerably less 17.6 percent).

Braggarts Need Not Apply

Of the guys having sex, honesty seems to be an underlying trait. No bragging rights or raging machismo here. Witness: 51.6 percent rated their own sexual technique as "adequate." Not earth-shaking or world-ending, but adequate. What's more, 65.3 percent thought their penis size was average (56.9 percent thought the average penis was six inches). And, when asked to rate their ability to meet their partner's emotional needs during sex, 45.2 percent of respondents felt they were—again—adequate. Not above average, but adequate.

This means there's room for improvement. Other numbers bore this theory out. For example, 15.4 percent felt their sexual technique was below average, while 16.6 percent felt they were below average in meeting their partner's emotional needs during sex. Again: Read this book. Cover to cover. Chapter by chapter. Then get out there!

Or perhaps it's your partners who should be reading this book. Only 6.9 percent of survey respondents said that their partners initiated sex; 42.2 percent said they have to get the ball rolling, so to speak. So, there's room for improvement on both sides.

Spanking the Monkey

Regarding the topic of masturbation, 29.2 percent of survey participants said they masturbate two or more times a week, while 12.3 percent showed remarkable restraint, citing that they never masturbate at all. On the flip side of the restraint scale, 11.8 percent said they crank the frank at least once a day; 5.1 percent were randier, claiming they had spunk sessions twice or more a day. However, survey respondents mentioned that when they have sex regularly, they masturbate less frequently or not at all. Makes sense.

A Sign of the Times

Perhaps the most eye-opening survey result centered on relationships. When asked to rank items in terms of importance in maintaining a relationship, survey participants ranked their partner's occupation and income as the most important thing to them. Not their shared interests or pastimes—that came in second. Or the partner's sense of humor—that came in fourth. Or the partner's intelligence, for that matter (that came in sixth). We're glad to see that physical appearance isn't that important—it ranked seventh—but it seems judging a person by their occupation and income is just as shallow as the age-old "judging a book by its cover." Sadly, friendship and companionship ranked dead last. As Jerry Maguire said: "We live in a cynical, cynical world."

> "... survey respondents mentioned that when they have sex regularly, they masturbate less frequently or not at all. Makes sense."

Chapter 7 sheds some additional light on the occupation and income drive as it relates to younger men. The good news: As men mature, their value systems shift. They seek out different types of relationships. Relationships built on friendship and common interests. On like-minded beliefs. On passion and sexuality. We intend this book to be a guide for those men—and all men—who want more out of life, more out of their sexuality and more out of their inherent maleness. Ultimately, this book is meant as a different type of eye-opener. It's one that shows men new ways of doing things—new ways of thinking—to create better sex, better relationships, and better health. Read on.

> "When asked to rank items in terms of importance in maintaining a relationship, survey participants ranked their partner's occupation and income as the most important thing to them."

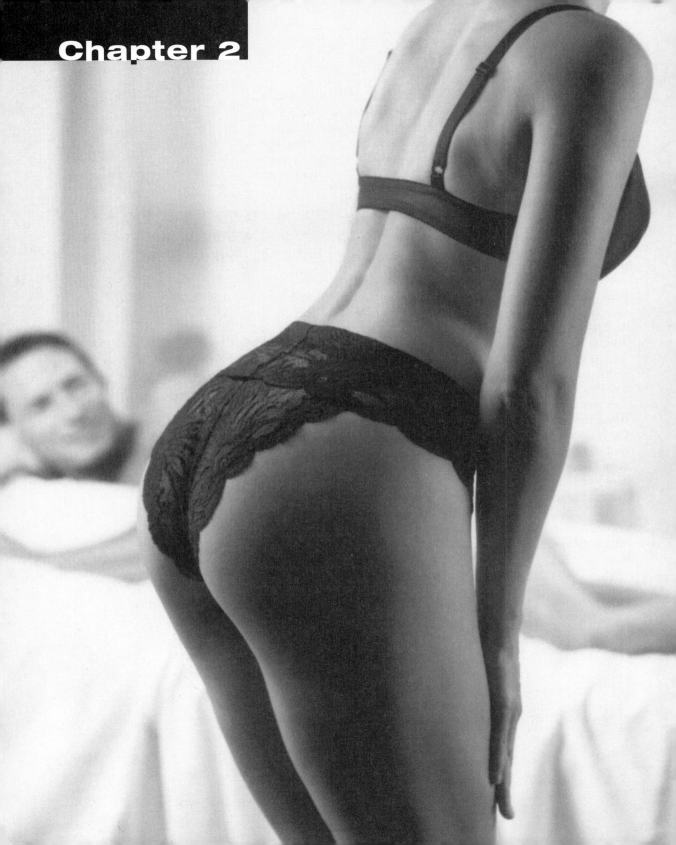

Chapter 2

hen was the last time you looked at your genitals? If you're like most adult males, you probably haven't taken a really close look since you were a kid—and that's completely normal, considering how uptight Americans are when it comes to sexuality. We're not encouraged to touch our "privates"—never mind explore them. But doing both is really an essential first step toward enhancing sexual pleasure. The more you understand your anatomy—and hers—the more fun you'll both have, in the bedroom, the kitchen, the bathroom, wherever.

So we begin our book with a little Sexual Anatomy 101. Here, you'll find the full scoop on the male and female genitalia, how they differ and how they're alike. We suggest grabbing a hand mirror. Though we offer some great diagrams, it's important for you to get up close and personal with yourself and your lover.

His Story
The Penis

No matter how hard you try, you can't miss this organ—especially when you're aroused. Watch a hard-bodied babe in a thong bikini pass by on the beach and the wrinkly, flaccid fellow could go full-mast in a matter of seconds. It's called an erection, a

boner if you will, but there are really no bones—or even muscles—in the penis. Blood vessels, and three long cylinders of erectile tissue, two on the back forming the *corpora cavernosa* and one on the front forming the *corpus spongiosum*, run down the length (or shaft) of the penis. When the penis is flaccid, these tissue fibers are contracted. During arousal, they relax to let more blood in. When fully engorged, the penis becomes erect.

The most sensitive part of the penis, rich in nerve endings, is the head or *glans*, particularly the *corona*, a ridge of flesh that connects the glans to the shaft of the penis, and the *frenulum,* a strip of flesh on the underside of the corona. When you ejaculate (or pass urine from the bladder), it travels through the *urethra* to the *urethral opening* at the tip of the glans.

The loose skin that covers the penis is called the *foreskin.* Hold your penis in your hand and notice how easily the foreskin slides over the shaft of your penis. At birth, the foreskin covers the glans and is retractable. When a boy (or man) is circumcised, the loose skin is cut off, exposing the glans.

Our best advice: Spend some time exploring your penis, alone and with your partner, to see which parts are the most sensitive to stimulation. And don't worry about size. It has no impact on virility or fertility. As many as 98 percent of all men fall within the normal range—two to four inches flaccid and

Body Talk

five to seven inches erect. Those on the small side grow proportionally larger, some even doubling in length when erect. Regardless, most women we spoke with said they'd run scared if you dropped your pants and revealed one of those Johnny Holmes 12-inchers. And if it makes you feel better, man does have (proportionally) the largest penis of all primates. Or, to paraphrase human anthropologist Dr. Desmond Morris: "We're apes with oversize dicks."

An Inside Job: Testicles, Scrotum, Prostate, and More

There's a reason why *testicles* are referred to as the "family jewels"—they're the glands that produce that priceless stuff called testosterone and sperm. The former fuels your sex drive and is responsible for the muscles, body hair, and other characteristics that make you recognizably male. The sperm, your reproductive material, enables you to multiply.

Size-wise, testicles (a.k.a. *gonads*) can vary greatly, from marble-sized to egg-sized. But on average, each weighs about 22 grams, and measures about two inches long by one inch wide. One usually hangs lower than the other, and they are situated inside the *scrotum*. This sac of skin beneath the penis protects the testicles from injury and extreme temperatures, which could inhibit sperm production. The optimum temperature for producing sperm is 8 degrees centigrade below normal body temperature. Next time you jump into a cold swimming pool, or start messing around with your girlfriend, notice how the muscles of your scrotum kick into gear, relaxing or contracting to keep the testicles at an ideal warming distance from your body.

Go with the Flow

Sperm follows a definitive route on its way out of your body, starting at the production site—the *semniferous tubules*. There are as many as a thousand of these tubules in each testicle and all create sperm nonstop, nourishing each one for more than a month in *Sertoli* (or nurse) *cells* attached to the lining of the tubules. Once the sperm gets its needed nourishment, it's released into the *epididymis*, a coil of tubing at the back of each testicle that's as long as a garden hose when straightened out. There, the sperm matures and is stored until its ready to pass through the *vas deferens* to the *semi-*

The penis is the primary sex organ responsible for male pleasure. But then we didn't need to tell you that.

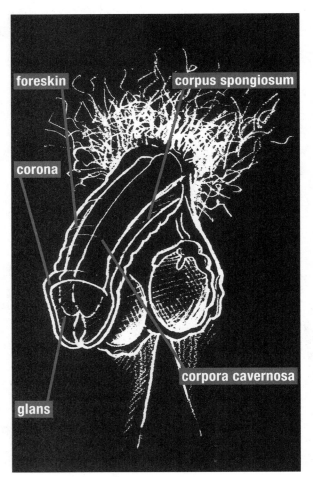

foreskin

corpus spongiosum

corona

corpora cavernosa

glans

nal vesicles. The latter produce semen, the sticky fluid that protects the sperm, playing the role of conductive medium as it exits the penis during ejaculation. Semen travels from the seminal vesicles through the *prostate gland* via the *ejaculatory ducts*. Most guys think of the prostate as that scary, cancer-prone part of their anatomy, but the role it plays in the sexual process is crucial. In addition to producing extra seminal fluid, the prostate squeezes shut the urethral duct to the bladder. This trick prevents urine from mixing with the semen during ejaculation, thus ensuring the essential pH balance necessary to keep sperm alive. The *Cowper's glands* also protect sperm by secreting a small amount of pre-ejaculate fluid into the urethra prior to orgasm. This fluid neutralizes the acidity that remains after you "drain the vein."

To give you an idea of how efficient this system is, healthy men produce sperm constantly throughout their lives, and release an average of 200 to 400 million sperm with each ejaculation. Each testicle is capable of producing nearly 150 million sperm every 24 hours. Note to all of you marathon men: if you come more than twice a day, it can take from five to seven days to replenish that "average" supply. That may not matter—unless you're trying to have children, in which case you should flip to chapter 6: Sexuality and Aging.

The Long and Short, and Thick and Thin, of It

If you've been hung up on your penis size since the first time you dropped trousers in the junior-high locker room, we'd like to say once again—get over it. A study conducted at the University of California–San Francisco by Dr. Tom Lue proved that most men fall within the normal size range—two to four inches flaccid and five to seven inches erect. Working with sixty men at ("Excuse me, may I measure

The portions of the male genitals illustrated here work behind the scenes, producing sperm and testosterone—the stuff that makes men men.

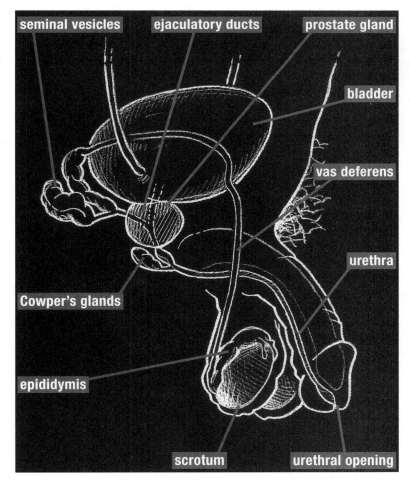

seminal vesicles

ejaculatory ducts

prostate gland

bladder

vas deferens

urethra

Cowper's glands

epididymis

scrotum

urethral opening

your member?") random, Lue found that the average flaccid penis was 3.5 inches long and 3.9 inches in circumference. Those stats jumped to 5.1 inches long and 4.9 inches in circumference during an erection.

If you absolutely must know where you fall on the charts, go ahead and measure your penis. According to Dr. Harold Reed, director of Reed Center for Ambulatory Urological Surgery in Bay Harbor, Florida, this is how it's done:

"As many as 98 percent of all men fall within the normal [penis size] range—two to four inches flaccid and five to seven inches erect. Those on the small side grow proportionally larger, some even doubling in length when erect."

While standing, get an erection. Gently angle your equipment down until it's parallel to the floor. Set your ruler against your pubic bone just above the base of the penis, and measure to the tip. (To get the most accurate reading, do not push the ruler into the skin on the pubic bone. There's a fatty pad there called the *mons pubis,* which could alter your measurement when depressed. And yes, measuring your unit from the underside will increase the numbers, but that's cheating.)

Of Knives and Men

There, are you happy? If not, you could always opt to have your penis enlarged. There are a couple of surgeries currently performed to increase penis size—ligament transections and fat injections. The first involves knives, the second needles, and both will drain your bank account to the tune of $4,000 to $7,000.

Still game? With the ligament transection, a razor-sharp knife (did we mention that it's really, really sharp?) is used to cut the suspensory ligament that secures the base of the penis to the body. You get about one-half to two inches of extra manmeat to work with; however, your penis will no longer be anchored to your body, so your erection will point forward, probably downward, rather than to the sky. Chances are, most women won't notice that change. But they will notice the pubic hair growing on top of your newly lengthened penis.

". . . if it makes you feel better, man does have (proportionally) the largest penis of all primates. Or, to paraphrase human anthropologist Dr. Desmond Morris: 'We're apes with oversize dicks.'"

As far as we're concerned, getting fat injected into the penis is off the gross-out charts. Here's how this "solution" works: Fat, removed from another part of your body—say your spare tire or your third chin—is injected under the skin of the penis shaft to make it thicker. Many doctors argue that the thickness of your gear—not the length—has the greatest impact on your ability to sexually satisfy a woman, an opinion supported by the late, great Alfred C. Kinsey's research. Apparently, Dr. Kinsey probed women with cotton swabs to determine their vaginal sensitivity. Fewer than 14 percent of his subjects could tell when the deep walls of their vagina were stimulated, but 97 percent of them could easily tell when their vulva and vaginal openings were probed.

Though we doubt a Q-Tip would stir the green-eyed monster in any man, we can understand the thickness issue. A plumper penis may indeed feel better to her. But for you, getting injections from your chubby chin to achieve a chubby has some serious side effects. Because the body absorbs a large portion of the injected fat, the procedure may have to be repeated several times. (That means more needles.) There's also reduced shaft sensitivity, a high risk of infection and, when all is said and done, you could end up with a lumpy dick. Yes, the injections can clump—and we guarantee women will notice that!

". . . healthy men produce sperm constantly throughout their lives, and release an average of 200 to 400 million sperm with each ejaculation."

How does the medical community feel about these procedures? Lue, the urologist who conducted the penis-size study we mentioned earlier, is not a fan. He was quoted in a medical trade publication saying, "I can save these patients a lot of money. I'll put their penis on a desk and whack it with a hammer. It will swell for about six months and then go down. They'll get the same results with fat injections."

In fact, only a handful of urologists throughout the country are willing to perform either of the penis-enlarging procedures, leading us to believe that most of Lue's colleagues share his sentiments; the Society for the Study of Impotence

"As far as we're concerned, getting fat injected into the penis [to increase its size] is off the gross-out charts."

has gone so far as to issue a statement warning that the procedures have not been proven safe or effective, and should be regarded as experimental. (Sorry, guys. That means no insurance coverage.)

Pump It Up

If you're still feeling inadequate, you may want to try a penis pump. This tubular vacuum device slips over your erection, pumping out the air and causing gravity to increase blood flow to the erectile tissue. The result: a bigger, firmer boner. Penis vacuums also come with small, circular rings that are placed where the shaft meets your body to hold the blood in place. The dangers: the ring can damage your urethra. Plus, overuse of the pump can cause chronic swelling and it can interfere with your ability to have a natural erection.

Our advice? See a therapist. If you're willing to go to such great lengths—so to speak—to increase the size of your penis, your problem may be bigger than merely having tiny equipment.

> "The Society for the Study of Impotence has gone so far as to issue a statement warning that the procedures [to enlarge the penis] have not been proven safe or effective, and should be regarded as experimental."

Another solution: Stay away from the hot fudge sundaes. As you gain weight, you also gain girth in an area at the base of the penis called the *prepubic panniculus*. For every 35 pounds above your ideal weight, you effectively lose an inch of penile length due to fat encroaching on the shaft. In other words, the leaner you are, the more effectively you can use your God-given tool—and the longer it looks.

Circumcision: Another Squeamish Subject

Chances are you didn't have much say about whether or not to have your foreskin removed. And chances are it's gone, because circumcisions used to be as routine as holding a newly born baby upside down and slapping him on his bottom. But that's changing.

For Jews and Muslims, the surgery has been performed for thousands of years as a religious ritual. But for Americans, it didn't become routine until the late 1800s, at which time prudish physicians claimed that removing the foreskin would inhibit masturbation, which they believed led to epilepsy, tuberculosis, and even insanity. Doctors in the forties debunked that theory (thank God), but still recommended a circumcision as a hygienic alternative with a variety of medical benefits—from preventing urinary tract infections to halting the spread of sexually transmitted diseases and cancer. Thirty years later, the American Academy of Pediatrics issued a statement saying there's no medical reason for routine circumcision. But in 1989, it had second thoughts, claiming that a task force found "reason to believe that the tissue that grows over the glans is predisposed to infection." The Academy cited a study showing uncircumcised infants have a ten times greater risk of urinary tract infections. And, Dr. James Roberts of Tulane University found that an intact foreskin provides an ideal growth area for P-fimbriated E. Coli, bacteria that quickly colonizes under the foreskin and then travels up the urethra, causing kidney infections.

Further, medical studies have shown that circumcision may contribute to a lifelong prevention of penile cancer. In the United States, there are approximately one thousand cases of penile carcinoma reported per year, which puts the risk to uncircumcised individuals at 1 in 600. There continue to be a number of loud voices opposing routine

Girl Talk

Sizing It Up

The experts agree that size of a man's member doesn't matter, but we wanted to give women a chance to speak for themselves. Here's what they had to say about one of the oldest questions to plague man since Adam and Eve dropped their fig leaves: Does size really matter?

"It's kind of like Goldilocks and the three bears: Too big and too small are a problem. I was once with a very well-endowed guy. While this size had its charms, I really felt like he was poking my spleen or something. Also, while I wouldn't mind if my husband was a tiny bit bigger, I would never in a million years let him know that. He gets the job done just fine."
—Jennifer, 28, married

"Size is just an added bonus if the guy is already responsive and aware. I need to be turned on by his creativity. If he's sexually athletic, and we're both totally into each other, size doesn't really matter. However, if he moves too fast and is focused on his own pleasure, whatever his size, it won't be fulfilling."
—Kelly, 34, single

"Size only matters in the extreme. Generally, if we're speaking about pleasure, I think thickness matters more than length. I've been with guys who were an inch or two above or below the average length, and I could never really feel much of a difference. Of course, size is not as much of an issue as how a man uses his penis. And let's not forget stamina. I don't want him drifting off to dreamland when I've only just begun!"
—Mindy, 28, single

"First, the bad news: Of course it matters. And the good news: The range of acceptable sizes is relatively large. The bottom line is that small (and I'm talking tiny) is horrible. It's hard to overcome your extreme embarrassment for the guy. Trust me, I saw one of these once . . . and then it was over. Too big is scary and uncomfortable, too. You find yourself wondering if his picture is on a porn video box in some dimly lit back room of a video store. It's like really large breasts on a woman—you can't help but stare, though you don't necessarily find it appealing."
—Sue, 28, single

"Not in the way most men think. For example, bigger is not better, it's just painful. I'd say the best size is average. What's way more important is how well he pays attention to my preferences. I like to see if he pays attention to, and remembers, where I like to be touched, in what way, and for how long. It shows an appreciation of sharing the moment, not just getting in, getting what you want, and getting out."
—Christine, 30, single

"No, as long as it's within what the medical community calls 'normal limits,' which probably includes about 99 percent of the male population. Men should keep in mind that length is pretty much irrelevant; if any dimension is important, girth would be it. The longest one I ever had a firsthand experience with was pretty much wasted because its owner was uninspired (and uninspiring) and lazy. There's something to be said for trying harder. As someone once sang, "It ain't the meat, it's the motion.""
—Miriam, 29, divorced, long-time cohabitator

circumcision, and the person with the largest forum may be Dean Edel, a respected medical doctor with a national health- and medicine-based radio program. Edel routinely stresses that the science in this area is still not solid enough to recommend wholesale cutting of a male's penis. Even the American Academy of Pediatrics has not come up with outright support for the practice. The last paragraph of its *Report of the Task Force on Circumcision* cautions, "Newborn circumcision has potential medical benefits and advantages as well as disadvantages and risks. When circumcision is being considered, the benefits and risks should be explained to the parents and informed consent obtained."

Today, the majority of infant boys are still circumcised, but the percentages have dropped significantly. Whereas 90 percent of American baby boys were circumcised in the eighties, according to the National Center of Health Statistics, that number has fallen to 59 percent. Partly responsible for these reduced statistics are vocal opponents, who argue that 85 percent of the world population is uncircumcised, with few related health problems. These anticircumcision crusaders also note that the foreskin is rich in nerve endings and removing it diminishes sexual pleasure during intercourse.

"Whereas 90 percent of American baby boys were circumcised in the eighties, according to the National Center of Health Statistics, that number has fallen to 59 percent."

And then there's the pain issue.

Many parents and medical professionals "pooh-pooh" the notion that a child will remember anything that occurs so early in life. But according to a report in *American Baby*, a new study conducted by Canadian researchers suggests that early instances of pain do indeed have long-lasting effects.

The study involved 87 baby boys 20 days old or younger, who were divided into three groups. The members of the first group were circumcised after being treated with a topical anesthetic cream. The second group of boys was circumcised with no anesthetic. And the third group was uncircumcised. Four to six months later researchers revisited the babies and recorded their reactions as they received routine vaccinations. Boys who were circumcised without anesthesia showed a much greater response to pain than their counterparts. The uncircumcised babies showed the least pain response of all.

"The study demonstrates that pain experienced in the newborn period can affect pain behavior later on," says study leader Dr. Anna Taddio, of the Hospital for Sick Children in Toronto.

The best thing new parents can do is consider the options *before* the baby is born. Once delivery day arrives, there's not a lot of opportunity for discussion and it's not a decision that should be made in lightly or in haste. And if you opt against the circumcision, be sure to practice proper hygiene and pass the need for it on to your son.

When Boys Become Men

A circumcision—or the lack of one—doesn't have to be permanent. There are steps you can take to alter the choice that was made for you. Thousands of men, for example, are taking steps to restore their bodies to a natural state with a process called "foreskin restoration." Sometimes it involves surgery—skin grafts, for example—to replace the foreskin. But it can also be done in a do-it-yourself manner with tape and weights that stretch the skin remaining on the penis.

In an article in *Sexlife* magazine, R. Wayne Griffith, cofounder and director of the National Organization of Restoring Men, recounted the steps he took to restore his foreskin and says the effort was worth it. "The glans is an internal organ . . . like the inside of the mouth or the vagina. The corona of the glans, with the movement of the foreskin over it, is the most pleasurable of sensations that I didn't know existed most of my life."

For more information on how you can go about restoring your foreskin, pick up a copy of the 1995 book by Dr. Jim Bigelow titled *The Joy of Uncircumcising!* or contact NORM at 510-827-4077.

Adult Circumcision: One Man's Story

Some men also opt to be circumcised as adults. "Allowing a man to approach my penis with a razor-sharp instrument was not a decision I took lightly," said Mike, a Chicago-based advertising executive. "But, in the end, getting circumcised when I was 19 years old was a necessity."

As a first-generation American, Mike endured a number of suspect traditions handed down from his Eastern European ancestors, the most life-changing of which was the belief that circumcision made a person less worthy. "Frankly, my father—and his father before him—thought circumcision was something only Jewish people did . . . and there was a significant anti-Semitic sentiment in my father's adamant proclamation that no son of his was to be circumcised," Mike said. "My father proudly talked of arguing with the nursing staff at the hospital about it, and how 'he had won.'"

Still, for all his father's posturing, Mike said no real hygienic education took place in his household. "My father thought only lesser people got circumcised, but he never really did anything to ensure that I learned proper cleaning procedures to lessen the risk of infection," he said. "So, from an early age, I was left to figure out things for myself. Worse yet, my father didn't realize that—unlike the old country—the majority of men in America are circumcised. . . . I felt like an oddity in the grade school locker room."

As Mike reached puberty, things worsened. He unknowingly suffered from phimosis, a condition that affects about 10 percent of all males in which the foreskin is overly tight, adhering to the glans it covers. "As I began to discover myself sexually, I found there was a very significant problem . . . if my foreskin was retracted when my penis was flaccid, the resulting erection would be unbearably painful," Mike said. "It was almost like tying off the head of my penis with a rubber band—my penis was so blood-engorged that it swelled to freakish proportions, and the only way to reduce the pain was to stop the arousal process. Try that as a horny teenager—no amount of thinking about baseball is going to help when you're at a girl's house and her parents are away. The only way to solve this was to keep the foreskin covered over my penis during the initial phases of the erection, so the head of my penis was covered. It took all spontaneity out of sex . . . imagine a woman drumming her fingers along the headboard, waiting for you to reposition yourself."

Covering the penis head with his foreskin presented another problem—bacteria—which led to a series of urinary tract infections. "It was almost like clockwork," Mike said. "I'd experiment with a girl—a quick romp, oral sex, whatever—and a few weeks later I'd be doubled over in pain. The real ridiculous thing about my situation was that it went on for *years*. It was only after I went to a new family practice practitioner—outside the realm of my parents' approved list of Slavic physicians, did I find a final solution to my persistent urinary tract infections."

Not that hearing a doctor talk of snipping at your penis was a welcome solution. "I must admit that I was really nervous when the doctor began talking about circumcision as a treatment option," Mike said. "I was in college at the time, so I did what any college student would do . . . I basically ran to the library and immersed myself in research." He soon found that adult circumcision is a common procedure, often used for the very maladies Mike faced. "During what I called my research phase, I was really blown away by some of the articles I found that documented cases of guys undergoing the surgery for aesthetic reasons," Mike said. "Sure, I was different in the locker room or in the shower at the gym, but if there wasn't a medical reason for someone to whack at you, why do it?

"What I did find, however, was that men were incredibly curious about the procedure. When I told some of my friends that I was considering the surgery, the reaction was always the same: they would mock-wince in a macho kind of way . . . then draw closer for all the 'gory details.' It's as if their circumcisions happened to them at such a young age that they didn't get some sort of experience out of it."

Mike checked into a hospital for the procedure, though his doctor mentioned that the surgery, in some cases, could be done on an outpatient basis. Prior to the procedure, his public hair was trimmed back. Then he was taken to the surgical suite.

"I remember being wheeled into the room, where I was transferred to an operating table. The nurse casually lifted my gown and swabbed my groin down with antiseptic. Then the realization sunk in—a resident spread my legs and strapped each one down to the table with a restraint." Mike's doctor said this minimized risk of an involuntary spasm hampering the surgery. "That's when I really realized that someone was going to go at me with a scalpel . . . and that there were significant consequences if there was a slip," Mike said.

The surgery required general anesthetic, and Mike soon found himself fighting sleep. "I remember feeling people touching my groin . . . then I drifted off," he said.

He awoke with a start. He was back in his room, his hospital gown back in place. Tentatively, he looked down. And . . . there it was. His penis, the head swathed in gauze. Then his doctor came in and slowly unwrapped the gauze. "He was brutally honest with me," Mike said. "He mentioned that my penis would look decidedly different right after the surgery. . . . I think he even used the word Frankenstein." With good cause, it turned out, because the surgeon resected the tight portion of the foreskin, slicing fully around the penis. Then, he reattached the two looser pieces of skin together. The resultant penis shaft had dissolvable stitches ringing it.

"First, it felt really numb," Mike said. "Then the pain set in." Despite the soreness, he was released the next day, with a handful of painkillers and a regimen of nightly warm-water baths to ease the swelling and discomfort. Gradually, the swelling subsided, the incisions healed, and the stitches dissolved. Then came the big test.

"I consciously tried to avoid any stimulating materials for the first few weeks after the surgery, because I was afraid of the consequences," Mike said. "I had visions of stitches popping everywhere. But after two weeks, I was so stir-crazy that even the mother on old *Who's the Boss?* reruns began looking sexy to me. So I went out. Got a handful of porno magazines and went to my room to see if 'things were all right.' I'll forever remember that first post-surgery erection, how I sat there dumbfounded, not knowing what to expect. And how different I looked. But since then, I haven't experienced another infection." Or another woman drumming her fingers along the headboard.

Her Story
The Vulva

What the penis is to a man, the *vulva* is to a woman—the external sexual organ. A woman's vulva consists of several parts. The *mons veneris*, Latin for "Hill of Venus," the Roman goddess of love, is a sex-

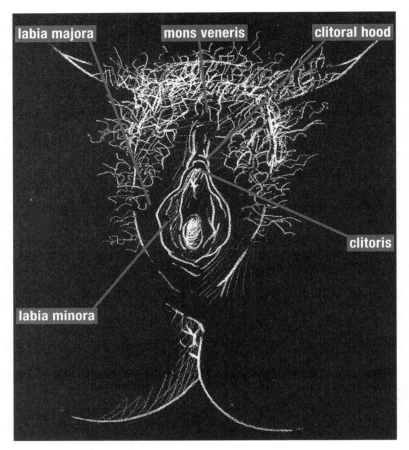

labia majora

mons veneris

clitoral hood

clitoris

labia minora

Vulva. We love the way that word just rolls off the tongue. We also love the way it responds to the tongue. The vulva, after all, is the external portion of the female genitalia containing the clitoris, a button of nerves dedicated exclusively to sexual pleasure. Get to know it . . . well.

ually sensitive pad of fatty tissue that covers the pubic bone, protecting it from the impact of sexual intercourse. The outer lips of the vulva are called the *labia majora*. These pads of fatty tissue are usually covered with pubic hair, contain numerous sweat and oil glands, and give off a scent that some feel is sexually arousing. Within the labia majora are the *labia minora*. Thin stretches of tissue that protect the vagina, urethra, and clitoris, the labia minora vary widely in appearance from tiny lips that hide behind the labia majora to large ones that protrude. Both the inner and outer labia are highly sensitive to touch and pressure.

Even more sensitive is the *clitoris*. This small, white mass of spongy tissue, located between the top of the labia majora and the *clitoral hood,* often extends during arousal, making it more accessible. There are several similarities between the clitoris and the penis. As pointed out in the *Lovers' Guide Encyclopedia*, "both were formed from the same lump of tissue in the embryo, the head and shaft of the clitoris and the penis are made up of sensory tissue, the small head of the clitoris and the glans of the penis contain the same number of nerve endings and their size and shape are no indication of their capacity to give or receive sensuous pleasure." In fact, the clitoris ranges from very small to quite large—and doubles in size during arousal. If you've ever seen a Vanessa Del Rio porn flick, you'll understand how lengthy this organ can become. If not, imagine a flesh-toned, French-style greenbean. (We should note that a severely enlarged clitoris is often one of the side effects of taking testosterone and anabolic steroids.)

That's what the clit and penis have in common. Where they differ is functionality. Whereas the penis does double duty as a passage way for urine, the clitoris exists exclusively for sexual pleasure. Plus men become aroused quickly and noticeably. For women, it's a gradual process and the visible signs are much more subtle.

**"If you've ever seen a Vanessa Del Rio porn flick, you'll understand how lengthy [the clitoris] can become.
If not, imagine a flesh-toned, French-style greenbean."**

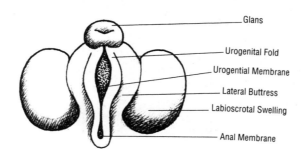

Glans
Urogenital Fold
Urogential Membrane
Lateral Buttress
Labioscrotal Swelling
Anal Membrane

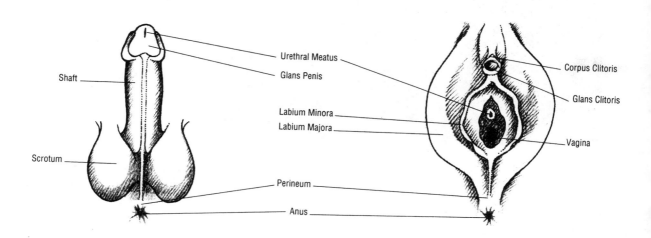

Shaft
Scrotum

Urethral Meatus
Glans Penis
Labium Minora
Labium Majora
Perineum
Anus

Corpus Clitoris
Glans Clitoris
Vagina

Fetal Genitalia: San Francisco sex therapist Patti Britton said we are sexual beings from cradle to grave. We'd like to amend that: We're sexual beings from about four to seven weeks of gestation. That's when the fetus's external genitalia begin transforming from the gender-neutral structure (pictured top) to male or female specific. The glans becomes either the penis (bottom left) or the clitoris (bottom right). The urogenital membrane ultimately develops into the urethra and the labioscrotal swelling forms either the scrotum (male) or the labia (female).

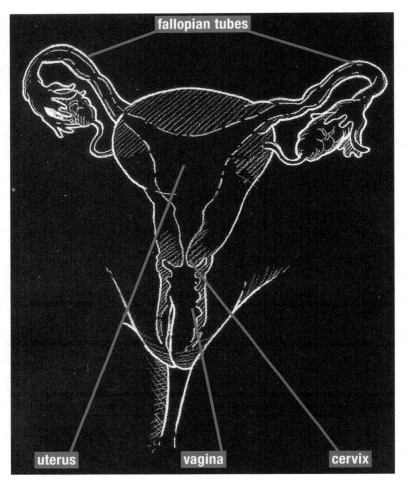

fallopian tubes

uterus

vagina

cervix

The vagina is a long muscular canal that connects a woman's uterus to her external genitals. Nerve endings concentrated at the opening of this organ provide significant sexual pleasure.

The Vagina

The vulva, labia majora and minora, and the clitoris are the female sex organs that meet the eye. But as with men, there's a lot that goes on behind the scenes.

Take that old telltale sign of virginity—the *hymen*. This membrane, which is present at birth, partially covers the vaginal opening (located just below the urethra). Though an intact hymen is a symbol of purity—a sign that a woman has never done the deed—it's so thin that it can easily "bust" during a vigorous round of *Buns of Steel* or when a tampon is inserted. So if your bride claims virginal status, but you discover her hymen isn't intact, cut her some slack. She was probably working out extra hard to please you.

Beyond the hymen is the *vagina*, a muscular, tubelike passageway that leads from the vulva to the *cervix*. As Kinsey's research with the Q-Tips indicates, the nerve endings in the vagina appear to be concentrated near the opening of the organ, with sensitivity decreasing as you get closer to the cervix. But beyond its role in providing sexual pleasure, the vagina is the path sperm take to enter the *uterus* and *fallopian tubes* to fertilize an egg, as well as the way out for menstrual fluid and a baby.

There are two types of muscle in the vagina. The smooth muscle within the vaginal wall relaxes and stretches involuntarily during sexual intercourse. It's these muscles that give credence to the claim that penis size doesn't matter; they'll expand and contract to accommodate any man. The muscle fibers surrounding the outer third of the

"Though an intact hymen is a symbol of purity—a sign that a woman has never done the deed—it's so thin that it can easily 'bust' during a vigorous round of *Buns of Steel* or when a tampon is inserted."

vagina are controllable, allowing a woman to grip the penis by tensing the pelvic floor muscles. During childbirth, the latter muscles are often damaged, but can be repaired through an exercise called the Kegel (explained in chapter 7: Troubleshooting).

"The smooth muscle within the vaginal wall relaxes and stretches involuntarily during sexual intercourse. It's these muscles that give credence to the claim that penis size doesn't matter; they'll expand and contract to accommodate any man."

You've probably noticed that when a woman is sexually aroused, the vagina produces a fluid that varies in thickness, stickiness, scent, and color, depending upon where she is in her menstrual cycle. Aside from serving as a natural lubricant, this fluid also aids sperm into the cervix when a woman is most fertile. (It becomes thin, clear, and super stretchy at that time of month—the ideal swimming conditions. If you're planning to have a child—or not—you can use this fluid as a guide.)

If you've felt the cervix, chances are you also heard a painful "youch" from your partner when it happened. This organ tends to move up and back, out of harm's way, during arousal, but sometimes can come in contact with your penis (during an especially deep thrust). Though reaching this spot may make you feel extra manly, it's not a technique you should attempt to perfect. The cervix is tender. When jabbed, it can hurt—whether a woman tells you so or not.

The Hot Zones
Learning to Touch

"Ultimately, the whole body is an erogenous zone," says Collin Brown, director of The Body Electric, an Oakland, California, school that offers classes and retreats for couples and individuals interested in enhancing their sexuality. "In our culture we tend to focus on the genitals and the nipples, forgetting that there are all these other erotic pleasure points."

If you want to really turn on a woman, for example, you should consider massaging her feet. "It's one of the most sensitive parts of a woman's body," Brown says. "But to know this, you have to be willing to explore."

There we go again. Exploring the body. It sounds so obvious, but few of us conduct tip-to-toe touch tests with our partners to see what feels great. It's not our fault. We've been conditioned to zero in on those spots that

We call them the hot zones—sensitive spots on the body that are great focal points during foreplay. Run your fingers lightly over her abdomen, then let her indulge you. It's the beginning of the dance.

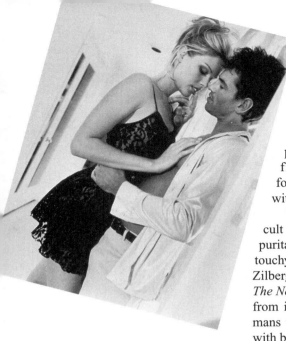

we know will get a response, and appreciate the sexual experience partly for its efficiency.

But what if you could slow down the lovemaking process —keep that average fifteen-minute romp going for hours? It's possible and has a payoff, according to Brown. You and your partner will enjoy a more intimate relationship. You'll have firmer erections and your orgasms will be more powerful. But before any of that happens, you need to become better acquainted with your own body and what you like.

To do this, you have to be willing to touch—which can be difficult for many Americans. After all, we're carrying some significant puritanical baggage. Our forefathers didn't exactly encourage a touchy-feely society. Males, in particular, suffer from what Dr. Bernie Zilbergeld calls "sensory starvation—a lack of nonsexual touching." In *The New Male Sexuality*, he points out that touch is a vital human need, from infancy through old age. It's been proven that animals and humans who miss out on comforting touch early in life often grow up with both serious physical and emotional problems. Yet parents still are afraid that too much affectionate touching—or "mothering"—will turn boys into sissies, writes Zilbergeld. "Physical contact is acceptable only in sports, in roughhousing and in sex."

The Art of Self-pleasure

Well guys, it's time to move on. Forget everything you learned from your parents about touching and sex. It's a new day. An opportunity to start fresh and travel light—without the baggage.

The first thing on the agenda? Touch *yourself*.

Yup. The experts agree: You'll become a more sexually satisfied guy if you learn to masturbate. Okay, so you've probably spanked the monkey on at least a couple of occasions. But we're not talking about some quick and quiet session in the bathroom over a copy of *Penthouse* magazine.

As cornball as it sounds, you need to learn to have a loving relationship with yourself. Take a warm bath or shower, run your hands gently (or not so gently) over your body. All over your body. Or when you're dry, elevate the senses with lotions, oils, or even cornstarch, suggests Brown. "Cornstarch has a silky, sensuous feel against dry skin. Every brush of the finger feels incredible." The point is to gain a better understanding of how things feel—behind the ears, at the nape of the neck, along the back of your thighs. If you become aroused, satisfy yourself. But this exploration can take place without going anywhere near the penis.

In fact, when you bring your partner in on the fun, Brown recommends that the two of you intentionally avoid the genitals. "In order to discover the other pleasure points of the body, you have to get past the obvious," he says.

Brown calls one great couples exercise Conscious Breathing. "Lie on the floor, breathing deeply in and out, so you're fully aware of the movement. The longer you work at your breathing, and learn to feel the rhythm of your body, the more you'll appreciate the heightened sensitivity."

"The longer you work at your breathing, and learn to feel the rhythm of your body, the more you'll appreciate the heightened sensitivity."

When you're ready to start exploring your pleasure points, Brown suggests looking at sex toys. Get a catalog like the one offered by San Francisco's Good Vibrations. "Don't buy anything right away; you need to use your hands, lips and tongue first. But see what's out there."

Brown also recommends instructional videos. "I'm personally not a fan of porno movies; they tend to desensitize sex. But I think the videos that take a conscious, more how-to approach to the experience can be extremely helpful."

And, of course, you have to talk. "The conversation is all important," Brown says. "If you're uncomfortable with the mere idea of something, say anal stimulation, you need to be able to communicate that, and your partner must appreciate that you've drawn a line.

"Opening your mind to new things is a huge step toward enhancing your sex life. But you and your partner need to agree up front that if something feels bad, you can say 'stop' at any time."

Fun with Fingers and Toes

Instead of just dispensing advice, we thought we'd give you some starting points. Everyone has their preferences when it comes to being touched, but there are some common (nongenital) areas of the human body that, when stimulated, can lead to arousal. Taking it from the top, the list includes:

- **The face:** Your mouth, cheeks, eyebrows, temples all respond to light touch and gentle kisses.

- **The ears:** Blowing softly into the ear, or licking the earlobe gently, can be a major turn-on for some men and women.

- **The neck and shoulders:** This highly sensitive area responds extremely well to kissing, licking, light touch, soft nibbling, and gentle massage.

- **The armpits, arms, and insides of the elbows:** Most of us don't think of our armpits as a sexual body part, but you need only run a finger in a circular movement there to know how tingly terrific it can feel. Likewise, the arms—particularly the forearms—can feel awesome when kissed, licked, and touched. Be aware, though, that this can be a ticklish zone for some.

- **The breasts:** We don't have to explain much here. Men love women's breasts. Women love men's pecs. Men's nipples are highly sensitive; women's are even more so. In fact, some fortunate females can reach orgasm via nipple stimulation alone. You can tweak them, kiss them, suck them. Have a blast. But be gentle. And don't worry, we'll discuss this subject in greater detail later.

- **Abdomen:** You need only look at the cover of men's and women's fitness magazines to know that washboard abs are a major turn-on these days. But whether yours are rock-hard or sensuously soft, they'll respond to touch. Go slowly. This area, too, tends to be ticklish.

Girl Talk

Pubic Hair: Point/Counterpoint

In researching this book, I was interested to learn that some cultures believe pubic hair provides insights into a woman's sexual demeanor: Stubborn women, they claim, tend to have black, feathery pubic hair. Generous women have brown, gold-tinted hair and women with thick, bushy hair are passionate. So what does a shaved bush say about a woman? It says that she's willing to go to great lengths to please her partner. For some reason, guys are turned on by the bald or semibald look. A quick glimpse through girlie magazines proves this point. But this isn't fun—and anyone who says it is a liar. Sure, I occasionally trim the jungle, but I do this for the same reason I wear clean underwear—to avoid being embarrassed by my extra-long tresses in emergency situations. But to agree to a total shave. I say, "No thank you." Aside from it being kind of creepy in a prepubescent way, it's a hassle and a pain. If you think women take long to get ready for dates now, prepare for an even longer wait. Going bald would add at least an extra half-hour to the average woman's daily routine. And we would have to shave our pubic hair daily, because it itches like hell growing back. And that's the tolerable part. Let me ask you this, boys: if you had hair on the shaft of their penis, would you shave it off? I think not. The thought of running a razor over Mr. Happy is probably sending shivers down your spine. So think about the sensitive spots that might get nicked by our Bics. And don't bother with that "How do you know you won't like it, if you're not willing to try it" crap? Let's just say its a gut instinct. After all, I don't have to eat cockroaches to know they probably wouldn't make my favorite foods list.

—B.T.

B.T. needs to lighten up. Sure, it's uncomfortable to let pubic hair grow back. And it's time-consuming to shave it daily. But if it heightens the sexual experience, I say go for it. My boyfriend and I shave each other's pubes. It's fun and sensual. And it's a great way to gain trust in your partner. What better way to show your faith in a lover than to let them take a razor to your genitals.

—Bernie, 25, beautician, San Diego.

- **The hands:** Nothing like a hand massage to elicit moans and groans of pleasure. The fingertips and palms are especially sensitive to firm, yet gentle touch.
- **The back:** Women primarily respond to kissing, touching, and massaging this area. Exploring the base of a woman's spine can be particularly arousing.
- **Buttocks:** Kiss them. Lick them. Knead them gently. You'll get a great reaction. Take our word.
- **The legs:** As much as women complain about their thighs, they're a source of great pleasure. Thin or thunderous, they respond to fingertip touching, kissing—the gamut. Men aren't particularly sensitive in this area, unfortunately.
- **The feet:** Another area where massage works wonders. Give a woman a foot massage and she'll doing anything for you. Well, almost anything. Rub a man's toes and he's yours—at least for the night.

The Seriously Hot Spots

Once you discover your more unexpected pleasure points, you're ready to move on to more familiar territory. Although we've already discussed the anatomy of the genitals, it's time to talk about them in terms of pleasure. There's no doubt, for example, that a man's penis and a woman's clitoris have the most erotic potential. But other areas of the genitalia can also feel exquisite to the touch.

The *prostate,* sometimes referred to as the "male G-spot," for example, is surrounded by numerous nerve bundles, making it one of the most erotically charged parts of the male body. Unfortunately, many guys never get to experience the organ's sexual potential because it requires stimulation of the *anus.* "Men tend to associate sexual pleasure derived from the anal area with homosexuality. It's hard for them to get past that," says Brown. "There's this massive taboo with the anus, which makes no sense.

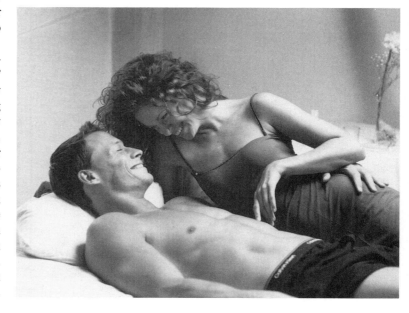

We've been evolving for millions of years, and still have hundreds of highly pleasurable nerve endings there. Why should we deny that?"

We shouldn't. But if you're uncomfortable with anal penetration, you should know that the organ can be stimulated internally as well as externally. For internal adventurers, we suggest that your partner insert a lubricated finger (protected by a latex glove, if you wish) into your anus (also lubricated). Have her press her finger toward the front of your body. She'll know she's reached the prostate if she feels a firm (chestnut-sized) lump. Massaging it gently may very well lead to orgasm.

> **"There's this massive taboo with the anus, which makes no sense. We've been evolving for millions of years, and still have hundreds of highly pleasurable nerve endings there. Why should we deny that?"**
> **—Collin Brown, director of The Body Electric**

If you prefer to sample the pleasures of the prostate from the outside, ask your partner to press the base of her thumb into your perineum, the spot between the scrotum and the anus. Taoists called the perineum "the Gate of Life and Death" for its role in preventing male ejaculation. According to Mantak Chia and Douglas Abrams Arava, authors of *The Multi-Orgasmic Man*, pushing on the perineum when you're about to come can stop the ejaculatory reflex. Pushing on it during arousal squeezes more blood into your penis, making it throb pleasurably.

Some guys love this, others find it uncomfortable. Either way, the perineum responds best to stimulation when you're fully erect and highly aroused. If your partner is exploring the spot, but you're not feeling anything, move on to other areas and come back.

The "female G-spot" requires a little more effort to locate. This erogenous zone made major headlines back in the early eighties with the publication of *The G-Spot and Other Recent Discoveries about Human Sexuality* by Drs. Alice Ladus, Beverly Whipple, and John Perry. (The "G" in G-spot is actually short for Grafenberg, the German obstetrician who first described the erotic trigger back in the forties.) Reportedly, the G-spot can be

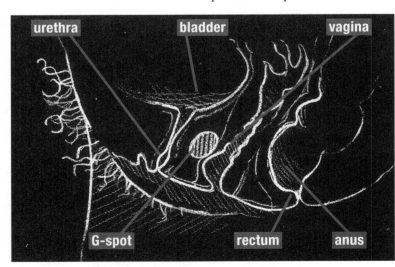

urethra   bladder   vagina

G-spot   rectum   anus

The G-spot

Searching for Hidden Treasure

If you're determined to find that elusive G-spot, San Francisco sex therapist Patti Britton says to try these two techniques:

Feel Your Way

Have your partner lie down on a bed (or floor) with some pillows under her hips. With her legs spread as wide as possible and her bottom slightly elevated off the pillow, straddle her torso, facing her feet, and support most of your body weight on your knees. Slowly and gently, stimulate her clitoris until she's aroused. Then slip two fingers into her vagina, keeping your hand palm-side up so your fingertips can brush against the front, top part of her vaginal wall. If she has a G-spot, you'll feel a small knob of firm flesh about the size of a bean or two. As you stimulate her bean (or two), don't be surprised if she goes wild and gushes fluid. Many women say orgasms stimulated from the G-spot are more consuming than clitoral orgasms.

Get Into Position

You can attempt to stimulate the G-spot through proper intercourse positions, too. The woman-on-top positions and nearly all rear-entry ones tend to work the best, as they allow the head of your penis to contact the vaginal wall.

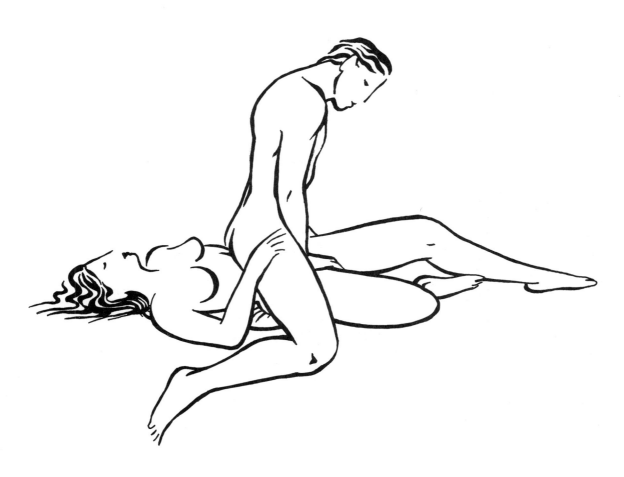

found about two inches beyond the vaginal opening, just behind the front upper wall.

Women who know it's there claim the G-spot can produce incredible orgasms that feel different from ones resulting from clitoral stimulation. They also claim to "ejaculate" a clear fluid during a G-spot climax. But even with the help of diligent partners, many women are unable to find their G-spot, making them wonder if it exists at all.

Consequently, controversy over the existence of the G-spot has many medical professionals divided. On one hand, there are physicians, psychologists, and sex therapists who feel it's nothing more than wishful thinking—a push-button option that appeals to our quick-fix society, yet has no real scientific backup. In fact, if the renowned research of Kinsey holds up, the interior walls of the vagina aren't supposed to have much feeling at all. Remember the cotton swab survey?

Ladas, Whipple, and Perry claim that the women in Kinsey's study showed minimal reaction because the G-spot responds best to firm, deep continuous pressure. It's tough to find, they claim, because the size of the G-spot varies considerably among women. Plus it has to be stimulated properly to really be felt. Then, they say, it can swell to dime or even silver-dollar proportions.

Our take: It doesn't hurt to try to find your partner's G-spot, as long as you go about the quest knowing that you might turn up empty-handed. There's no clear-cut proof that the G-spot exists, so don't be disappointed. Have fun.

Breasts

Breasts aren't just an erogenous zone—they're a worldwide obsession. Why else would Russ Meyer have sustained an entire career based on making movies starring women who consider a D cup flat-chested? And why else would the massive, uh, thespian talents of Pamela Anderson Lee captivate legions of testosterone-addled youngsters?

> **"Breasts aren't just an erogenous zone—they're a worldwide obsession."**

Ironically, breasts seem to be more of an erogenous zone for men (who suckle, lick, squeeze, and kiss them) than they are for women—according to various sex surveys, only a small percentage of women actually find their breasts a source of sexual stimulation. Still, the breasts play an important role in mating rituals, as the areolas (the darker, raised circular area surrounding the nipple) and the nipples themselves flush with blood during periods of excitement. They, in turn, swell, giving the woman's sexual partner the outward indicator that the woman is aroused. Either that, or the room is too cold.

While the breasts aren't often a source of sexual excitement for women, they certainly are for men. And because of that, women tend to allow men to fixate on their breasts in and out of the bedroom.

The advent of such technological advancements as the breast implant (just look at any B movie or something from the current crop of pornos) has increased men's adoration of these mounds of mammary. Even though breast implants significantly dull a woman's breast sensation, women continue to flock to such procedures, in part because breasts are tied to a woman's self-esteem, and in part because women realize an erogenous zone doesn't necessarily have to be erogenous to them.

Of course, we mustn't forget to mention the female breasts' life-sustaining function. Men may love to fondle them, women may love to dress them up, but to infants, they're lunch. And we're not talking about the average boxed variety. It's truly amazing to learn that a mother's breast milk is uniquely designed for her child. As the baby's nutritional needs change, so too does their mother's milk. And it's loaded with antibodies that prevent a host of ailments, from ear infections to allergies. So the moral of this story, guys: If you love breasts as a single man, you'll love them even more when you're a dad. They're miraculous. (And they can get pretty bodacious when nursing, too!)

The Chemistry of Lust

After a hard day's work, you're looking forward to a relaxing evening with your girlfriend. You'll get a bite to eat, agree to a couple hours of Chick TV, and fantasize about the great sex you'll have later on.

In theory, it's a foolproof plan. But, before you can flip on *Ally McBeal,* it happens. You say something—whatever it is, it's the wrong thing—and now the two of you are headlong into an argument. It must be her time of the month, right? Maybe.

Before you check her calendar, though, consider this: It might not have been her hormones that ran amok; it could have been yours. Studies show that men's testosterone levels fluctuate every 15 to 20 minutes and may have a profound effect on behavior. If yours were running high at that moment, you may have been the one with the problem.

And that's just the tip of the iceberg. There are other hormones like oxytocin, prolactin, and vasopressin racing around through your system, and some experts theorize that everything you do—particularly when it comes to sex and love—is profoundly affected by the constantly fluctuating tides in your body. All these substances have varying effects on one another, and the range of hormonal combinations and behavior possibilities is dizzying.

Make eye contact with that beautiful brunette across the bar and phenylethylamine courses through your brain. Engage her in a conversation, and levels of testosterone and endorphins—so-called "feel-good" chemicals—soar. Share a dance, and your levels of the touchy, feeling hormones—dopamine and oxytocin—leap. Think you're in control now? "By the time all that's happened, you're emotionally 'stoned,'" says Theresa L. Crenshaw, M.D., who writes about the effects of hormones and other body chemicals in *The Alchemy of Love and Lust*. In fact, she says, there's a good chance you're headed for a one-night stand. "And the next morning you're thinking, What did I go to all that trouble for?" Crenshaw adds.

Chemical Cocktails

Modern research into the effects of hormones and other naturally occurring chemicals on male and female sex drives didn't really bloom until the early forties, but centuries ago shamans and witch doctors used animal sex organs, particularly animal testicles, as active ingredients in love potions and aphrodisiacs. Oddly enough, they unwittingly were closer to true love chemistry than they might have thought. Though there's no proof that noshing on dried testicles has any effects after ingestion, they do manufacture some of the hormones responsible for sex drive.

> "... centuries ago shamans and witch doctors used animal sex organs, particularly animal testicles, as active ingredients in love potions and aphrodisiacs."

Still, scientists concede they're only beginning to understand how hormones and other chemicals operate in men's bodies. "It's a new area of research, so there are only a dozen researchers actively working on it," says Alan Booth, Ph.D., professor of sociology and human development at Pennsylvania State University. Booth believes a number of studies presently underway will soon shed more light on the issue. "I figure in three or four years we're going to know a whole lot more than we do now," he says. Hopefully, that research will reveal if and how these sex-related hormones and chemicals are affected by diet, supplements, exercise, and, perhaps, other lifestyle factors. Right now, here's what we know about them.

- **Dehydroepiandrosterone (DHEA):** DHEA made headlines a couple of years ago for its anti-aging benefits. In terms of sexuality, it's a hormone typically manufactured in the adrenal glands, which sit atop the kidneys, and in the testicles and brain. It's known as the basic building block of other sex hormones, in that enzymes acting on the DHEA molecule spin off to form other hormones. So there is more DHEA in the human body—both male and female—than any other hormone. And since it is the basic building block, it can easily transform itself into other hormones.

DHEA produces pheromones, which emit our personal scents—or olfactory markers—through the skin (more on pheromones later in this chapter). Interestingly, DHEA also acts on our brains to receive the specific scent of females, as a way of affecting mating choices. In short, if you're attracted to a woman completely outside the realm of your usual type and you can't figure out why, DHEA may be the culprit. More importantly, research has suggested that DHEA increases sexual desire in both males and females.

- **Phenylethylamine (PEA):** According to Crenshaw, DHEA may be the basic hormonal building block, but PEA can be thought of as the "molecule of love." PEA is a natural amphetamine that floods the brain when romance ensues, furthering sexual excitement and stimulation.

  While DHEA triggers the secretion of pheromones and taps into what some scientists believe is an innate sense of smell for use in sexual pursuit, visuals—like that blonde in the crop-top by the bar—trigger a release of PEA into the bloodstream. That, in turn, quickens your pulse and begins a domino effect of other hormonal and chemical triggers. So PEA makes you believe in love—or lust—at first sight.

  PEA is also a potent antidepressant—that's why people in love feel like they're on top of the world. It's no wonder that a box of chocolate has high levels of PEA . . . hopeless romantics the world over have often used the sticky sweets to win over the hearts of their intended. And countless women say they have turned to the Whitman Sampler on lonely Saturday nights, trying to create a sense of love in their lives.

- **Oxytocin:** A chemical secreted by the pituitary gland, oxytocin promotes bonding of individuals through touch, sensitizing a person's body to tactile senses. So while DHEA affects the sense of smell through pheromone secretion and recognition, and PEA affects the sense of sight, oxytocin gives people an overwhelming desire to reach out and touch someone—an all-important element in courting and mating rituals. After all, you can't forget your first schoolyard crush, and how something as simple as a girl reaching out her hand to innocently hold yours sent electric shivers throughout your body. Ultimately, oxytocin is the chemical that makes people affectionate. So when your mate wants to cuddle after lovemaking and you want to watch the news, blame oxytocin.

  In women, oxytocin causes uterine contractions during orgasm.

  "... when your mate wants to cuddle after lovemaking and you want to watch the news, blame oxytocin."

In fact, contact between the penis and the vagina releases oxytocin into a woman's bloodstream, creating a overwhelming need to be filled—that is, to continue having sex.

On the male side, oxytocin increases penile sensitivity. That's good! It also speeds ejaculation. That's bad! Further, studies on rats showed that oxytocin improved erections. Researchers have also found that increased oxytocin levels jacks—no pun intended—the amount of ejaculate in test subjects. It also increases sperm count. In Europe, researchers are even investigating using oxytocin nasal sprays to treat impotence and orgasmic disorders.

- **Testosterone:** The granddaddy of them all, this hormone is responsible for a man's aggressive sex drive. In essence, it's what makes a man a man. Or, more precisely, it makes you want to watch football, fix things, and never ask for directions. The presence of testosterone accounts for an adolescent male's deepening voice and broadening shoulders. It also works as a natural antidepressant, giving men an optimistic attitude and self-confidence. In fact, testosterone levels surge after a man has won a contest or closed a deal.

"Studies show that men's testosterone levels fluctuate every 15 to 20 minutes and may have a profound effect on behavior."

According to Crenshaw, its frequent fluctuations (every 15 to 20 minutes) may affect your moods. We know much more about what affects testosterone than we do about the more recently discovered chemicals. For instance, exercise raises testosterone by as much as 27 percent, while stress, an unbalanced diet (too much protein, carbohydrate, or fat), excessive drinking, nutritional deficiencies, and having too little body fat (under 5 percent) may lower it. And, to the eternal embarrassment of vegans all over the world, eating meat—eating red meat—increases testosterone levels.

On the sexual side, testosterone increases lustful thoughts and fantasies. And, while it doesn't impact on a man's ability to maintain an erection, it does increase a man's urge to masturbate. Masturbation is a forceful impulse that originates from a natural hormone. According to Crenshaw: "Almost everybody masturbates and almost everyone feels bad about it. Catholics do it, and then confess to God about it. Orthodox Jews become bed masturbators. They turn on their stomachs and thrust against a pillow or mattress without using their hands. If

"In essence, [testosterone] is what makes a man a man. Or, more precisely, it makes you want to watch football, fix things, and never ask for directions."

they don't actually touch themselves, how can it be their fault? Evangelists get prostitutes to lend them a hand, and Southern Baptists don't masturbate at all. They get possessed by the devil, who does it for them. It isn't Satan. It's just testosterone."

Okay, okay. Testosterone isn't evil; it's just misunderstood. Sure, it gives man his aggressive sex drive. And sure, it makes him want to lose his "precious bodily fluids." But it also promotes touching. It surges when we're caressed, spikes during orgasm, and, over the long haul, leads couples to bond.

- **Dopamine:** A neurotransmitter, or brain chemical, that experts believe inspires action, dopamine causes us to perceive pleasure and boosts our sex drive. More importantly, it is commonly found in drug and alcohol addicts. It's what makes a person crave a long-lasting high. And dopamine addicts one person to another—more commonly known as romance. In essence, it makes a person feel pleasure through sex and contact. Without it, sex is just a bodily function.

- **Prolactin:** This is a hormone that escalates during orgasm. High levels can lead to impotence. High levels also decrease a man's testosterone level, which, in turn, decreases sex drive.

- **Vasopressin:** A chemical that helps us think clearly and read sexual clues, vasopressin allows men to stay in the "here and now" instead of daydreaming all the time. According to some researchers, vasopressin may also keep men's emotions in check and even promote monogamy because it discourages sexual extremes.

- **Serotonin:** This hormone decreases sexual drive, plain and simple. Prozac is a serotonin booster, which explains why so many in the Prozac nation would rather talk incessantly about how cool Prozac is than have sex. Serotonin also inhibits premature ejaculation.

Hormonal Possibilities

With this information, Crenshaw offers some interesting educated guesses to explain the crazy ways men and women often behave. None of this should diminish the importance of social, environmental, and emotional factors in our behavior, Crenshaw says, but it should help highlight some of the chemical possibilities.

Consider these theories:

- Love at first sight may not be such a far-out idea after all. Phenylethylamine, Crenshaw says, may explain why some people go head over heels after a brief glance.

- Men and women in their twenties are ill-suited for one another in bed, chemically speaking, that is. Young women are mainly influenced by estrogen, Crenshaw says, which leads them to want romance and caresses. Men, on the other hand, are driven mainly by testosterone. As a result, they're focused on their genitals and preoccupied with orgasms. All too often, that preoccupation comes at the expense of romance.

- Men and women in their thirties may also run into problems related to body chemicals. Men in their thirties are more inclined toward commitment, possibly because of the influence of vasopressin, which Crenshaw calls the "monogamy molecule." Ironically, women are feeling more independent because they're experiencing a greater testosterone influence. This testosterone shot increases the likelihood that a woman will have affairs if she's unsatisfied in bed, according to Crenshaw. Fortunately, she says, chemicals converge and relationships improve by the time men and women reach their forties.

- Touching keeps couples together. Simply touching at the beginning of a relationship can lead to strong, long-lasting bonds due to the influence of oxytocin. After you've known your girlfriend a while, oxytocin will surge at the mere thought of her. Be warned: You can bond chemically with her and possibly think you're in love, even if you feel only lukewarm about her in other ways.

Into the Future

All this talk of hormones can make life and love seem like nothing more than a giant lab experiment—with our heads and hearts at the mercy of some freaky guy in a white coat. But according to Crenshaw, there's no cause for alarm. "This is not going to take away from the romance and the highs that people enjoy," she says. "If anything, you can enhance those highs."

One easy way to do that, Crenshaw says, is to stop what you're doing during the day and simply think about your wife or girlfriend. Your oxytocin level will surge, she says, making you feel more affectionate. While you're at it, plan a sexy evening and even fantasize about your plans. You'll ride a testosterone high, too. When you're together, stroke your partner's hair or caress her shoulders, even if you're just waiting for a restaurant table. You'll enjoy a complimentary oxytocin boost with your appetizer. Or, if the two of you are home watching television, sit close together, letting your bodies touch, and you'll also experience an endorphin surge.

Finally, consider your fluctuating testosterone level. By knowing that it peaks every 15 to 20 minutes, possibly increasing the likelihood that you'll want to be alone, you can avoid snapping at your wife or girlfriend when you're feeling moody, Crenshaw says. Instead, go for a walk, or change the oil in the car. You'll avoid a testosterone-induced argument and still have time to relax—watching Ally and her pals' angst on TV instead.

A Rose by Any Other Name

As mentioned earlier, we each have a unique scent—or pheromone—that's triggered by the hormone DHEA. Researchers have long known that animals emit pheromones to repel or attract others in the species. But when it comes to the function of human pheromones, the scientific community is divided. On the one hand, some scientists consider man to be an evolved animal—one that has moved away from base forms of communication, like giving off a scent for attraction, sexual desire, or fear. Then there's a portion of the scientific community that recognizes the production of human pheromones. The problem here: scientists know human pheromones exist, but don't necessarily know how this olfactory information is processed.

To this end, research into the vomeronasal organ (or VNO) has begun anew. Scientists have known about this tiny organ located in the nasal passageways for approximately 100 years, but common thought—until recently—was that the VNO was a nonfunctioning link to our evolutionary past, similar to the coccyx, or tailbone. However, research using "distant cousin" mammals—such as mice and rats, who have similar genetic heritages to humans—has shown that pheromones are an active part of their information-gathering processes. More interestingly, researchers determined that the receptor and processor of these scents was the VNO.

Since the VNO gave mammals a "sixth sense," some scientists now believe that a similar phenomenon takes place within humans. Indeed, autopsies on humans have shown that nerve bundles lead to the brain from the VNO, and research being conducted at the laboratories of the University of Utah by Erox Corporation suggest that these bundles are also active electronic passageways.

Dr. Clive Jennings-White, consultant to Erox, is a bio-organic chemist who was able to isolate the human pheromones and re-create their molecular structures. Working in collaboration with Drs. David Moran (whose research proved that humans still possess a VNO) and Lewis Monti-Block (who measures the electrical responses of pheromones on humans), Jennings-White tested the effects of synthesized pheromones using a group of 40 people. The nasal cavities of each participant were outfitted with an apparatus that measured electrical responses of the VNO. The first 20 had the synthesized human pheromones delivered directly into their VNO, while the remaining 20—the control group—received puffs of plain air. Before and after the test, study subjects answered a psychological questionnaire describing how they felt. The group that received the pheromone had a decrease of negative thoughts, while the control group showed no significant change.

Based on the findings, Jennings-White and Erox Corporation used the first pheromones as the basic building block of Realm and Inner Realm fragrances.

"The pheromones in both fragrances increase a person's sense of openness," he says. "The wearer becomes more mellow and comfortable . . . which opens up all kinds of possibilities. They may relate better to a spouse, a date, strangers, or even their boss.

"Pheromones are gender-specific—the ones in our fragrances are designed to appeal to the wearer, not the opposite sex." That, Jennings-White says, allows a person to become more relaxed, exuding a sense of calm that is picked up by other people. In essence, the more relaxed and self-confident one becomes, the more attractive one becomes to others.

Research into human pheromones and the VNO continues. Jennings-White and his team of researchers have already isolated an additional 20 pheromones. As more neurological pathways are explored, some scientists believe that our "sixth sense" will be the explanation for untold situations that have, up until now, been chalked up to such ethereal things as karma, fate, or just plain luck.

So the next time you hear of an officeful of females that mysteriously all get their periods at the same time, month after month after month, don't be astonished. It may just be the pheromone communication system working overtime.

And speaking of a woman's menstrual cycle, Moran says the Realm fragrances were just a logical first application of Erox's research. The company actually has much bigger fish to fry. By the time this book goes to print, there may be a pheromone-based product on the market that combats the symptoms of premenstrual syndrome. "It's going

Sexbit 1

Next time you spot your honey munching on Good & Plenty candies while slicing a cucumber, you may want to consider jumping her bones. According to Alan Hirsch of the Smell & Taste Research Foundation in Chicago, a mix of those aromas enhances a woman's sex drive by increasing vaginal blood flow by as much as 13 percent. Hirsch, who has been putting his nose to the grindstone to find out what scents spark the male and female libido, also found that women who call themselves "multiorgasmic" are turned on by the smell of baby powder, while whiffing cherries and charcoal-barbecued meat tends to leave them cold. What scents get men charged up? A combination of lavender and pumpkin pie. Dr. Hirsh has yet to find an odor that inhibits male desire.

through the FDA approval process, which takes a few years," says Moran, adding that there are numerous pharmacological uses of pheromones. Moran says he also doesn't doubt that humans produce a pheromone for sexual attraction. "We just haven't been able to isolate it yet. It's such a new frontier."

Waiting to Inhale

The human sense of smell is hardly a new frontier, but over the past decade, there's been a renewed interest in fragrances, bath products, and candles based on scents that arouse. According to scientists, man-made fragrances actually work by appealing to the psyche. "You smell something and it conjures up a memory, thus appealing to your emotions," Moran says. But supporters of homeopathic medicine believe that essential oils, herbs, and other by-products of nature have a direct impact on our desires. "They can take away everything from an aching heart to aching muscles," writes Mary Muryn in *Water Magic*, a book that contains bath recipes "for the body, spirit, and soul."

Though a number of medical professionals say this is all mere placebo—you think something will happen so it will—aromatherapy is being taken seriously these days by individuals and businesses. Many retailers pipe uplifting scents into their stores that—in theory—energize shoppers and subconsciously get them to spend more.

Although there's no proof that holistic techniques will improve your sex life, it doesn't hurt to try to set the mood with a little scents-appeal.

Fit for Sex
Body Image and Sexuality

It's no great revelation that a person's body image affects his sexuality. When you feel good about yourself, it shows, in your posture, your mood, your dress—and especially your willingness to undress.

Overall, women tend to be more sensitive about their physical appearance than men—and who can blame them? Turn on the television, or flip through any fashion magazine, and you'll see page after page of the American "ideal"—young, gorgeous, exceptionally thin women. "I know most men don't expect to date supermodels," says Janelle, a 25-year-old accountant from Denver, Colorado. "But they sure do strain their necks when one who fills the bill walks by. It makes us 'average' women feel as though we will never measure up as a date—never mind as a lover."

According to sex therapist Joel Block, author of *Secrets of Better Sex*, a combination of self-image issues often inhibit female sexuality. They include:

Weight: Most women think they would be desirable "if it weren't

Scentsational Sex

Next time you're out shopping, look for bath oils, candles, lotions, or other products containing these essential oils. Alone, or in combinations, they are said to enhance possibilities for romance and to stimulate sexual desire and passion.

Arabian musk
cedar
frankincense
ginger
jasmine
magnolia
nutmeg
patchouli
rose oil
sandalwood
ylang-ylang

for those five to ten extra pounds." Men, on the other hand, tend to feel that this so-called "ideal" is a bit on the skinny side. "I like a woman with curves and a little extra flesh on their bones," said James, a 28-year-old stockbroker from Chicago.

Breast size: Women who are busty wish they were smaller. Women who are tiny are often willing to pay big bucks to have a more heapin' helpin'. But rare is the woman who thinks she's just right.

Aging: Thirty was once the age at which women began to fret about wrinkles and saggy flesh. But these days, it seems to be starting much earlier. "I'm 21 and spend about $200 a year on moisturizers and anti-wrinkle creams," said Samantha, a senior at New York University. "By the time I'm 60, I'll have spent a fortune to fight a battle that's probably beyond my control."

Thighs: They can't be thin, or hard, or cheese-free enough for most women.

Scars from pregnancy and childbirth: Worse than the stretch marks is the realization that sex will never be quite the same. "I expected my vagina to be stretched out after having my baby," said Elizabeth, a 27-year-old mom from San Francisco, "but the look on my husband's face the first time we attempted intercourse confirmed it—and then some."

If you're thinking that this all sounds quite neurotic, be assured: men are not immune. Though guys are less likely to link their body image with sexuality, Block says they have nagging concerns of their own. Chief among them are:

Penis size: For women, those extra five pounds are one of the main obstacles to great sex. For men, it's too few inches. Even though most guys fall within the normal range of penis size, they seem to think there is no such thing as big enough. "It's not just that we want to be larger for women, there's a need to measure up in the locker room," said Joel, a 35-year-old New York writer.

Balding: Hair loss can be devastating for some men. Millions are spent each year on remedies to combat balding, from hair transplants to bizarre paintlike sprays that conceal bare patches of scalp.

Aging signs: Many women say that they think men with graying hair are sexy. But in the business world, where youth has become an asset, men are beginning to feel that the salt-and-pepper look seems weathered. Consequently, guys are coloring their hair in increasing numbers and they're investing big bucks in skincare products to keep the wrinkles at bay.

Stomach: The old spare-tire scare usually starts in the mid-twenties—and doesn't let up. "It doesn't matter how many crunches, reverse crunches, or full sit-ups I do," says Rodger, a 30-year-old computer software developer from San Francisco. "I can still pinch way more than an inch around my abdomen—and chicks notice this."

Height: "He had a really cute face, and we had a great time on our date," said Marie, a 32-year-old administrative assistant from New York City. "But he was, like, shorter than Michael J. Fox." Men love petite women, but the reverse is not always true. That's why short men (like super-tall women) often have height complexes.

The Anatomy of Attraction

The good news, gentlemen, is that most of these self-image issues are addressable. Sure, you can't do anything about your height, or the fact that your father, your father's father, and your father's father's father all had love handles by the age of 35. But you can work on enhancing your assets—a great step toward feeling better about yourself.

In our opinion, eating right and exercising regularly is the best means to that end. Yes, this is where we make our fitness and nutrition pitch. But anyone who has lost even a few pounds the smart way—by working out and making sensible dietary changes—will agree: If you feel good about your body, you feel good period. Height, bald spots, aging. They don't really matter, as long as you're in shape.

Interestingly enough, research conducted at the University of New Mexico shows that there is, indeed, a direct link between a person's shape and his sex life. The study, which was designed to determine the affects of body symmetry on human attraction, was conducted by Dr. Randy Thornhill. A behavioral ecologist, Thornhill learned, through a previous study, that female Japanese scorpion flies were turned on by the male flies who had the most symmetrical tails. To see if humans had similar tastes, Thornhill examined the sexual histories of 122 students and measured their feet, ankles, ears, hands, hips, and waists. During the first round of his study, he found that the respondents whose measurements were the most symmetrical enjoyed two to three times as many sex partners in their lifetime as those with less body symmetry. It didn't matter if the women, for example, were slightly overweight, as long as their hips-to-waist ratio was balanced (i.e., 38–28–38), which men instinctively prefer.

Also interesting was Thornhill's finding that men who had the most

"I used to look forward to having sex with my husband; our relationship was intensely passionate and I always felt extremely comfortable getting naked. But that was before I had a baby. Now I have this beautiful little boy, but I've lost myself. I'm 30 pounds overweight. My once-firm breasts hang down to my knees. None of my clothes fit me. How can I feel sexy when I'm disgusted by my own reflection in the mirror?"
—Cindy, 32, married, Atlanta

No Sex High

Sure, having sex is a great way to release endorphins—chemicals that are the key components of the runner's high. But you don't have to enjoy a roll in the hay to experience a great natural buzz. Go for a run, a swim, a hike, or a good bike ride. If you work out regularly, you'll probably start to feel a rush after about 20 or 30 minutes of aerobic exercise, when your brain begins to release endorphins. The secret, experts say, is to exercise moderately and not push yourself to exhaustion. "As soon as you start overdoing it, the endorphin release tapers off," says Lee Berk, Ph.D., a researcher at Loma Linda University Medical Center in Southern California. "Then your body moves into a distress response." Not only will you enjoy regular highs by exercising moderately, you'll also feel better when you do have sex, says Bryant Stamford, Ph.D., author of *Fitness Without Exercise* and a member of the *Men's Fitness* Advisory Board. "When you're doing a reasonable amount of training, chances are good that hormone production is up and your sex life is healthy."

symmetry started having sex as much as four years earlier than their asymmetrical counterparts. And women who were with the most symmetrical men claimed to orgasm more—75 percent of the time compared to 30 percent for women who were with the lopsided guys. Plus more couples were able to enjoy simultaneous orgasms if the guy's body parts matched up.

Certainly, genes play a role in man's physical makeup. But a few days a week at the gym will go a long way toward enhancing just about anyone's symmetry. And it provides an immediate psychological boost. "When I'm working out, I feel better about myself. It's like I can do anything. And when I'm having a rotten day, 60 minutes at the gym can turn that around," says Michael, a 40-year-old Iowa construction worker.

In fact, that "feel-good" sensation Michael talks about can last several hours after exercise and is the result of real hormonal fluctuations in the body. As rigorous movement raises the temperature in the muscles, the autonomic nervous system—the part that deals with the unconscious regulation of the body—kicks into gear, just as it does in response to stress. Epinephrine (a.k.a. adrenaline) and other hormones are released to prep the body for the physical (or mental) challenge. And just to ensure we stay mentally in check, the nervous system releases calming neurotransmitters, such as beta-endorphins and serotonin, simultaneously. This mix of hormones is what results in the "runner's high" we so often hear about. And it's also responsible for the improved mood and increased energy we get from exercise.

Some guys say working out actually makes them horny. "The adrenaline and endorphins start pumping. It's a total turn-on," says Davis, 29, of New York City. "Sex is an awesome release."

Moreover, an improved lean body mass (i.e., more muscle), improves overall metabolic response. That means you'll burn calories faster—even when you're not exercising.

When women get fit, they often become less inhibited in the bedroom. "I love to show off my buff body in sexy lingerie or doing private stripteases for my husband," says Liz, a 34-year-old Chicago writer. "Plus I can enjoy sex more when I'm fit, because I'm not wondering—in the middle of the deed—if my husband is grossed out by cellulite on my butt or extra chub on my thighs."

It's true that strength and cardiovascular training will enhance your sex life, according to Chicago personal trainer Christa Eskridge, who holds a Master's of Science in Exercise Physiology from Kansas State University. "There's the obvious mental benefits of being in shape," she says, "but being in shape also means you'll have greater stamina and endurance as well."

To that end, Eskridge recommends working out aerobically at least three times a week for at least 20 minutes "on a treadmill, exercise bike, Stairmaster . . . it doesn't matter, as long as you exercise within your target heart range." Most fitness experts recommend working out in a training zone ranging from 60 to 80 percent of your maximum heart rate. To determine your maximum heart rate, first subtract your age from 220. Then multiply that rate by 60 percent and 80 percent to arrive at your zone. For example, a 31-year-old man's maximum heart rate would be 189 beats per minute. To get the best results he should work out between 113 and 151 beats per minute, monitoring his pulse periodically with a heart rate monitor or the old-fashioned way using his fingers and a clock.

The acrobatics of sex also require strong muscles and flexibility, says Eskridge, "so weight lifting and stretching are essential, too." But don't go nuts, she warns. "Exercising alters your hormonal balance, and too much of anything is never good." Women who train too rigorously, for example, often stop menstruating and note a marked change in their libido. "It's your body telling you to slow down," Eskridge says.

Sexercises

If exercising is a new concept to you, Eskridge recommends a strength training program that works assorted muscle groups that are particularly important during sex. You need a strong upper body for the missionary position, for example, and powerful glutes mean more powerful thrusting ability. You can do any of these exercises at home using only a set of dumbbells (and if you're in the gym you can use dumbbells and/or their gym-equipment equivalents). "Perform each of the movements slowly—at least two seconds on the upward motion and four seconds while returning to the starting position," Eskridge says. "Don't forget to exhale as you're working the muscle and inhale as you release. Follow the repetitions I've outlined and use a weight that causes muscle fatigue (the momentary inability to continue) at the final rep. Finding the appropriate weight to reach muscle fatigue will take several workouts before you dial it in." And as always, check with your physician before beginning any exercise routine.

Standing Alternate Dumbbell Curl (biceps or front of arms)

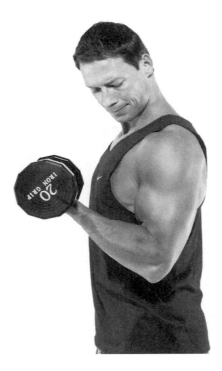

The move: Standing with your feet shoulder-width apart and your knees slightly relaxed, grasp a dumbbell in each hand. The dumbbells should hang at your sides, with palms facing forward. Slowly curl one dumbbell (let the other hang) toward your shoulder. Make sure that the elbow of your working arm remains tucked at your side. After curling to the top, slowly lower the dumbbell to the starting position. Repeat the process with the other dumbbell.

Reps: One set of 12; a second set of 10.

Advice: For an alternative version, curl both arms simultaneously. If you can easily get through both sets, increase the weight of the dumbbells. To maximize the movement's potential, you can start with the palms facing in, and then slowly rotate the wrists (as soon as you start the exercise) until the palms face forward.

Triceps Dips (back of arms)

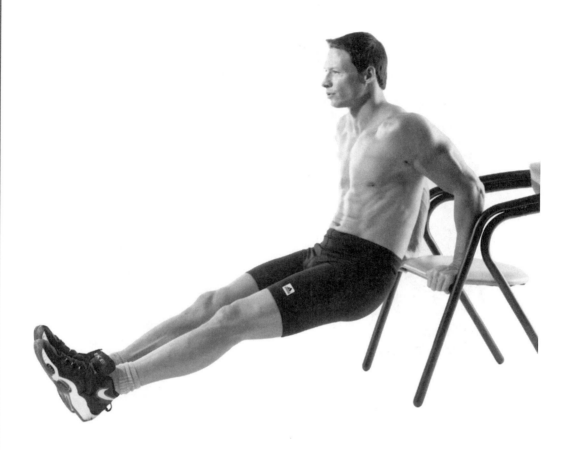

The move: Sit on the edge of a sturdy coffee table or chair with your legs extended straight out in front of you. Without locking your elbows, straighten your arms, place your hands shoulder-width apart, and firmly grip the edges of the table or chair. Slide your butt just off the front of the table or chair so your torso is pointing straight down toward the floor. Keep your abdominals contracted and your spine straight. Bend your elbows and lower your body in a straight line toward the floor. When your upper arms are parallel to the floor, push yourself back up to the start.

Reps: One set of 12; a second set of 10.

Advice: To make the exercise easier, bend your knees (instead of extending your legs out in front of you). To increase the intensity, position your feet horizontally on another table or chair in front of you.

Overhead Shoulder Press (deltoids)

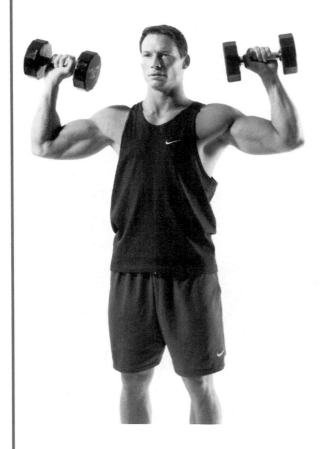 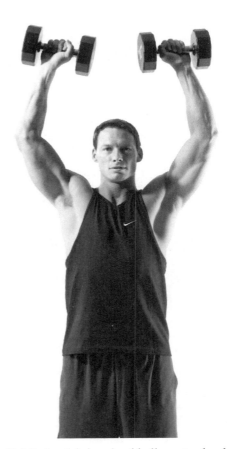

The move: With your legs hip-width apart and knees slightly bent, bring dumbbells up to shoulder height with your palms facing forward. Exhale, slowly lifting your arms straight up until the weights almost touch directly over your head. Then inhale, while returning to the start position.

Reps: One set of 12; a second of 10.

Advice: To make the exercise easier or more difficult, alter the weights accordingly.

Upright Row (for upper back and shoulders)

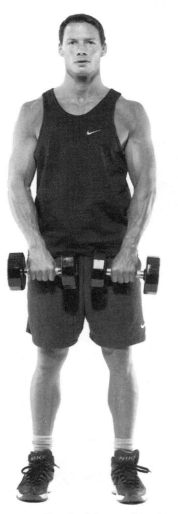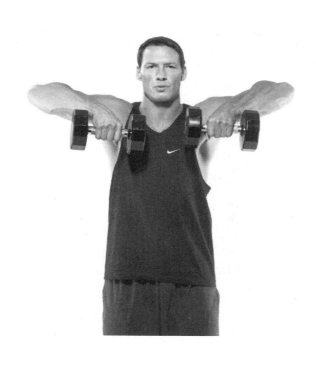

The move: Stand with your legs hip-width apart, knees slightly bent. Hold weights about an inch apart in front of your thighs, palms facing toward your body. Inhale, lifting the weights straight up to the top of your chest (about four inches apart), with your elbows pointing out at the sides and slightly upward. (Make sure your wrists do not point downward.) Then exhale, lowering the weights to the starting position.

Reps: One set of 12; a second of 10.

Advice: To ease up, lift each arm individually, alternating the arms until you finish your reps. To make the move more difficult, lift each arm individually, completing all reps on one arm before moving to the next.

Pushups (arms, chest, back)

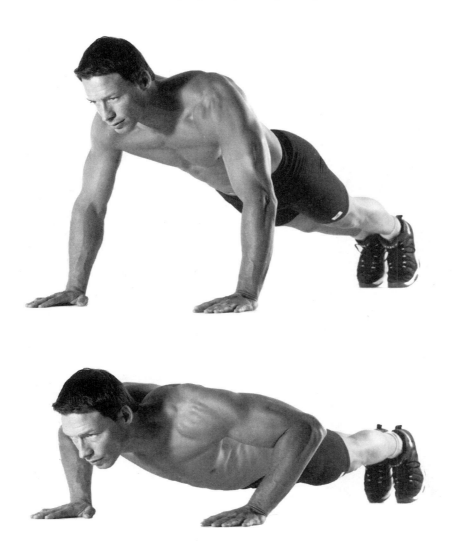

The move: Lie on your stomach with your legs straight out, feet flexed, toes on the floor. Bend your elbows and place your hands on the floor at the shoulders. Lift your body off the floor by straightening your arms. Hold in your abs on the way up and keep your butt down and your back straight.

Reps: Do as many as you can until it hurts like hell.

Advice: Bending your knees (the "girl" way) makes pushups easier. Using one arm—military, or Jack Palance–style—ups the difficulty level tenfold.

Squats (front thighs and glutes)

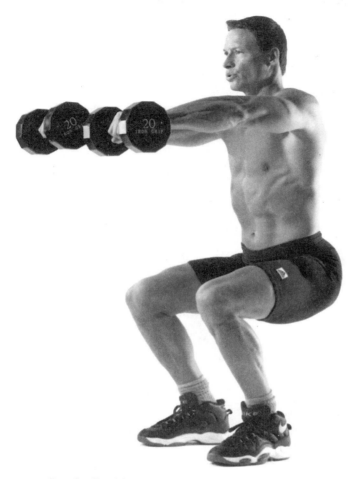

The move: Stand tall with your feet shoulder-width apart, dumbbells at your side (palms facing rearward). Pulling your abdominals in toward your spine to create a natural curve, sit backward and downward until your thighs are nearly parallel to the floor. To maintain balance, simultaneously lift the weights forward to shoulder height. Hold the position for a few seconds and then return to the start by pushing off your heels. Squeeze your butt on the way up.

Reps: One set of 25; a second set of 15.

Advice: An alternative exercise that works the inner thigh muscles is the wide-stance squat, which is identical to the standard squat except that the feet are slightly wider than shoulder-width apart. Holding the dumbbells at shoulder height makes either of the squats more difficult. Lose the dumbbells altogether to make the exercises easier.

Lunges (thighs and hips)

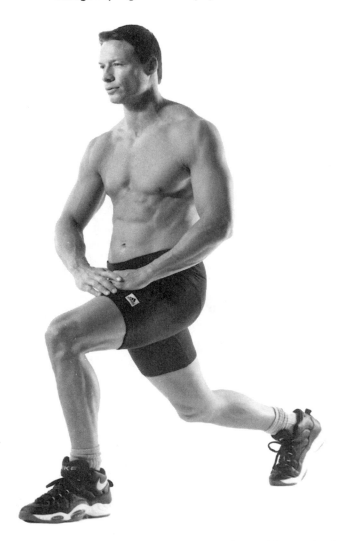

The move: Stand tall with your feet shoulder-width apart. Leading with your heel, step forward with your left foot, bending both knees so that your left thigh is nearly parallel to the floor and your right thigh is perpendicular to it. Press off the ball of your left foot and spring lightly back to the start position. Don't allow your knee to go beyond your toes. Alternate legs until you've completed 20 lunges on each side.

Advice: Add weights held atop your shoulders to add difficulty. You can also hold the weights at your sides at arm's length. Lessen the lunge to simplify.

Crunches (for upper abs)

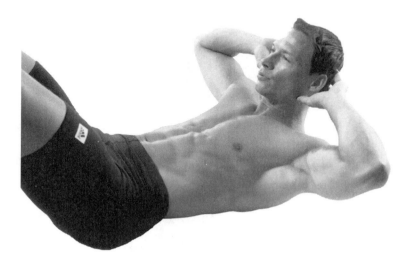

The move: Lie on your back with your knees bent and your feet flat on the floor, shoulder-width apart. Place your hands behind your head, elbows pointing outward (for support only!). Round your lower back into the floor by pulling your abs in, slowly curling up and forward, lifting your head, neck, and shoulder blades off the floor. Exhale on the way up and inhale as you lower to the start position. Don't pull your head forward toward your abdomen, or lift your lower back off the floor.

Reps: Two sets of 35.

Advice: Go slow for the maximum benefits.

Reverse Crunches (for lower abs)

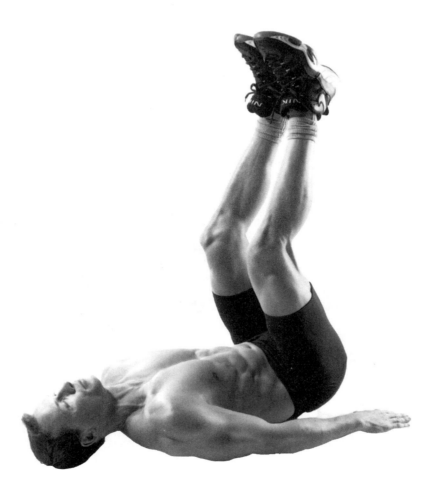

The move: Lie with your back on the floor, legs raised to a 90-degree angle, and your arms straight along your sides. Exhale as you lift your tailbone one to two inches off the floor and your feet straight upwards. Hold at the top of the movement for a few seconds before returning to the start position.

Reps: Two sets of 20.

Advice: Again, slow and steady gets the maximum benefits.

Lower Back

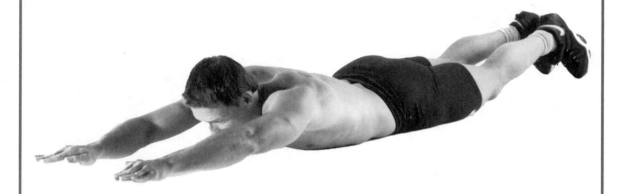

The move: Lie with your stomach on the floor and your hands out in front of you. Push your upper body up off the floor. Hold for about ten seconds and lower to the start position.

Reps: Repeat four times.

Advice: If you have a weak lower back, start with a single set and work your way up to four.

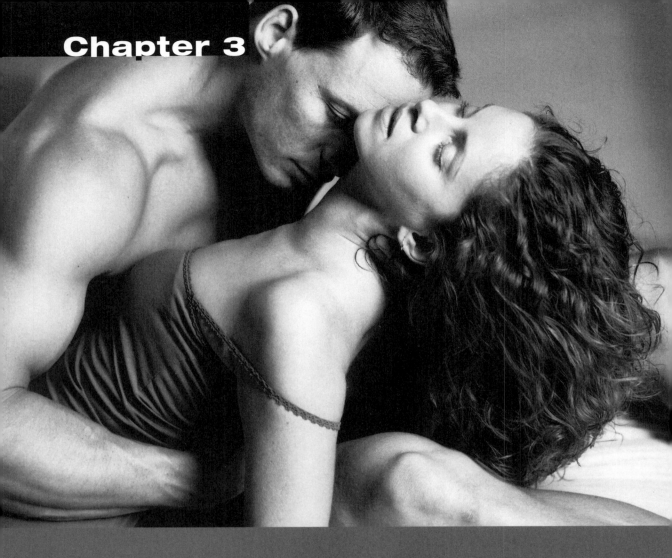

Chapter 3

Responsibility

Ah, the seventies. The Me decade was brimming with hedonism. Drinking—hard drinking—was in vogue, showcased on every nighttime sitcom and emulated at every nightclub. Drugs? Name your poison—heck, a coke spoon even became a fashion accessory, dangling from a chain on every hairy-chested body slinking through the crowds at Danceteria or the 2001. And sex . . . well, sex was pursued, lusted after, hunted down, bagged, grabbed, shared, and snared. Women were looking for Mr. Goodbar, and men . . . men were looking for *anybody*. The worst thing about sex in the seventies was the pestering would-be girlfriend (called stalkers nowadays) and an occasional scorching case of syphilis—which, by the way, was cleared up with a quick needle poke in the posterior.

What a difference a generation makes.

Thinking of drinking? Don't drink and drive. Drugs? Just say no. And sex? Mister, sex can positively kill you.

Nothing took the edge off the bacchanalia that was the seventies like the go-go eighties, a decade that saw the number of AIDS cases rise as quickly as the stock market riches of the Gordon Gecko wannabes on Wall Street. And in a postfeminist culture, women are demanding a new type of man in the boudoir—one who uses his head as much as his hands.

Indeed, the watchword for the next millennium is responsibility. Responsibility in relationships, in sexual encounters, and in sexual practices. The days of diving headlong into a night between the sheets with a Sally or a Monique or a Tiffany you just met are officially over.

But all is not doom and gloom, friend. Responsibility may be a watchword, but you can still explore your sexuality. You just have to do it safely. And that's where this chapter comes in.

Sexually Transmitted Diseases

There once was a time when the worst thing that could happen after a brief encounter was a bout with the dreaded "venereal disease" (VD being a catch-all phrase for the double whammy of syphilis and gonorrhea). It was the scourge of every sailor visiting too many ports, if you know what we mean. But even then, the risks were small, the fatalities rare. Sure, Al Capone may have died from VD, his mind slowly rotting away until he spent his last days babbling to himself—but hey, he was a villain . . . that's what happened to "those" types of people decades ago.

These days however, sexually transmitted diseases (or STDs) affect more than just villains and wayward sailors—STDs affect a significant segment of the U.S. population, and the category itself has grown from syphilis and gonorrhea to a wide variety of maladies—more than 20 STDs (such as herpes,

and Protection

chlamydia, and genital warts) are recognized by the medical community. All of them are contagious and dangerous. It's a very risky time, indeed.

How risky, you ask? One in four Americans will catch a STD in their lifetime. That means 50 people on that airplane you took home for the holidays may have been percolating with some form of nastiness.

Want some more sobering news? According to the National Herpes Hotline, an estimated forty million Americans have genital herpes. Every year, four million new cases of chlamydia crop up. A million men and women get gonorrhea in the U.S. each year. Then there's AIDS. It's incurable, like genital herpes, but unlike genital herpes, at the time of this book's printing the prognosis for AIDS carriers is ultimately death.

"Indeed, the watchword for the next millennium is responsibility. Responsibility in relationships, in sexual encounters, and in sexual practices."

Which brings us to this point: We hope the stats make you scared straight . . . straight into acting more responsibly and safely. After all, the vast majority of STDs can be prevented by engaging in safe sex (see Safer Sex later in this chapter).

"Not Me" Psychology

Given the vast number of Americans contracting STDs, the majority probably believe this is something that "happens to other people," not them. For example, the fastest growth segment of those afflicted with AIDS are heterosexuals; while homosexuals have taken safety precautions to decrease risks, heterosexuals engaging in risky, unprotected sex see themselves as invincible. And therein lies the crux of the problem: STDs can affect anyone—you, your friends, coworkers, even unborn babies. It's better to venture forth well-armed with knowledge regarding STDs and prevention. Sound preachy? Too bad. Read on.

The Most Common STDs
Chlamydia

Chlamydia has been called the "silent epidemic"—a majority of men and women who have the bacteria-based disease show no symptoms; they don't even know they have contracted it. So even though four million cases are reported per year—making it the most common STD—that number is probably low, given that you can't report what you don't know you've got.

Chlamydia is spread through vaginal or anal intercourse. Symptoms start as early as seven days after sexual contact and include a puslike discharge from the penis, as well as a burning sensation when urinating. Burning or itching around the opening of the penis and swelling in the testicles are also common symptoms.

Women are more susceptible to getting chlamydia, as well as other STDs. The fact is, they receive bodily fluids from men and their moist, warm genitalia are perfect breeding grounds for bacteria-based STDs. Additional symptoms for them include lower abdominal pain and bleeding between menstrual cycles. In the long run, untreated chlamydia can lead to pelvic inflammatory disease, a leading cause of infertility in women.

"Chlamydia has been called the 'silent epidemic'—a majority of men and women who have the bacteria-based disease show no symptoms; they don't even know they have contracted it."

Testing involves a simple cotton-swabbing of the penis tip to collect a fluid sample, which is analyzed for bacterial growth. Single-dose antibiotics then can be used to successfully treat the disease.

Gonorrhea

Typically, people who contract chlamydia also contract gonorrhea. Like chlamydia, gonorrhea is caused by a bacterium. And, like chlamydia, gonorrhea is spread through direct sexual contact and exchange of inflected bodily fluids, most typically through the penis and vagina, but also by way of the mouth and rectum. Typical symptoms, which begin two to seven days after infection, include a discharge from the penis, a sore throat (or difficulty swallowing), testicle tenderness or pain, and a sharp burning sensation when urinating.

If left untreated, gonorrhea progresses first as simple joint pain, then advances through the blood stream, causing infections of the heart, joints, skin, and brain, as well as disorders of the central nervous system, arthritis, and sterility.

Treatment is simple. Antibiotics are used to cure gonorrhea. Penicillin, which was the drug of choice for all those sailors, has been supplanted by newer medicines, such as ceftriaxone, since gonorrhea strains have become resistant to penicillin's charms.

Syphilis

You wander into a smoky gin joint. The place is packed. The band is playing a jumping little swing number, so you pull the snap brim on your fedora down a bit more and venture into the zoot-suited crowd. It looks to be a good night. It's a postwar boom time. You're flush with cash. And the place is crawling with Skirts. Dames. Broads. You pick the creme of the crop—a little filly with the never-ending gams—and head out to the dance floor for a quick jitterbug. Later, you'll head out to your place for a little Sinatra on the Victrola. In the morning, she'll be gone.

In a few weeks, you'll be reminded of her again. When the sores start to appear.

The scenario could have taken place in the 1940s . . . or just last month, given the resurgence of Swing. And the resurgence of syphilis. According to Planned Parenthood, infectious syphilis is at its highest level in 40 years. It's still the granddaddy of sexually transmitted diseases. And it still is considered a very serious disease. Ironically, syphilis has all but disappeared in most industrialized countries—except in the U.S.

". . . syphilis has all but disappeared in most industrialized countries—except in the U.S."

Syphilis has three stages. In the first stage, painless sores may appear where the syphilis bacterium entered the body (usually on the head of the penis or in the mouth). This typically occurs some 10 to 90 days after sexual contact with a carrier.

The sores may disappear on their own . . . but that doesn't mean the disease has run its course. The bacterial infection is just lying dormant, waiting for stage two, which usually occurs three weeks to three months after the initial stage. This period is marked by flulike symptoms (sluggishness, headaches, sore throat, swollen glands, fevers) and potential patchy hair loss. The second stage can also be marked by rashes on the palms and soles of an infected person's feet, which means that microbes are traveling through the bloodstream into the lymphatic system, which functions as a bacteria filter. That's trouble . . . because the lymphatic system serves the entire body and affects every organ. So, the infection is nesting throughout the body.

Unfortunately, since the rashes heal (leaving no outward signs or scars) many people chalk up the rash to allergic reactions, athlete's foot, or a similar malady. And since the disease can again lie dormant for anywhere from a few years to a lifetime, infected people may again think that whatever's ailing them has run its course. But then comes stage three.

Stage three of untreated syphilis is marked by a host of wicked symptoms: skin lesions, blindness, loss of balance, mental deterioration, shooting pains through the body, heart disease. Stage three syphilis attacks the central nervous system, destroying bones and joints, as well as interrupting the supply of blood to the brain. In short, untreated syphilis can be a death warrant.

The good news, however, is that syphilis is easy to detect and treat. A simple blood test is used to identify the disease, and antibiotics (usually long-acting forms of penicillin) are used to destroy it. It should be noted that these medications work for the first two stages; stage three, and the resultant damage to bodily systems, cannot be treated successfully with antibiotics.

Genital Warts

Spread through unprotected vaginal, oral, or anal sex, genital warts—caused by the human papilloma virus (HPV)—affect approximately two million Americans a year. The warts, which look like small bumps or cauliflower-like clusters, appear on the genitals, inside the vagina, on the anus, in the throat or urethra. The warts often itch and can block openings to the genitals, throat, or anus.

There are a variety of treatment methods: chemical treatments by way of topical ointments; freezing the warts with liquid nitrogen; laser therapy to burn off the warts; and cauterization treatments to rid the body of the wart. It should be noted that, even though the outer wart can be easily removed, the virus remains in the layers of the skin. Because of this, more than one treatment application may be needed to fully get rid of the wart. Unfortunately, because the virus remains in the host body, more warts can develop at any time.

Hepatitis B

Hepatitis B is an infection of the liver caused by a virus that is passed through blood or bodily fluids of carriers. Aside from sexual contact, kissing and even sharing the same toothbrush or razor with someone who is infected puts you at tremendous risk of getting the virus. Three hundred thousand Americans get hepatitis B each year; approximately 10 percent of adults who catch the virus go on to become lifetime carriers, with increased risks of liver disease and liver cancer.

Symptoms include sluggishness, fever, yellow skin and eyes, dark-colored urine, extremely light colored feces, and vomiting. There is no known treatment for hepatitis B; typically, a person's own immune system works to eradicate the virus. In some extreme chronic cases, interferon (an immunological drug often used to treat cancer) is used to combat the virus.

Ironically, there is a preventive vaccine for hepatitis B—the Centers for Disease Control in Atlanta currently recommends that sexually active teenagers and young adults get inoculated. Three shots is all it takes.

Pubic Lice

Remember that one kid in elementary school—the one that disappeared for a few days and came back with a closely shaven head? Ah, the rampant playground talk. Talk of cooties. Or technically speaking: lice.

Lice, small insects that live on the skin, can be transmitted from one person to another through sexual contact—the little buggers simply see a better "ride" and hop on. More typically, they are picked up by using the same bed linen, towels, or clothes as an infected person . . . which often happens after a close encounter with the opposite sex.

Pubic lice infect the hairy parts of a person's body: the groin area, underarms, and head. Here's where it gets really gross—lice lay eggs. On you. These eggs can be seen on the hair close to the skin, where they hatch and create more little buggers in five to ten days.

Typically, the symptoms of lice—and its close cousin, scabies (or itch mites)—is itching, the driving-you-up-the-wall kind of itching. There's lots of it, too.

If you have lice, you don't have to subject yourself to a trendy hairstyle (read: shaved). Treatments abound for the critters . . . just check the local pharmacy for the shampoos, special combs, and creams specially designed to rid oneself of lice. Here's one note, however: The lice may still live in your clothing and surroundings, so repeat infestations are possible. It's best to clean all suspect garments, towels, and bed linens with extremely hot water or dry-clean and press them with a very hot iron.

Herpes

In the early 1980s, a number of articles appeared in newsmagazines describing a new epidemic: the herpes epidemic. It was the one sexually transmitted disease that truly frightened people, heralding the end of the free-love era. It was incurable. It stayed with you forever.

You probably have herpes. Most people do. Before you go postal, however, know this: you probably have *herpes simplex virus I*, a virus that is quite similar to the sexually transmitted genital herpes, or *herpes simplex virus II*. Did you ever have a fever blister or a cold sore? Did you ever feel a tingling sensation on your upper lip when you're stressed out before that first date, only to find a blister there a day later? You've got herpes simplex virus I.

Unfortunately, a huge number of Americans also have herpes simplex virus II—an estimated forty million people have genital herpes, with some 500,000 new cases reported every year. And that number may actually be lower than the true number of people getting infected. According to the Herpes Resource Center, 75 percent of individuals with genital herpes have no idea they're infected, because a good deal of them show no symptoms.

When signs of illness do show up, they're often confused with other conditions. Flulike symptoms are often mistaken for the flu. Genital itching may be assumed to be simple jock itch. Sometimes there's urination pain or lower back pain, which may mean a kidney infection.

Perhaps the most telltale sign of genital herpes is an "outbreak"—a flare-up of red bumps on the genitals or buttocks that turn into painful blisters. After a few days, these bumps become blisters, and the blisters crust over (often within several weeks), heal, and subside. Sometimes another flare-up isn't seen for years—or ever. Or flare-ups occur frequently, depending on a person's physiology.

Diagnosis of genital herpes is difficult, because a sample from blister fluid must be extracted to determine if the virus is present. The problem comes if a person never has a flare-up, because there are no blisters from which to take fluid. It can be very tricky, indeed.

"According to the Herpes Resource Center, 75 percent of individuals with genital herpes have no idea they're infected, because a good deal of them show no symptoms."

Moreover, a person doesn't necessarily have to have an outbreak to pass the virus along to someone else. Unprotected oral, vaginal, or anal sex can transmit the disease. Transmission is further complicated by this fact: a person with herpes simplex virus I can give a person genital herpes by engaging in oral sex during an outbreak of a fever blister or cold sore.

Aside from playing havoc with an infected person's body, genital herpes can put a significant strain on relationships. For example, a monogamous couple could have been together for years, when suddenly one partner is diagnosed with genital herpes. It isn't a sign of infidelity on one person's part, but the fact that the virus had been dormant for a long time, possibly decades.

Safe sex is also complicated. Using a condom has been shown to be ineffective if an outbreak of lesions is near, but outside, the area covered by the condom. Also, if a female is infected, her bodily fluids may spill over the condom. In the case of genital herpes, the only safe measure is abstinence when an outbreak occurs. And, as mentioned earlier, the virus can be passed along even if there isn't a visible outbreak.

The good news? The duration of genital herpes outbreaks can be shortened through administration of antibiotics like acyclovir. And herpes vaccines are currently being tested in the U.S.

AIDS

Myth number one about AIDS: It's a new plague—a scourge that struck out of nowhere in the eighties, scorching the hedonism of the sexual revolution into cinders overnight.

In fact, frozen blood and tissue samples screened for HIV (the virus that leads to AIDS) in 1988 fixed the date of the first probable American AIDS death much earlier. A sexually active 15-year-old black male, known in the medical files as Robert R., succumbed in St. Louis in 1969 after a 16-month illness. And according to Drs. Lyn

Frumkin and John Leonard in *Questions and Answers on AIDS* (Health Information Press), stored blood samples from central Africa taken in 1959 showed HIV infection. So, the explosion of new cases that began in the late seventies and early eighties with ominous reports of a "strange wasting disease" among gay men in New York, Los Angeles, and San Francisco was really only the flare-up of an epidemic that apparently had been smoldering unseen for decades.

This "strange wasting disease" actually was a failure in (initially) men's immune systems to eliminate microorganisms that pose no threat to healthy people. This inability to respond to infections—and battle illness—was dubbed acquired immunodeficiency syndrome (AIDS), quite simply because that was the crux of the problem: the bodies of those infected had a deficiency in their immune systems, acquired from an outside source. That is, this disease wasn't genetic. Ironically, it wasn't AIDS that was killing off great numbers of men at the time, but the opportunistic illnesses that their bodies couldn't fight off. This includes illnesses like pneumonia and rare cancers.

HIV's Role

Researchers believe AIDS is caused by human immunodeficiency virus (HIV), a virus that kills lymphocytes—cells in the bloodstream that fight bacteria, fungi, and viruses. After all, HIV is present in the blood of almost all AIDS patients. And HIV is found most often in the groups most susceptible to getting AIDS—homosexuals, bisexuals, intravenous drug users, heterosexuals engaging in risky sexual practices.

In truth, the only way researchers could be universally sure that HIV causes AIDS is to infect individuals with HIV and monitor the progression of the virus. That did happen—sort of—when HIV-tainted blood was unknowingly donated at blood banks across the country in the early eighties; people outside of the AIDS-associated risk groups, such as children and the elderly, who received the blood contracted AIDS.

"HIV is transmitted one (or more) of three ways: through sexual contact; through contact with HIV-contaminated blood; and through transmission from mother to child at birth."

HIV is transmitted one (or more) of three ways: through sexual contact; through contact with HIV-contaminated blood; and through transmission from mother to child at birth.

Still, with all that's known about HIV and AIDS, the disease is elusive. AIDS, scientists discovered early on, isn't like other infections. For example, the cellular actions of something like a staph (staphylococcus bacteria) infection or gonorrhea can be charted and usually halted. While the overwhelming evidence is that HIV does indeed cause AIDS, scientists also know it's not HIV that makes you sick.

Rather, the virus serves as the doorway to a host of opportunistic invaders that otherwise healthy people would have no trouble defeating. It's not HIV that gives you a typical (and often fatal) AIDS-related pneumonia, but a fungus, *Pneumocystis carinii,* that exploits the vulnerability HIV creates. Another microbe, cytomegalovirus, lives in most humans as a harmless parasite. Unleashed by HIV, it can cause fever, uncontrollable diarrhea, liver failure, and blindness. Kaposi's sarcoma, a rare cancer marked by purplish lesions, previously was seen only in elderly Mediterranean men; it is now commonly diagnosed in young AIDS patients.

Also atypical is the long delay between initial infection and the first tangible symptom of illness. Most studies suggest a median lapse of ten years. But some HIV-positive people have remained symptom-free for as long as 15 years and counting—encouraging if you're HIV-positive, but a conundrum for epidemiologists, since statistics lag behind the virus by more than a decade.

Cold Statistics

According to the Centers for Disease Control, there were 548,102 reported AIDS cases as of June of 1996. Of these cases, more than 540,000 were adolescents or adults; more than 7,000 were children. According to statistics from the HIV/AIDS Surveillance Report, 51 percent of these cases were men who had sex with other men, 25 percent were heterosexual intravenous drug users, 7 percent were men who had sex with other men and were intravenous drug users, and 8 percent were persons who acquired the disease through heterosexual contact. One percent contracted the disease from an infected blood transfusion; hemophiliacs made up another 1 percent.

Although the heterosexual numbers seem low, the statistics are deceptive. In the early days of the AIDS epidemic, fully 90 percent of AIDS cases were homosexual men. That number has dropped, while the number of heterosexual cases has dramatically increased. And according to the book *Questions & Answers on AIDS,* 15 percent of the heterosexual population is currently at risk—through sexual practices, drug use, or the like.

Ever wonder why HIV isn't easily transmitted through a kiss? Turns out that saliva contains a sugar protein called thrombospondin that helps heal wounds, and has anti-HIV properties. This groundbreaking discovery was made at Cornell University. Human trials of TSP-coated condoms are expected to commence in 1999. If the new prophylactics prove to further inhibit the spread of HIV, you can bet FDA approval will follow promptly.

One more cause for concern in the heterosexual population: According to *Questions & Answers on AIDS,* AIDS cases in Africa—spread primarily through heterosexual contact—have also dramatically increased, showcasing how easy it is for a traditionally low-risk group to become a high-risk one. According to the World Health Organization, in Uganda alone, there are 1.3 million estimated cases of HIV. There are 900,000 in Zimbabwe; 840,000 in Tanzania; 650,000 in Malawi. All in countries with no significant homosexual populations. Ultimately, AIDS isn't just a "gay" disease.

> **"Indeed, Magic Johnson's claim in 1991 that he'd been infected by HIV through heterosexual intercourse suggested that the virus doesn't discriminate by sex or sexual preference."**

Indeed, Magic Johnson's revelation in 1991 that he'd been infected by HIV through heterosexual intercourse suggested that the virus doesn't discriminate by sex or sexual preference. Heterosexual AIDS, whatever its prevalence, is no myth.

Which distills to a harsh conclusion: AIDS is here; it's staying; get used to it. As far as you can see into the future, it'll be licking its lips, peering speculatively into bedrooms, snuggling up to anybody whose behavior encourages its spread. Barring a miracle, which nobody in the field is expecting, sobering AIDS statistics are going to form a hard-to-swallow part of our national diet for the foreseeable future.

Fear . . . or Fearless?

Are we defenseless? Emphatically not. Remember, a great deal is known about HIV infection, enough that you can somewhat accurately assess—and substantially lessen—your risk.

The fact is, regardless of whether you're straight or gay, you're vulnerable if you're sexually active. And once an individual's infected, HIV can be found in virtually all body fluids. Kissing seems safe—though no one can be sure that it's never been responsible for transmitting a case of HIV. And AIDS plainly can't be spread through a sneeze, touching, using the same toilet seat, or any other casual contact—one fact that Americans finally seem to understand.

But blood, semen, and vaginal fluids are dangerous; evidence is overwhelming that they're the major factors in the spread of the disease among humans. Contaminated blood, of course, is the main vehicle for HIV infection through intravenous drug use and accidental needle sticks among health workers; it's also a potential danger if it gets onto other, less widely feared implements, like tattooing needles or ear-piercing equipment.

When it comes to sexual transmission of HIV, semen and vaginal fluids are plainly the major culprits. In hetero sex, women, some experts contend, may be more vulnerable, both because semen carries a larger load of the virus and because of anatomy. Barbara Starrett, M.D., a New York physician with a large AIDS practice, both gay and straight, explains it. "Consider men's plumbing," she says. "A penis is generally well protected, with good skin around it. The urethral opening is small. Whether it's placed in a vagina or an anus, its potential for [becoming infected with] HIV is much smaller than (that of) the anal or vaginal canal."

Don't breathe a sigh of relief yet. "The insertive male is at less risk," Starrett adds, "but not at nonrisk." While estimates of the relative danger to men and women vary, studies clearly have shown that women can and do pass the infection to men during "normal" sex.

"Far too many males deny they're at risk from having sex with women," D. Peter Drotman, M.D., assistant director for public health in the CDC's Division of HIV/AIDS, says. "I don't think you can easily quantify the relative risk for men and women, but I'd say they're about equal." The Centers for Disease Control doesn't assume sex differences are a factor. "Unless preventive measures are taken," Drotman adds, "the next wave of infection will be from women to men. In a bizarre way we'll have equality, though I wouldn't characterize that as an achievement."

Frustrations and Hope

Almost 20 years into the AIDS epidemic, researchers are newly optimistic, encouraged that AIDS will be transformed from a death sentence into a manageable chronic illness like diabetes. A few have even suggested that AIDS might be curable.

Such thinking represents a major change of heart. When HIV, the virus that causes AIDS, was identified in the early eighties, researchers gamely predicted that a protective vaccine would be developed within a few years. But unlike most viruses that carry their genetic blueprint as DNA, making vaccine development comparatively straightforward, HIV is a retrovirus that carries its genetic code in the related RNA molecule. No RNA-virus vaccine has ever been created.

Their hopes for a vaccine dimmed, researchers focused on developing antiviral drugs that could control, if not actually kill, HIV. Azidothymidine (AZT), introduced with great fanfare some years ago, keeps the virus from subverting host-cell DNA, but AZT's benefits are

In New Jersey, knowingly penetrating a person while infected with a sexually transmitted disease other than HIV is a fourth-degree crime, punishable by up to 18 months in prison and a fine of $7,500. Doing the same to someone while infected with HIV will get you three to five years behind bars.

The HIV Test: One Man's Story

"I'm not gay. I've never had a blood transfusion. The closest I've come to shooting up is listening to Nirvana. So I always figured I wouldn't have to bother getting an HIV test, that it was for people with legitimate concerns.

"Then I found myself enjoying the post-sex glow with Sherry, whom I'd only known for a few months, and she was asking me if I had ever been tested. What difference does it make now? I thought. But I didn't want to ruin the moment by saying it, so I mumbled something about how I'd slept with just a handful of women in my life, all of them the girl-next-door type, whatever that means.

"'All it takes is one time,' she answered, an annoyingly cliched remark that instantly keyed in on my apprehension. 'I'd feel better about us if you got tested,' Sherry added.

"Apprehension gave way to offense: Was she implying I'd had sex with just anyone I could get my hands on, that I had lied to her about all my partners being the 'wholesome' type? No, I hadn't worn a jimmy every time I did the deed, but what guy could stay under wraps for seven years? 'What about you?' I responded.

"She looked at me like I'd just called her a whore, then defended her sex partners as I had mine. Frankly, I wouldn't have minded calling it a draw and dropping the matter altogether. For some reason, even though I'd stamped myself low-risk and undamaged, I really didn't want to get tested. But I did want to continue getting laid, and since Sherry said I couldn't have one without the other, the matter was settled.

"On my drive over to the community HIV-testing center, I started accounting for all the women in my past. Upon closer reflection, I realized that any one of my partners could have infected me with HIV. People can go years without experiencing any symptoms. Worse, I could have picked it up and passed it on to someone else.

"I parked across the street and down several blocks away from the testing center because I didn't want people speculating about why I was there. When I entered the harshly lit lobby, someone immediately ushered me back to a waiting room. Promptness was good: I wanted this whole thing to be over as quickly as possible. I wanted to get on with my life, to find out whether I'd have the chance to raise a family and pursue all the things I'd begun putting on hold in my mind.

"A volunteer medical counselor took me into his office and asked me several questions: Had I ever had unprotected vaginal sex? Anal sex? Oral sex? Had I ever injected drugs, had sex with a prostitute, been exposed to blood on the job? He explained to me how HIV is transmitted (all ways I had already heard or read about), then handed me a vial and an ID number.

"Several minutes later, a guy wearing latex gloves called me into his office and took some of my blood. A spot splattered my arm. 'Dark blood,' I said, trying to make conversation. 'Good blood,' he said blandly. We'll see, I thought.

"He told me to call back in ten days to see if the results had arrived. When they did, I'd have to come in to get them, along with some mandatory counseling. They don't give results over the phone for two reasons: one, in case someone gains access to your ID number and poses as you; and two, so they can give you counseling and, if necessary, a repeat test to confirm the results.

"As happy as I should have been that they were making such a big deal of maintaining anonymity, the secrecy disturbed me: It just drove home again how serious the matter was.

"With all that buildup, it's no wonder that I felt edgy the day I returned for my results. I was about to come face-to-face with my past, maybe my doom. When I sat down in the counselor's office, he said, 'You're definitely nonreactive.' I just about lost it. All I heard was that I 'definitely' had something. My God! I thought. Really? Then he explained that 'nonreactive' means the test detected no HIV antibodies. That was the extent of our little session. Walking out, I didn't know whether to cry for joy, or for the people in the lobby who may have tested positive.

"On our next date, Sherry and I exchanged results. She wasn't too thrilled about getting tested, either, but we agreed that the immediate discomfort paled in comparison to the thought of living with AIDS.

"Will I have unprotected sex again? I already have on several occasions—but with a woman who I now know is 'definitely nonreactive.' I'd like to say my reasons for getting tested were less selfish, more noble. I wish I could say I did it for my health and hers. But I was thinking with the wrong part of my body again. For once, though, it was giving me some sensible advice."

only temporary because the virus typically becomes resistant within a year or two. Other antiviral drugs can prolong AZT's effectiveness, but at best they're stopgap measures.

Recently, however, a promising new class of drugs that prevent HIV replication—protease inhibitors—was introduced. The first, saquinavir, won FDA approval in December 1995. Since then, two more—indinavir and ritonavir—have arrived, and they appear even more potent. In a four-month study, a combination of indinavir, AZT, and the antiviral 3TC controlled the virus in 24 of 26 people with high blood levels of HIV, to the point where it was no longer measurable. No other AIDS treatment has ever achieved such remarkable results. At the very least, the success of protease inhibitors combined with other drugs shows that HIV has vulnerabilities that future treatments might exploit. And at best, says HIV codiscoverer Robert Gallo, M.D., protease inhibitors just might make AIDS curable. More research is needed, however.

Safer Sex

Want to free yourself of the thought of acquiring a life-threatening STD? Unfortunately, there's no such thing as "safe sex." The only true protection against STDs is total abstinence from sexual activity. But for a large portion of the population—okay, almost all of us—that's impossible. So there's safer sex ... precautions you can take to ensure that you are as well protected as technology and science allows, while still affording you the pleasure you crave and deserve.

First and foremost among safer sex alternatives is an age-old method: communication. Talk with your partner to gauge your comfort level with various safer sex techniques, gadgets, and gizmos. Communication also allows you to get a frank understanding of your partner's sexual experience. That goes a long way toward achieving a more intimate relationship. Indeed, the safest sex is sex performed with a long-term, monogamous, uninfected partner. And honest communication can determine whether your significant other fits the bill.

Just looking for a one-night stand instead of a "more intimate relationship?" Then prepare to do battle with a host of bacteria and the like. Just do it with latex. As in latex condom. Be aware that condoms don't offer the be-all and end-all in protection. They break. They leak. And then there's that matter of oral sex. Using a condom is great for vaginal or anal sex, but often people forget that STDs can be transmitted orally, too.

Still, viruses and bacteria can't pass through latex—as they can with lambskin condoms, which have tiny imperfections in the skin membrane through which bacteria can creep.

Latex condoms are convenient, affordable, and readily available. Just walk into your corner grocery, liquor store, pharmacy, or even bowling alley. There are some things to be mindful of, though. Use a new condom for every sex act, not every session. For you ten-hour tigers out there, that means a reload with each new withdrawal and reposition of your mate. And be aware, latex can cause an allergic reaction in some men and women. Please note that there are plastic condoms on the market—these are effective birth control devices but aren't deterrents for STDs. The reason: they have a breakage rate four times that of latex condoms. If you're allergic to latex, try using a plastic condom with a latex condom layered on top of it.

Only use fresh condoms. Check the expiration date on the box. No expiration date? Then throw your stuff away and tell your partner your lack of a raincoat means a rain check. You probably bought a novelty condom or one that isn't under FDA approval. And that means there were no manufacturing regulations.

> "Use a new condom for every sex act, not every session. For you ten-hour tigers out there, that means a reload with each new withdrawal and reposition of your mate."

Also, check that condom for any grittiness. It's a telltale sign that the latex is too old—it's started to break down. It's also a sign that you don't get laid enough.

When unfurling the flag, so to speak, make sure that you open the condom package gently . . . and use the condom once you open it. That way, an opened package isn't lying around as you tussle. Less exposure means less potential damage to the rubber.

Hate condoms because they dull your sensitivity? Here's a trick: place a bit of water-based lubricant such as K-Y Jelly inside the condom before you put it on. That will heighten sensitivity. Be careful though. Slippage may occur. If you're not skilled at keeping a condom on—or if you don't know that the average sex-toy store has condoms of different sizes—avoid this trick altogether. If the condom is way too big—it happens—try pulling the base over your testicles to maintain coverage. Or, get the Mentor condom. It has adhesive around the rim to secure the condom to the base of your penis.

Want to increase security? Try the spermicide Nonoxynol–9. Nonoxynol–9 has been found to inhibit HIV growth in lab experiments. However, please note that Nonoxynol–9 by itself is not an effective barrier. It should be used in conjunction with a condom. Also be aware that Nonoxynol–9 has been known to cause genital irritation for both men and women.

Once the deed is done and you ejaculate, hold the condom at the base of your penis to prevent slipping and spillage of seed.

Then there's the female condom. Made of polyurethane, the female condom consists of two flexible rings inside a condom-shaped pouch. Inserted into the vagina, the female condom has proven to be an effective means of preventing STDs. (More on the female condom under Barrier Methods later in this chapter.)

Is oral sex your specialty? Two words for you: dental dams. These incredibly thin pieces of latex were originally used by drillers of a different sort—dentists used them to isolate teeth being repaired. But apply some water-based lubricant to one side, stretch that side over

Girl Talk

The AIDS Effect

We asked a group of women who work for *Shape*, our sister publication, to tell us what effect AIDS has had on their sex lives. Is it bringing back romance or killing it? Here's what a few of them said:

"It's bringing back lust."
　　—*Ann, 25, newly single*

"AIDS has kind of put the boot on my sex life—you know, like that thing they put on parked cars. I used to get to know people by sleeping with them. Not anymore."
　　—*Linda, thirty-something, single*

"It's bringing back an active fantasy life. It's very scary. I'm tired of serial monogamy, and that's why I'm 'kissing around' now instead of going farther. I'm kind of glad we're being forced to slow down, though. It's forced me to look at men in a completely different way. You get to know them without sex being part of the relationship."
　　—*Meredith, 29, single*

Condom Concern

The FDA has considered banning novelty condoms, such as glow-in-the-darks and flavoreds, from store shelves. The reason: Some of them are not subject to effectiveness tests and therefore may not provide adequate protection against pregnancy and sexually transmitted diseases.

When purchasing condoms for protection, read the package. It can only claim to provide protection if the brand is individually tested in conformity with FDA guidelines. Conversely, untested brands must stipulate on the package that they are not for disease or pregnancy prevention.

Unfortunately, some recent studies have cast serious doubts about the efficiency of even the most well-known condom brands. Responding to the studies, the Centers for Disease Control recently asserted, in strong terms, that condoms, when used properly and consistently, have an efficiency rate approaching 100 percent.

your partner's genitals, begin your oral sex routine, and she'll never think of a dental visit the same way again.

Dams have become so popular that a number of manufacturers are marketing them to the public—the sex-minded public, so you don't have to spirit some away when you go in for your six-month teeth cleaning. Gylde Dams are purportedly the thinnest and come in a variety of colors. And Lixx Dams come in strawberry and vanilla flavors—in case the taste of rubber doesn't turn you on. Or you can use a regular dam and spike it with a flavored water-based lubricant, like strawberry-flavored Motion Lotion.

Some sex education researchers even recommend the use of latex gloves during lovemaking, to further reduce the risk of contracting an STD. Just remember: no oil-based lubricants, such as Vaseline, on latex, as they break down latex properties. And remember to clip those fingernails.

Population Control

When you're in the midst of a glorious orgasm, and your body is quaking, shaking, and begging for more, it's easy to forget that intercourse actually has an evolutionary purpose—to propagate the species. Yup. Sex is the means to an end, and that end is reproduction. Making babies. The pleasure is merely a bonus . . . or insurance to keep the Homo sapiens population flourishing.

Fortunately, modern science makes it possible for us to have awesome sex without resulting in offspring—if we're careful and use the proper protection. These days, the majority of birth control options are for women. Though some complain that this minimizes the man's responsibility, others (including the female coauthor of this book), welcome the control. "It's not that I don't trust men," says Denise, a 29-year-old nurse from Detroit. "I just trust myself more."

Of course, even if both partners share the birth-control responsibility, there's still a risk that a pregnancy may occur. With the exception of abstinence, none of today's methods of preventing conception come with a 100-percent guarantee. The human body is an amazing machine that often surprises even the most highly trained medical experts.

What we do know is that the female reproductive system follows a pattern each month. Though we can't call it a predictable one—something as simple as a stressful day can throw off a woman's cycle—understanding the pattern provides greater insight into how the various birth control methods work.

The Anatomy of Female Reproduction

You know from your lesson on the female sexual anatomy in chapter 2 that the cervix is the opening through which sperm can enter the woman's uterus to fertilize an egg. The uterus, also known as the womb, is a muscular chamber where the fertilized egg implants and matures throughout a pregnancy. At the time of conception, the uterus is typically the size of a pear, but can expand to accommodate a growing baby.

Eggs are released from a woman's ovaries, two walnut-sized organs located on either side of her uterus. Each produces

"With the exception of abstinence, none of today's methods of preventing conception come with a 100-percent guarantee."

hormones and holds thousands of immature eggs. The fallopian tubes, which measure about four inches long and have an inner passageway that is no wider than the head of a pin, connect the ovaries and the uterus.

When you hear a woman refer to her "monthly cycle," she's talking about the hormonal process that prepares her body for a pregnancy. The cycle begins every 28 to 32 days following the onset of menstruation. Women have lots of nicknames for this weeklong span—from their "period" to their "friend" to "surfing the crimson tide." Whatever the preference, menstruation is usually a good indication that a woman has not become pregnant. Menstruation, after all, is the shedding of the uterine lining, which builds up each month to receive and nourish a fertilized egg.

Ovulation

As the uterine lining thickens, several egg follicles begin to mature on each ovary. Somewhere between days 12 and 18 days (on average), one follicle will rupture, releasing a fully developed egg. (In the case of multiple births, more than one egg may be released.) The egg is picked up by the nearest fallopian tube, through which it travels to the uterus. If Miss Egg happens to meet Mr. Spermatozoa along the way, fertilization will occur. Although millions of sperm are released during ejaculation, only one diligent fellow needs to penetrate the egg for a pregnancy to occur. At this point, the fertilized egg becomes an embryo and travels down to the uterus where it implants and begins to grow.

For couples trying to prevent pregnancy, it may be helpful to know that a woman is fertile for only a few days in each menstrual cycle—two to three days before ovulation, the day ovulation occurs, and one day afterward. Researchers have learned that once an egg is released, it's viable for only 24 hours. Sperm, on the other hand, can survive for several days inside of a woman, in her fallopian tubes or in one of the hundreds of glandlike cervical crypts. Having intercourse any time during that five-day window could result in a pregnancy.

One Small Schtupp for Man . . .

Peruse the aisles of your local pharmacy or sex-toy shoppe and you'll notice a bewildering array of prophylactics. Something in every size, shape, and color. In order to make sense of our condom culture—and condom couture—we sent New York–based stand-up comic Lee Frank on a mission. His goal: to find the condoms that were the most pleasurable. STD prevention didn't factor into his "road test." Bear that in mind, when you read his report:

I hate condoms. I know all about AIDS, I know all about herpes and syphilis and gonorrhea and chlamydia, too. I know if I'm not careful, my link to future generations might shrivel up and fall off.

Yes, I'm educated. And maybe education equals safe sex. But let's not kid ourselves: No one wants to have safe sex; and our occasional lapses in judgment have nothing to do with awareness. The truth is that denial, in many ways, is integral to the sex act, and AIDS is just one more item added to the list of things you don't want to think about. We know the risks. We choose pleasure. We tell ourselves AIDS is fatal but not serious.

So when I was asked to sort through the condoms on the market and find the one that feels the best, I thought maybe they meant the one that feels the least bad. Nevertheless, what I

discovered amazed me: I learned that while I've been bitching and moaning about Trojans, science has been busy improving the condom. I also learned that my girlfriend, God bless her, can be very supportive. Together we tested more rubber than Charles Goodyear.

Clipboard and pen at my bedside, I begin my evaluations with the three market leaders: Trojan, Ramses, and LifeStyles. I also try some other big sellers, including Gold Coin and Prime. I hate them all. Prime maybe a little less. My joystick feels rubberized, like I just slapped on a few coats of Weatherbeater. My girlfriend says it's like having sex with the Michelin Man. I make a note on my clipboard.

Disheartened, I return to my makeshift lab bearing a selection of Japanese-made latex condoms produced by two companies, Sagami and Okamoto. Eureka. The Sagamis, in particular, are noticeably thinner and more transparent than the others I've tried. The company's Excalibur condoms (apparently, whoever names these things finds inspiration in the Arthurian legends) is fine, but I mostly like their Vis-A-Vis, which is contoured and ultrathin, and their Type E, which is form-fitted with ribs and tiny bumps and tinted green. My girlfriend says it's like having sex with a Martian. I make a note on my clipboard.

I try one of the Okamotos, a style that has been mysteriously dubbed Beyond 7. This is one tight condom. I don't like it. I feel like Cinderella's fat stepsister squeezing her foot into the glass slipper and going for a jog. I also don't like the Snugger Fit condom for the same reason. I'm huge. What can I say?

But not that huge. I wish I could report that the extra-large condoms—Magnum and Maxx—are my size, but they hang off me like loose-fitting sweaters and have all the sensitivity you'd expect from a cardigan. Somehow the Magnum feels better than the Maxx. My girlfriend says it's like having sex with a man possessed of shattered dreams.

The Rough Rider condom is studded "for her pleasure." But she says she can't feel a thing, so I turn it inside out and make it studded for *my* pleasure. Ummmm. Not bad. Where is that clipboard?

I also try a Tuxedo Condom, which is colored black. I love the name. It's like formal wear—for when you're not having casual sex. I fantasize that I am Linc from the Mod Squad.

At this point, I'm beginning to suspect that in the field of condoms, as with automobiles and electronics, the Japanese have once again left America in the dust. And indeed, while these products have not yet caught fire on our shores, Jerry Sachs,

Sagami's eastern district manager, tells me that the brand is already the number-one seller just about everywhere in the Western world except America. Don't laugh; 20 years ago you probably couldn't even pronounce "Toyota."

Not willing to see America take a beating from foreign competition, a New Jersey surgeon went back to the drawing board a few years ago and came up with the first major condom innovation in 30 years. Lookit: When you wear a conventional condom, the only way to feel friction is through the latex barrier, but A.V.K. Reddy, M.D., solved the problem. His Pleasure Plus condoms have a small pouch on the underside. The idea is that the latex moves around right beneath the head of your trouser-trout, stimulating the most sensitive area. This ties for first place in my search for the best-feeling condom. Yeah, I like it. My girlfriend says she, too, is thoroughly satisfied. Reddy says women generally rate this one high because the latex bunches up into small wrinkles at the base of the condom, within striking distance of the clitoris. The Pleasure Plus condom is marketed by Reddy Distributors in Windsor, New Jersey.

My choice for a first-place tie surprises even me—it's the Reality female condom. Yup, that tubular monstrosity we've seen on all the talk shows. I am shocked to discover that despite its alarming resemblance to a Hefty Cinch-Sack, it actually feels great—to me, anyway. I ask my girlfriend how she likes it, but she's peering over my shoulder at the Yankees game. To get her attention, I put another condom on myself. "Do you smell rubber burning?" she asks.

The big reason the Reality feels so pleasurable is that it's made of a soft, heat-conducting plastic, rather than latex, which has insulative properties. But in terms of aesthetics, forget it. The female condom is not a pretty sight: It dangles out of her like her guts are falling out.

The material used in Reality is similar to what's being developed for the new plastic male condoms. At least one company, Tactyle Technologies of Vista, California, hopes to have a product made of what they call thermoplastic elastomer on the market by the time this book is published. It's a real bitch getting hold of a demo model, but I'm glad I finally get to sample it. I place it in a three-way tie for first. That's right, there are three world's-best condoms. If that's not definitive enough for you, well, have pity. I'm getting sore, and my girlfriend is getting annoyed.

In addition to transferring heat, a plastic condom is twice as strong as latex, so it can be made thinner. You can use oil-based lubricants on it (which would dissolve latex). And for the 3 percent of the population who are allergic to latex, the Tactylon is a godsend. "Hmmm, plastic," my girlfriend says. "This must be like having sex with a Ken doll." Damn, I've got to find that clipboard.

I also sample some novelty items, which, for the most part, turn out to be disappointing. You want a taste sensation, eat a Peppermint Patty. The flavored condoms, my girlfriend says, are more on the order of "sucking on a mildly flavored hockey puck." They don't do much for me either, though we both rate Kiss of Mint slightly higher than the flavored Malaysian condoms designed to simulate Trader Vic's-style cocktail punch.

There is also a glow-in-the-dark condom with a hand on the end. It's made with more rubber than the Hindenburg and lights up like somebody pumped radium into Mickey Mouse's arm. Again, it falls way short in terms of sensitivity, but my girlfriend says the little fingers are tickling her G-spot. If I could figure out which finger, I'd be a millionaire.

I think the key to scoring with willy-wear is learning to have fun with it. Because, in truth, I find that there is no condom that feels exactly like nothing at all. But a few come really close—close enough so you no longer have to sacrifice pleasure for safety.

There, I said it. I've learned to stop worrying and start loving condoms.

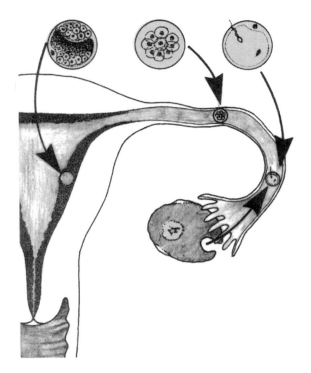

Fertilization: All it takes is one sperm in the right place (a fallopian tube) at the right time (between 12 and 24 hours after ovulation) to fertilize the egg. Almost immediately, the fertilized egg, known as the zygote, begins to divide, making its way to the uterus, where it implants (within about four days) and begins to grow into an embryo. That embryo takes about ten months to grow into a bouncing baby, who then takes about 12 years before growing into an obnoxious teenager.

Contraception Methods

So that's the bare-bones scoop on reproduction. What follows is a summary of the methods of preventing it from happening, the effectiveness of each option, and the pros and cons of each. Make sure you consider your lifestyle when choosing contraception and discuss your preferences with your partner. If spontaneity is important, for example, Mr. Happy may lose his enthusiasm quickly if your girlfriend has to run to the bathroom to insert her diaphragm. And if you're having casual sex—that is, sex with individuals you don't know very well—you should always use a condom. As mentioned previously, it's the only method of birth control that also greatly reduces your risk of catching—or passing—sexually transmitted diseases. As morose as it may sound, the condom should be viewed as a preventer of both life and death. Single guys should keep a stash on hand at all times.

With that said, contraception basically falls into five categories—hormonal methods, barrier methods, natural family planning, sterilization, and abstinence. Here are the options.

Hormonal Methods

Hormones are chemical substances that the body secretes to control the various organs. Birth control methods that fall into this category involve the use of synthetic hormones that control the functioning of the female sex and reproductive systems. First introduced in the sixties—and now available in pill, injection, or implant form—hormonal-based contraception is among today's most popular means of preventing pregnancy.

The Combined Pill

How it works: Combined oral contraceptives are birth control pills that contain estrogen and progestin, two hormones produced by the body during pregnancy. This one-two punch attempts to prevent conception primarily by stopping the ovaries from releasing an egg. It also makes the lining of the uterus thinner. The latter is a kind of safety net. If the estrogen doesn't do its trick—and an egg is released—the thin uterine lining prevents the embryo from thriving. There are three types of combined pills, called mono-, bi-, and triphasic. Monophasic pills contain the same level of hormones, whereas the other two vary the amount of each hormone to follow the body's natural cycle more closely.

How it's used: One prescription pill is taken at about the same time each day for 21 days, then no pill (or a sugar pill) is taken for 7 days during menstruation. The sugar pill is an inactive pill useful for women who have trouble remembering to take medication. Physicians recommend using a backup method of birth control when a pill is missed, or when a woman is on antibiotics, which can reduce the effectiveness of the hormones.

Effectiveness: About 99 percent when used to the letter; about 97 percent otherwise.

Pros: The Combined Pill . . .

- can be used by most women, up to the onset of menopause if they remain healthy (and have regular pelvic exams) and are non-smokers;
- has been proven to decrease a woman's risk of developing ovarian and uterine cancers as well as ovarian cysts and benign (noncancerous) breast masses;
- decreases symptoms of premenstrual syndrome, including tender breasts, menstrual pain, and cramping;
- regulates a woman's menstrual cycle;
- reduces menstrual bleeding and the risk of developing anemia;
- reduces acne flair-ups (one variation, Tricyclen, is often prescribed as an acne treatment);
- does not interfere with lovemaking;
- tends to heighten a woman's sexuality because she is confident she won't get pregnant.

Cons: The Combined Pill . . .

- does not protect either partner from the spread of HIV or other infections;
- has to be taken every day;
- can cause nausea, breast tenderness, midcycle bleeding during the first few months, as well as weight gain, mood swings, headaches, and skin problems;
- can cause serious complications such as blood clots, but this is very rare;
- has been known to promote the growth of breast cancer—but not to cause it;
- can be obtained only by prescription, although some clinicians will provide three to six months of pills without a pelvic exam.

Average cost: Between $25 to $45 per month.

The Mini Pill

How it works: This variation of the Pill contains only one hormone, progestin, and works by thickening the cervical mucus so sperm cannot reach the egg, and thinning the lining of the uterus to prevent implantation (in case conception does occur). The Mini Pill also affects ovulation in some women by preventing the ovaries from releasing an egg. However, using only one hormone decreases the effectiveness of the Mini Pill somewhat.

How it's used: A woman takes one pill a day for 28 days and then starts a new pack.

Effectiveness: Works 96 percent of the time when taken according to prescription.

Pros: The Mini-Pill . . .

- has fewer side effects than the Pill—that is, nausea, breast tenderness, midcycle bleeding, weight gain, mood swings, headaches, or skin problems are less likely to occur;

- can be used by nursing mothers, preferably after the baby is six weeks old.

Cons: The Mini Pill . . .

- does not provide protection against HIV or other infections;
- can cause menstrual irregularity (a woman can go several months with no bleeding at all), as well as spotting in between periods;
- must be taken every single day to be effective;
- has a slightly higher failure rate than the combined Pill;
- requires a prescription.

Average cost: Between $25 and $45 per month.

Contraceptive Implants

How they work: Norplant implants are six small (matchstick-like) tubes that are surgically implanted into a woman's upper arm. It takes about seven to ten minutes to perform the relatively painless procedure. Once implanted, the tubes slowly release small amounts of levonorgestrel, a synthetic form of progesterone that keeps the ovaries from releasing eggs, thickens the cervical mucus, and inhibits the thickening of the uterine lining.

How to use them: Women typically schedule a doctor's appointment to have them inserted—and then forget about them. Norplant implants offer the benefit of not thinking about birth control for five years. During that time, if a woman decides to have a child, the implants can be removed and fertility returns immediately.

Effectiveness: Works 99 percent of the time.

Pros: Norplant . . .

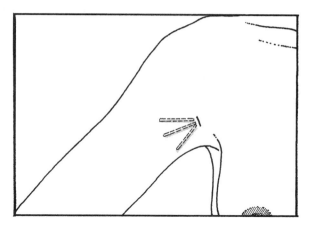

- is highly effective (only one woman in a thousand becomes pregnant during the first year of use);
- provides protection within 24 hours of insertion;
- protects against uterine cancer;
- can be safely used after childbirth and during breast-feeding;
- reduces menstrual bleeding;
- is a low-maintenance form of birth control, requiring nothing more than an annual doctor's checkup for five years;
- allows for spontaneous lovemaking.

Cons: Norplant . . .

- does not prevent the spread of HIV or other infections;
- has been known to cause irregular bleeding and prolonged periods (though blood flow is often light);
- can have wicked side effects, including weight gain, hair loss, headaches, acne, and depression;
- can lead to a decreased sex drive;
- can cause arm discomfort and discoloration of the skin surrounding the implants (and the tubes are often visible);
- must be inserted and removed by a trained clinician. (Not all doctors offer Norplant.)

Average cost: Between $450 and $900 for insertion, and $100 to $200 for removal. Some docs require payment up front; others permit financing.

Injections

How it works: The birth control shot contains a drug called Depo-Provera, which functions much like progesterone—preventing the release of an egg, thickening cervical mucus, and inhibiting the growth of the uterine lining.

How it's used: A woman takes a trip to her health-care practitioner once every three months (or 13 weeks) and rolls up her sleeve for the injection.

Effectiveness: Works 99 percent of the time, provided the woman gets her shots on schedule.

Pros: Depo-Provera . . .

- often results in lighter periods, less menstrual cramping, and reduced PMS symptoms;
- protects against uterine cancer;
- can be used by nursing mothers;
- permits spontaneous lovemaking.

Cons: Depo-Provera . . .

- does not protect against HIV or the transmission of other infections;
- is not recommended if pregnancy is desired within one to two years (fertility can take up to 24 months to return after a depo injection);
- causes irregular periods; menstruation may cease entirely after three injections (which is safe);
- can cause bloating and weight gain, headaches, and depression;
- requires a visit to the doctor every three months;
- may cause allergic reactions (although this is rare);
- is not a logical option for women with aversions to needles;
- may lower your estrogen level, causing bone mineral loss. (Though this is not certain, doctors recommend that women on Depo-Provera take calcium supplements and exercise regularly.)

Average cost: $30 to $65 every three months.

Emergency Contraceptive Pills (ECPs)

How they work: Approved last fall by the FDA, ECPs (commonly referred to as morning after pills and packaged under the label Preven) are essentially two large doses of ordinary birth control pills given to women after unprotected intercourse. Due to the potency of the double dose, an anti-nausea drug is often administered simultaneously. A synthetic steroid called Damazol also is used as a morning after pill. Both options alter a woman's hormonal patterns, either preventing fertilization or stopping a fertilized egg from implanting in the womb. Prior to FDA approval, ECPs were prescribed primarily to victims of rape. Under normal circumstances, physicians did not offer the drugs unless requested by a patient. With the new government sanction, Planned Parenthood expects doctors to feel more comfortable prescribing morning after pills, thus revolutionizing efforts to reduce the need for abortions.

How they're used: A first batch of pills (which can vary from two to five tablets depending upon the type used) is taken within 72 hours after unprotected intercourse, and the second batch 12 hours later.

Effectiveness: Statistics on the effectiveness of emergency contraceptive pills range from 75 percent to 95 percent. The controversial drug RU-486, currently available only in France, Britain, Sweden, and China, is 100 percent effective.

Pros: Emergency contraceptive pills . . .

- are a viable means of preventing unwanted pregnancy should a condom break, or a diaphragm or cervical cap become dislodged, or following unprotected sex;
- are safe for women who can't take birth control pills on a regular basis;
- can prevent abortions and are a more affordable means of terminating a pregnancy;
- can be left in your medicine cabinet in case of emergency.

Cons: ECPs . . .

- cause nausea in at least 50 percent of women and vomiting in about 20 percent of women;
- can cause bleeding, breast tenderness, and headaches for days;
- have rare side effects, including blood clots, heart attacks, stroke, liver problems, and high blood pressure;
- may cause birth defects if pregnancy occurs.

Average cost: Between $25 and $45.

Barrier Methods

The name aptly describes this type of birth control: barrier contraceptives are designed to block the sperm from reaching the egg. Many individuals favor this option because it doesn't involve medication—or even a prescription in some cases. Others feel that the various barrier methods of preventing pregnancy—the diaphragm, the contraceptive sponge, and the condom, for example—lack spontaneity and take the sizzle out of sexual encounters.

Though the latter may be true, particularly in newer relationships, most of your choices in this category also provide some protection against sexually transmitted diseases. The way we see it, spur-of-the-moment sex is a small price to pay for a lifetime of great safe sex. The condom, in particular, is the most effective means of protection against STDs, particularly the HIV virus. We'll discuss the prophylactic's usefulness as a birth control option here; however, we have devoted an entire section of this chapter to its role in safe sex.

Intrauterine Devices

How they work: There are two types of intrauterine devices: the Copper T and the Progestasert IUD. Both must be inserted by a physician into a woman's uterus. The Copper T is T-shaped (there's a no-brainer) and releases small amounts of copper into the uterine cavity to stop sperm from making their way up into the fallopian tubes. The Progestasert is similarly T-shaped, but contains progesterone, which thickens the cervical mucus so that sperm cannot reach the egg. Both types of IUD prevent an embryo from implanting in the uterus should fertilization occur. And both have tampon-like strings that hang down from the cervix into the vagina.

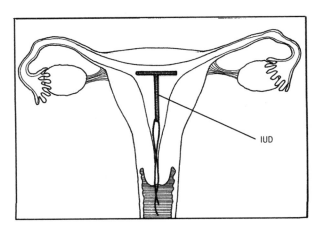

IUD

How they're used: IUDs are inserted by physicians, generally at the time of a woman's period. They can be left in for as many as ten years, but require that a woman check for the string after each period. This ensures that the device is in place and still providing protection against pregnancy.

Effectiveness: The Copper T works 99 percent of the time; the Progestasert 97 percent.

Pros: The Copper T . . .

- is the most effective reversible method of birth control currently available in the United States;
- needs to be changed only every ten years;
- prevents ectopic pregnancies;
- can be used while breast-feeding;
- may be inserted immediately following the delivery of a baby, or immediately after an abortion;
- does not interfere with lovemaking.

Pros: The Progestesert . . .

- provides effective contraception for one year;
- decreases menstrual cramping and blood loss;
- can be used while breast-feeding;
- encourages spontaneous sex.

Cons: The Copper T . . .

- does not protect against sexually transmitted diseases;
- may cause cramping, pain, or spotting after insertion;
- may increase menstrual cramping as well as the number of bleeding days;

- may fall out without the woman's knowledge, thus putting a couple at risk for an unplanned pregnancy;
- must be inserted by a doctor, nurse practitioner, nurse-midwife, or physician's assistant;
- may cause an allergic reaction in some women.

   Cons: The Progestesert . . .

- commonly causes irregular periods, increasing the number of bleeding days but not the flow of blood;
- causes menstrual flow to stop completely in some women (which could be viewed as a plus, depending upon her mindset);
- may cause cramping or pain at the time of insertion;
- must be replaced after one year;
- may fall out without the woman's knowledge, thus putting a couple at risk for an unplanned pregnancy;
- must be inserted by a doctor, nurse practitioner, nurse-midwife, or physician's assistant;
- can be costly to remove and insert an IUD each year.

   Average cost: Insertion of the Copper T costs $250 to $750 every ten years; the Progestesert costs $200 to $400 annually.

The Diaphragm

   How it works: The diaphragm is a shallow latex disk with a flexible rim that a woman places into her vagina to cover her cervix. A coating of spermicide jelly is applied to the inside of the diaphragm and around the rim; the combination, when used properly, effectively blocks and immobilizes the sperm in its sprint to enter the uterus.

   How it's used: Diaphragms come in different sizes—just like the women who use them. In order to ensure that the contraceptive fits properly, a physician will take an internal measurement and provide a prescription, along with—ahem—hands-on instructions in inserting and removing the device. As weird as it sounds, it's best for women to get their practice with experts. After all, the springlike rim of the diaphragm has been known to rebel, sending the device careening across the room. Better that this happens at the doctor's office than in the bedroom, where rocketing prophylactics could take the spark out of the most ardent romantic.

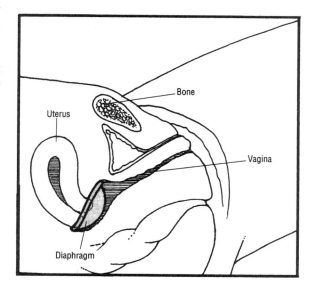

As for the spontaneity debate, the diaphragm can be inserted up to six hours before intercourse. So if a woman thinks she might get lucky, she can be prepared. After the deed has been done, the diaphragm must remain in the vagina for six to eight hours. (It can be left in place for up to 24 hours; however, if marathon sex is in order, an extra dose of spermicide is necessary for each go-around.)

Effectiveness: Between 82 and 94 percent, according to Planned Parenthood, with real-world stats leaning toward the lower end of the range.

Pros: The diaphragm . . .

- can be put in several hours before sexual activity, so it doesn't necessarily eliminate spontaneity;

- is easy to insert—with a little practice;

- cannot be felt by either partner when inserted properly;

- contains no hormones, which means no bloaty, headachy, crampy side effects like with the Pill;

- can provide some protection against sexually transmitted diseases, including chlamydia and gonorrhea.

Cons: The diaphragm . . .

- must be fitted by a physician;

- requires repeat fittings following a pregnancy, or a weight loss (or gain) of more than ten pounds;

- can be messy to insert;

- may disrupt lovemaking;

- may become dislodged when certain positions are taken (such as the woman on top), thus increasing the risk of an unwanted pregnancy;

- must be left in for at least six hours after intercourse;

- must be washed thoroughly after each sexual encounter;

- may cause an increase in urinary tract infections;

- may cause an allergic reaction in women sensitive to latex;

- must be replaced periodically (because the rubber can deteriorate).

Average cost: Between $50 and $125 for an examination and fitting and about $13 to $25 for the diaphragm, plus an additional $4 to $18 for a kit of spermicide jelly or cream.

Cervical Cap

How it works: Think of the cervical cap as the diaphragm's twerpy sibling. Whereas the palm-sized diaphragm has a dome shape, the cervical cap looks like a thimble and is fitted more tightly to cervix. When coated with spermicide, it prohibits sperm from passing into the uterus and rendezvousing with an egg.

How it's used: Cervical caps come in four sizes and must be fitted by a physician. You can insert it within an hour prior to lovemaking and it will continue to provide protection for up to 48 hours without additional spermicide.

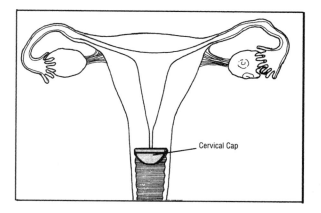

Cervical Cap

Effectiveness: Statistics vary widely: 64 percent to 91 percent effectiveness is cited. Planned Parenthood says the device is less effective for women who have had children than for those who have not.

Pros: The cervical cap . . .

- is small enough to fit in a purse;
- can be inserted an hour before sex and can be left in for up to 48 hours;
- allows you to have sex repeatedly over a 48-hour period without requiring additional spermicide, as long as you leave it in for at least six hours afterwards;
- cannot be felt by either partner if inserted properly;
- provides some protection against sexually transmitted diseases, when used with spermicides (though not as much as a condom).

Cons: The cervical cap . . .

- must be fitted by a physician;
- is more difficult than the diaphragm to insert and remove;
- can be dislodged;
- can cause urinary tract infections and allergic reactions in some women;
- can make oral sex less appealing;
- can cause an unpleasant odor when worn for longer periods of time;
- can deteriorate over time;
- must be refitted annually, as well as after pregnancy and a weight gain or loss of more than ten pounds.

Average cost: The cervical cap will make the same initial dent in the budget as the diaphragm, but because it has to be replaced more frequently, it's ultimately more expensive.

Spermicides

How they work: Creams, foams, vaginal suppositories, and vaginal film form a chemical barrier that either destroys sperm or makes it immobile and unable to pass through the cervix to meet the egg.

How it's used: Vaginal suppositories are inserted like a tampon and can take up to an hour to dissolve. Creams and foams come with applicators that place the product inside the vagina near the cervix. All forms of spermicide come with specific instructions, but in general must be in place within 30 minutes prior to intercourse.

Effectiveness: Spermicides prevent pregnancy about 80 percent of the time.

Pros: Spermicides . . .

- can be purchased over the counter;
- are relatively inexpensive;
- pose no known health risks;
- offer some protection against sexually transmitted diseases.

Cons: Spermicides . . .

- can be messy;
- are not considered reliable unless used in conjunction with other barrier contraceptives, such as a diaphragm or a condom;
- lack spontaneity;
- can cause vaginal irritation and allergic reactions;
- must be reapplied each time you have intercourse;
- require the woman to wait at least eight hours before bathing or douching.

Male Condom

How it works: A sheath of thin latex, plastic, or animal skin is worn over the penis to collect semen before, during, and after ejaculation to prevent sperm from reaching the egg.

How it's used: A condom should be unrolled over the shaft of an erect penis before the penis has any contact with a woman's vagina. Air bubbles should be smoothed out and a pocket (reservoir) must remain at the tip to collect sperm.

Removing the condom is a crucial step in ensuring the contraceptive's effectiveness. One partner should hold onto the rim of the condom in order to keep it on the shaft of the penis while the man withdraws his penis from the vagina. (A condom should also be worn during anal sex and when the man is fellated to protect against the transmission of HIV.) To minimize leakage, it's best to withdraw the penis before it becomes flaccid.

Effectiveness: Unfortunately, condoms can break and they can leak, so the figures for this contraceptive aren't the greatest. On the low end, it's cited as 80 percent effective, but when used in conjunction with spermicide, that figure jumps to 98 percent.

Pros: Condoms . . .

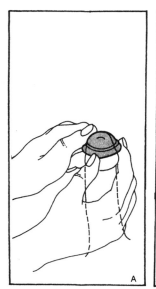
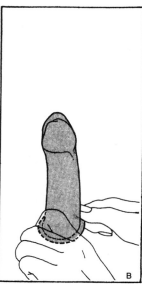

- in latex form, are the most effective means of preventing the spread of sexually transmitted diseases, including the HIV virus;
- allow men to take responsibility for birth control;
- can be worn by virtually all men (those who are sensitive to rubber may try plastic or animal tissue condoms, though these won't provide the same level of protection against STDs);
- can be purchased over the counter or via mail order for added privacy;
- comes in a variety of sizes and shapes to accommodate all types of men;
- can help relieve premature ejaculation;
- has no side effects for either partner.

Cons: Condoms . . .

- can potentially break or leak;
- in animal-skin and plastic form do not protect against STDs;
- can inhibit sensation for both partners;
- may interfere with spontaneity;

Give her a break—buy lubricated condoms. According to researchers at the University of Michigan, women whose partners use unlubricated prophylactics are 30 times more likely to developing their first urinary tract infection than those whose partners use no condom at all. The researchers' thinking? The unlubricated condoms cause greater friction during intercourse, giving bacteria a more direct route into the body.

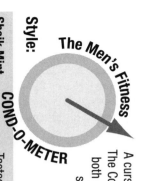

The Men's Fitness COND-O-METER

A cursory guide to condoms featuring actual quotes from our testers. The Cond-O-Meter is a subjective assessment gauging sensitivity, ease of use and range of pleasure provided to both partners. It's not meant to indicate a product's effectiveness in preventing pregnancy or disease. Our scale: 10=Orgasmic; 1=Are we having sex yet?

Style:	Boning Up:	He Said:	She Said:	Cond-O-Meter Rating:
Sheik Mint	Tastes better than rubber and is unlubricated, making it an excellent option for oral sex.	Here, honey, have some breath freshener.	Is this a hint?	3
Trojan Ultra Pleasure	Designed to enhance sensation.	Hey, when did you get here?	Get off me!	1
Handy Condom	Glows in the dark.	This looks like a light saber from Star Wars.	Come to the dark side, young Skywalker.	6
Pleasure Plus	Has a baggy pouch at the tip that massages the penis with each stroke.	Gaaaaa!	Gaaaaa!	9
X-Tra Pleasure	Oversized tip shaped to enhance friction and enhance sensation.	Gaaaaaaaaaaaaaaa!	Gaaaaaaaaaaaaaaa!	9.5
Gold Circle Coin	Unlubricated and packaged in a snazzy foil wrapper that can be opened by mouth. Look, mom, no hands.	Am I in yet?	Next!	1
Vis-a-Vis	Contoured and ultrathin condom from the Far East.	Tora! Tora! Tora!	Oh, God!	8
Tactylon	Fantastic Elastic Bubble Plastic for adults.	Ay caramba!	Kiss me, you mad, mad fool!	9
Reality Female Condom	It's for her.	Wow! Amazing!	Yuk!	9 (he) 2 (she)

- when used in conjunction with spermicides, may irritate female partners.

Average cost: Dry condoms start at about 25 cents a piece (cheap!); lubricated varieties are priced upwards of 50 cents; and condoms made of plastic or animal tissue, or those that are textured for extra sensitivity ("ribbed for her pleasure!"), can cost more than $2.50 each.

Female Condom

How it works: The Reality female condom works like an inverted male condom. Made of a thin plastic called polyurethane, it lines the vaginal walls, with the closed end positioned at the cervix and the open end positioned outside the vagina. Flexible rings on both ends keep the contraceptive device in place.

How it's used: The sheath is placed inside the vagina before coming in contact with the penis. A new condom must be used each time a couple has intercourse.

Effectiveness: Between 75 and 85 percent; slightly higher when used in conjunction with a spermicide.

Pros: The female condom . . .

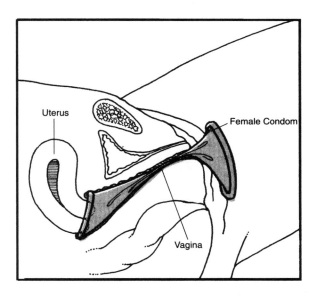

- provides protection against sexually transmitted diseases, including HIV;
- can be purchased over the counter and through the mail;
- is fairly sturdy and stays in place well;
- provides women with the ability to protect themselves against STDs.

Cons: The female condom . . .

- decreases vaginal sensation;
- requires advanced planning (as they're not as readily available as the male condom);
- can only be used once;
- looks funky—protruding outside of the vagina (if the male condom is a raincoat, this is a tent);
- tends to make strange rustling noises prior to intercourse (lubricants may help here);

- can be difficult to insert;

- are triple the price of most male condoms.

    Average cost: Between $1.50 and $3.50 each.

Natural Family Planning

How it works: The most successful method of avoiding pregnancy is to abstain from sex—that is, to not have intercourse at all. For those who are single—and whose religious faith dictates abstinence—this is the only birth control option until marriage. But even then, contraceptive devices may be frowned upon by the church. Sex in marriage, after all, is about being fruitful and multiplying. For these individuals, as well as for women who prefer to avoid hormonal or mechanical intervention, there's the fertility awareness method (FAM).

Commonly referred to as the rhythm method or natural family planning, FAM involves monitoring a woman's monthly menstrual cycle for signs that indicate when she is the most fertile. During these "unsafe days," couples either abstain from sex or use a barrier contraceptive.

Because a woman's cycle can vary from month to month, most physicians recommend professional training in the various FAM techniques, which include charting basal body temperature, observing cervical mucus, and charting the menstrual cycle on a calendar. Should a couple change their mind about having a baby, these efforts can help them conceive as well.

How it's used: To increase the effectiveness of natural contraception, most physicians recommend using all three of the FAM. Here's how they work:

- Charting basal body temperature: A woman's temperature goes up and down throughout her cycle. Beginning on the first day of her period, she takes her temperature before getting out of bed in the morning. Barring an illness, the temperature remains fairly consistent until just before ovulation, when it dips slightly and then rises between 0.4 degrees and 0.8 degrees Fahrenheit. It remains at that level until her next period or if she becomes pregnant. Conception may occur anytime during the six days prior to the temperature rise, so experts recommend completing at least three months of a temperature chart to note patterns and consistencies.

- Observing changes in cervical mucus: A woman's vaginal discharge also changes throughout her cycle. Generally cloudy and sticky, the mucus becomes clear and slippery a few days before ovulation, so much so that it can be stretched between the fingers. Slippery mucus is a key indicator of a woman's most fertile days, as it enables the sperm to race more quickly to the egg. Avoiding pregnancy means avoiding intercourse, or using an alternative form of birth control, when this change is detected.

- Charting on a calendar: With this technique, a woman charts her menstrual cycle on a calendar in an attempt to predict which day of the month she will ovulate. This only works for women who menstruate "like clockwork" every 28 to 32 days. It assumes that ovulation takes place somewhere between days 12 and 18 of the cycle and requires abstinence during the "unsafe" days. Because sperm can live for up to three days in a woman's body, using the calendar technique on its own would mean avoiding intercourse for at least half of the month. What fun is that?

Effectiveness: Planned Parenthood claims the fertility awareness method is between 80 to 99 percent effective. Achieving the higher end of the scale requires using all three methods simultaneously—without fail.

Pros: The fertility awareness method . . .

- has no medical or hormonal side effects;
- is accepted by most religions;
- is easy to use, with calendars, thermometers, and charts readily available.

Cons: The fertility awareness method . . .

- does not protect against sexually transmitted diseases;
- requires fastidious record-keeping;
- requires a cooperative partner, who won't pressure a woman to have sex on her "unsafe" days;
- can be negatively impacted by illness or lack of sleep (which cause body temperature to rise) and vaginal infections and douches (which alter the consistency and texture of cervical mucus);
- is ineffective for woman who have irregular periods or temperature patterns.

Average cost: About $10 for the thermometer, $2 for a notebook for charting temperature changes, and $5 for a calendar.

Withdrawal

How it works: "But honey, I pulled out." Those are often the famous last words uttered by men who prefer withdrawal—or coitus interruptus—as their method of birth control. The premise of withdrawal is that sperm won't get to the egg if the penis is removed from the vagina just prior to ejaculation. Though withdrawal is certainly better than doing nothing at all, it's still risky, as most men release pre-ejaculate containing enough sperm to cause pregnancy. And even if you're the tidiest guy in the world, your semen can spill on the vulva upon withdrawal, providing sperm with access to the vaginal canal. All it takes is one diligent swimmer to make a baby.

How it's used: At the point when a man feels he can no longer control or postpone his ejaculation, he withdraws his penis from the woman's vagina, being careful not to spill any semen near the vulva.

Effectiveness: Estimates indicate that one-quarter of the couples regularly using this method of birth control will become pregnant. In other words, it's reliable only 75 percent of the time.

Pros: Withdrawal . . .

- involves no medical or mechanical intervention;

- does not affect spontaneity.

Cons: Withdrawal . . .

- does not protect against sexually transmitted diseases;

- requires the man to have significant self-control (not always possible);

- is extremely risky if a man is prone to premature ejaculation.

Average cost: Zip.

Sterilization
Tubal Ligation

How it works: Tubal ligation involves surgically blocking, cutting, or tying a woman's fallopian tubes in an effort to prevent sperm from reaching the egg. The 30-minute procedure is generally performed on an outpatient basis under local anesthetic, or within 48 hours after a woman gives birth. Physicians often use a laparoscope, an instrument that's inserted through a small incision in the abdomen, allowing the doctor to see the tubes and either cut them or apply rings or clips to block them.

Worldwide, tubal ligation is the most commonly used form of birth control. Women choosing this option still ovulate and have monthly periods, and many report enhanced desire as they no longer fear becoming pregnant.

Effectiveness: Planned Parenthood rates tubal sterilization at 99.6 to 99.8 percent effective in preventing pregnancy.

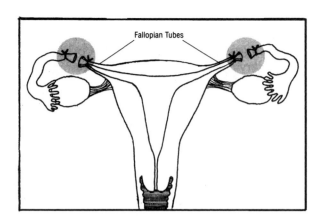

Fallopian Tubes

Pros: Tubal ligation . . .

- provides permanent protection against pregnancy;
- is ideal for couples who are finished having children and don't want to think about birth control;
- has no lasting side effects;
- involves a one-time expense that is relatively low compared to the lifetime costs of other birth control alternatives.

Cons: Tubal ligation . . .

- does not protect against STDs;
- involves a surgical procedure with possible complications, including bleeding, infection, and bruising at the incision site;
- is complicated and expensive to reverse (doctors offer no guarantees);
- occasionally does not work, or reverses itself. Pregnancies that occur under these circumstances are often ectopic (Greek for "out of place")—frequently in the tubes. Ectopic pregnancies can be extremely dangerous in that the tube can rupture, causing the woman to hemorrhage.

Average cost: Between $1,000 and $2,500 when performed on an outpatient basis with local anesthetics; more than double if general anesthesia and a hospital stay are involved.

Vasectomy

How it works: This surgical procedure for men involves cutting and tying the vas deferens—the tubes that carry the sperm from the testicles to where they are mixed to form semen. Hormones, sex drive, orgasm, and ejaculation are unaffected by the procedure; the only difference post-op is that the semen no longer contains sperm.

The vasectomy is performed on an outpatient basis under local anesthetic. In about ten minutes, you can be snipped and on your way. Because some sperm remain in the man's system following the operation, doctors recommend using an alternative form of birth control for at least 15 ejaculations.

Effectiveness: Does what it's supposed to do about 99.6 percent of the time.

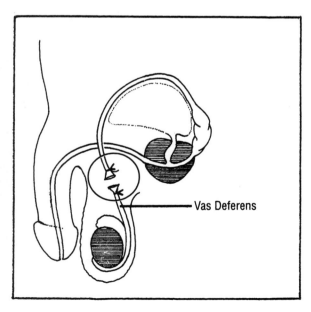

Vas Deferens

Pros: A vasectomy. . . .

- is intended as permanent protection against pregnancy;
- is a relatively painless procedure that is quick and effective;
- is less expensive and involves fewer complications than tubal ligation;
- has no known long-term side effects;
- is ideal for couples who do not plan to have children or have completed their families;
- does not diminish sex drive or inhibit spontaneity.

Cons: A vasectomy. . . .

- does not protect against sexually transmitted diseases;
- is not effective immediately (you must use a backup contraceptive until the sperm clears your tube, which takes between 15 to 20 ejaculations);
- involves surgery with possible short-term complications such as bruising, swelling, and pain near the testicles;
- is not easily reversed (the operation is highly technical, expensive, and offers no guarantees);
- can lead to small lumps (granuloma) near the testicles, which is formed by the sperm and sometimes requires medical attention;
- on rare occasions, reverses itself.

Average cost: Between $240 and $520.

The Unkindest Cut:
Writer J. Spencer Dreischarf Visits Snipland

After three careers, two divorces, zero offspring, and much contemplation, I still felt no biological imperative to help overpopulate the world. But after reading that the Pill might compromise her health, my partner did feel a biological imperative to discontinue taking it. Though using spermicide-coated condoms probably didn't pose a health risk, a chance of pregnancy still existed. So I decided to invest in permanent male birth control.

I called around to price vasectomies throughout the area, starting in Atlanta, near my home in Flowery Branch, and working outward into the suburbs. Not surprisingly, the farther from downtown the doctor was, the less the cost of the procedure—$1,100, $600, and then, as the receptionist put it: "Three hundred and fifty, up front."

I was afraid if I found anything cheaper, they would mail me a double-edge razor blade, a mirror, and written instructions. So just 50 miles from my starting point, my search was over.

Wanting to be an informed patient, I asked, "Do I need to fast or anything, before . . ."

"Nope, don't worry about it. Eat whatever you want."

"Is there any counseling? I've given this a lot of thought, and I don't think I need to talk to . . ."

"No, nothing like that to worry about."

"How about shaving? Do I . . ."

"No, don't worry about it. Come in on Friday. Should take 15, 20 minutes."

But I did worry about it, especially in the waiting room. I spent more time there than in surgery. In the midst of fending off a conversation with a gray-haired gentleman about his enlarged prostate, a very chipper nurse with a flowered laboratory coat fetched me from my seat next to the magazine rack.

"Mr. Dreeskarf, it's your turn," she chirped with the happy face of a Wal-Mart greeter.

"No, I think you skipped that guy over there."

"No, you were before him. Anyway, he's only ten. We'll get him later. Did I pronounce your name correctly?"

"Dry-sharf. But you gave it a good try," I answered.

At that she chortled much too gaily. I didn't think my name was funny at all, but she was really chipper.

She led me into a tiny examining room and assaulted me with her pre-op checklist.

"Here, sign this. Take off your clothes from the waist down. Sit up here and put this over you."

After I signed something stating I couldn't sue anyone no matter what, she handed me a paper sheet the size of a single square of toilet paper—my fig leaf, apparently—and flitted out of the room, humming. I did what she said, then perched on the end of an examining table, my thighs between two ominous, shiny stirrups.

When the nurse returned, I mentioned wishing that I'd brought a video camera. She laughed way too much in response and told me to scoot back and lie down. Fortunately, I didn't have to place my feet in the stirrups.

From this position, I couldn't see what was going on down there, but I could make an educated guess. The nurse swept away the paper sheet, neither gasping in awe nor snickering at what she saw. She placed folded blue towels around the area, leaving the surgical target exposed and looking like an oddly shaped UFO against an azure sky. I felt vulnerable.

Gingerly, she pinched the head of my penis between thumb and forefinger and lifted it so that she could butter my scrotum with Betadine, or iodine, or perhaps red dye number 3. It felt like a wet, cool breeze blowing up my kilt. I was not aroused.

All the while, she maintained a stream of banter about vasectomies, but I only remember her saying that my scrotum wouldn't be shaved and that if I didn't follow the post-op instructions, little vessels would rupture, tissue would swell, and I would either get "blue balls" or "bowling balls" or "blue bowling balls." There was no way I wasn't going to follow the post-op instructions. She exited again, this time whistling. I hoped I'd get the same drugs she was on before I went under the knife.

The tall, slender, bow-tied doctor came in soon thereafter. As he injected some sort of relaxant into my arm, he asked if I knew what the hell was about to happen. I told him I had a pretty good idea. After all, some years ago, when I was a trial attorney, I'd defended a doctor who'd performed a vasectomy on a man—one who fathered a healthy girl a year after his tubes were supposedly snipped. I was about to start my closing argument, when the doctor working on me shut me up by sticking a needle into my scrotum.

"See that knob?" He nodded toward a dark-blue plastic handle connected to the stirrups. "If you don't follow the post-op instructions, that will be the color of your scrotum, and it will swell to the size of . . ." He described various melons and pneumatic sports equipment. I renewed my vow to be steadfast in following the post-op instructions. "And don't have sex for five days. You know when you're told you can't have it, that's when you want it the most, but . . ." I know, I know: blue bowling balls.

With a scalpel, he cut a quarter-inch slit in my scrotum, a little below the base of the penis, and gave me a running commentary of his ministrations while I stared at the ceiling and silently repeated a mantra: "Please don't hurt. Please don't hurt. Please don't hurt." I felt some tugging as he stretched the opening to the size of a quarter and maneuvered the right testicle so he could breach its membrane. He pulled a tube, the vas deferens, through the hole. I sensed a squeezing as he clamped something. Using scissors, he snipped a half-inch section out of the vas and then cauterized the sliced ends with a pencil-size soldering iron.

"This will smell like barbecue," he said as wisps of smoke rose from my crotch. I did not salivate. Still, it wasn't so bad—a little discomfort, but no pain. Then some more tugging ensued as he made his way to the other vas. The squeezing followed, but it started to feel like a Vise-Grip tightening on my left testicle. So much for the mantra. "That hurts a teeny bit," I said calmly, a manly tear sneaking into my beard.

"Sorry. I'll just give it some more of this." He stuck the needle back into my scrotum, and the pain went away. A few minutes later, it was done. Not even a stitch was required to close. I thanked the doctor and told him it was the best vasectomy I'd ever had. He almost smiled.

"Very reasonable, too. You charge a lot less than the big-city urologists," I said, still lying on my back awaiting instructions.

"I make it up on the reversals," he said. "There's no discount for microsurgery to reconnect the faucets." He'd disconnected my plumbing for the duration, but I didn't want to disappoint him by saying so.

Within 20 minutes of entering the examination room, I was gingerly on my way back home. Only slight swelling and soreness developed, along with a new daily ritual: inspecting my wound with a five-power makeup mirror. The contortions required for viewing, if documented, could've gotten me onto *America's Funniest Home Videos*—maybe the adult version. Can you blame me for being curious?

Ice and immobility were the keys to recuperation. "Rocks on the rocks, neither shaken nor stirred," the nurse instructed me. I heeded her advice very carefully. In fact, I followed the post-op instructions for a few days beyond the prescribed time limit. I shuddered to think I might otherwise have to replace my jockstrap with a wheelbarrow.

Sure, it was a hassle. Sleeping with an ice pack strapped to your crotch usually is. Putting the fate of your manhood in the hands of a scalpel-wielding stranger isn't a winning experience, either. But having avoided the lingering pain and the blue bowling balls some vasectomies lead to, I have not a single regret or second thought about my decision.

Future Stuff

As long our birth control options remain less than 100 percent effective, researchers will continue to strive for the perfect contraceptive. Among the most anticipated is the "male Pill." This elusive method of birth control has been talked about for years, with scientists around the world striving to be the first to "invent" it. And why not? If it becomes a reality, it will be a veritable gold mine—not to mention a relief for both men and women. For guys, a male Pill means greater control and a resultant boost in confidence. "It's not as though I don't trust my partner," says Randy, a 28-year-old artist from Boulder, Colorado. "It would just be comforting to know that I remembered to pop my pill each day of every month rather than have to wonder if she did."

For women, the male Pill means greater parity—and less guilt. "As strange as this may sound," says Elizabeth, a 30-year-old businesswoman from Chicago. "If I were to get pregnant by a guy who was on the pill, I wouldn't be nearly as terrified to tell him. Birth control fails, but somehow, when I'm the one responsible for ensuring the protection—and it doesn't work—I feel as though I did something wrong. It's not that I want guys to feel this way; it just seems like they might be

We've Come a Long Way, Baby

Next time your girlfriend starts complaining that the Pill makes her feel bloaty, remind her how lucky she is to be preventing pregnancy in the twentieth century. Had she been living in Egypt four thousand years ago, that puffy feeling would have been the least of her worries. According to the *Lover's Guide Encyclopedia*, women in those days inserted tablets made of honey and animal dung into their vaginas to keep the offspring at bay, while Arabian women used a birth control concoction that included rock salt. What's more, historical records indicate that the idea for the intrauterine device actually came from an Arabic custom in which a stone was placed in the uterus of female camels to make them sterile. (Talk about giving new meaning to the term humping.)

Other interesting methods of preventing pregnancy in the past: Long ago in Persia, women were instructed to jump backwards nine times, then sit on their toes stroking their navel. And Japanese men wore sheaths made from tortoiseshell, horn, or leather. No wonder Chinese women didn't complain about foot binding.

more understanding of that margin of error if they were the ones taking the pill every day."

So what's the big holdup? First, it's a lot easier for scientists to find ways to control the release of one egg per month than the hourly production of millions of sperm. Scientists back in the fifties thought they had made some progress when a group of organic compounds proved successful at halting sperm production in the lab and in a test conducted on a prison population. But when the concoction was tested on the general population, the scientists learned that it caused side effects such as vomiting, chills, and shortness of breath when mixed with alcohol.

Other attempts have been made over the years. The Chinese thought an oil called gossypol was the answer, but it proved to cause kidney damage and sterility. The World Health Organization (WHO) introduced their own testosterone derivative, which caused the test subjects' sperm counts to drop considerably (a good thing), but also caused increased irritability and aggressiveness, as well as acne (not so good).

More promising is research that is being conducted stateside by the National Institutes of Health (NIH) in Bethesda, Maryland. There, scientists have developed a drug that controls the production of hormones responsible for sperm and testosterone production. An early form of the drug had to be injected weekly, but the NIH has come up with a formula like Depo-Provera for women, which requires an injection once every three months. Why a shot and not a pill? Because the hormones can cause liver damage when taken orally. That means the male Pill probably won't come in pill form—ever. And even the injection won't be available until after the turn of the century. According to a spokesperson at NIH, clinical trials have begun on the male hormonal contraceptive, but the process can take several years and requires Food and Drug Administration (FDA) approval.

But don't be discouraged. This alternative is inevitable. We suggest checking with your physician periodically for an update.

In the meantime, your partner may soon have a couple of new options. One, called the Vaginal Ring, is a hormonal method of birth control that's inserted into the vagina for three weeks of the month and removed during menstruation. While the Vaginal Ring is in place (next to the cervix), it releases hormones similar to the pill—but in lower dosages (which means milder side effects). The goal is to prevent the sperm from reaching the egg by thickening the cervical mucus. Although there's no date yet for the release of this promising alternative—it's still being studied—most gynecologists should be aware of its status.

Another hormonal method, presently available in Europe, is the Levonorgestrel IUD. T-shaped like the two types of IUDs used in the States, the Levonorgestrel variation releases a synthetic form of progesterone similar in a quantity to that given off by the Mini Pill. As with the Mini Pill, this IUD causes cervical mucus to become so thick that

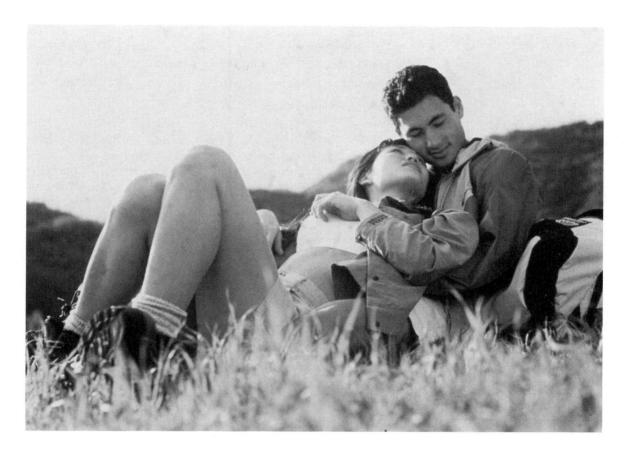

sperm cannot pass into the uterus. It's the most effective IUD available and has minimal side effects. Again, women should check with their physicians on availability.

When Nature Rules

If you've read the effectiveness ratings of the various forms of contraception, then you know none is perfect. Certainly the odds are in your favor. But unless you're abstaining from sex, there is a chance your partner will become pregnant. So what are your options should this occur?

There are several ways a scenario such as this can play itself out. Here are a few:

- You and your partner could have the child and raise it together.

- You could provide the mother with child support should you opt not to remain in the picture.

- You could flee the scene, get tracked down later, get thrown in the slammer for being a deadbeat dad, and be required to pay back child support for all the years you were missing. (Not advisable!)
- You and your partner could decide to put the child up for adoption.
- She could have an abortion.

Should you choose to put the baby up for adoption, you may be pleased to know that current laws favor the birth parents. In some states, you and your partner would have up to six months after the birth of your child to change your mind about giving up the baby. We've all seen the heartbreaking stories on television about couples who have adopted an infant only to have to return it to the birth parents four years later. This is a rarity, albeit a controversial one, that has some legal eagles attempting to change adoption laws. Until that happens, you may take comfort in knowing that there is a window of time before your decision becomes permanent. Contact the Planned Parenthood office in your area regarding your options. If you choose adoption, the office will provide you with information on adoption services in your area.

> "Of the one million-plus abortions performed in this country each year, 90 percent occur within the first 12 weeks of pregnancy, at a time when the fetus is no larger than a pea and cannot survive outside of the womb—even with today's sophisticated medical technology."

Unfortunately, if you're unmarried, you may not have much say in the matter. No court of law has ever forced a woman over the age of 18 to carry a child to term against her will. The landmark case of *Roe v. Wade* (1973) secured a woman's right to obtain a safe, legal abortion—and she can do so without anyone's consent.

There is no other issue in this country that is more emotionally charged than abortion. For many people, it is black and white, right or wrong. We will not get into that debate. The law provides women with the right to choose whether or not to terminate a pregnancy. For the purposes of this book, we will tell you how that is done in order to give you a clearer understanding of what your partner will experience if this is the route she chooses.

Of the one million-plus abortions performed in this country each year, 90 percent occur within the first 12 weeks of pregnancy, at a time when the fetus is no larger than a pea and cannot survive outside of the womb—even with today's sophisticated medical technology. Many abortions are performed surgically using a suction-type instrument that is inserted into the uterine cavity. This is called vacuum aspiration and is considered to be the easiest method for women psychologically, as the procedure is completed in about ten minutes. And physically, the only side effect may be mild cramping during and shortly after the surgery.

If the pregnancy has progressed fewer than 60 days, its also possible for a woman to take a combination of drugs called methotrexate and misoprostol. She'll receive an injection of the first drug and must return to the clinic five to seven days later for the second, which is inserted into her vagina in tablet or suppository form. Cramping begins in about 12 hours, and the pregnancy is terminated up to 24 hours later. Other side effects include nausea, vomiting, diarrhea, and, of course, bleeding, as the methotrexate and misoprostol effectively induce a miscarriage.

After 12 weeks, the fetus has grown larger, making an abortion much more complicated and risky. Doctors may recommend a dilation and curettage (D&C), which involves scraping the uterine lining. Some may perform an aspiration in conjunction with the D&C to ensure no tissue is left behind. A saline abortion is another alternative. In this case, a saline solution is injected into the uterine cavity, causing contractions that dispel the fetus. Late-term abortions are available, but these are rare and performed primarily when the mother's life is threatened.

Our final word on this subject: The decision to terminate a pregnancy is never easy one for anyone—particularly the woman. However, the sooner the choice is made the better it will be for the woman, as the health risks are minimal in the very early stages of pregnancy. The longer it progresses, the more difficult it becomes—both physically and emotionally.

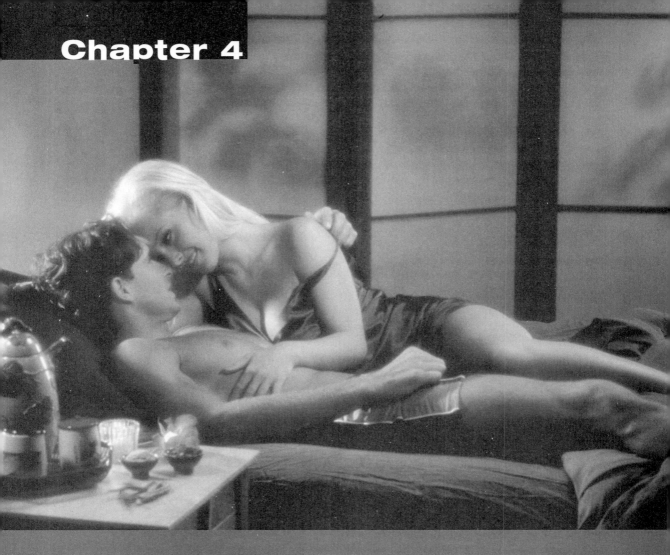

Chapter 4

The Whole Shebang:

et's not beat around the bush. Humans enjoy sex. In fact, we're one of the few members of the animal kingdom that get it on for fun rather than purely for procreation. Of course, adding enjoyment to the element makes us a bit more picky. Rather than hump a female purely because she's in heat, we tend to be selective about our bed partners. Okay, so after a few beers we're a little less selective. But, in general, men and women tend to require a certain amount of physical or mental attraction before they're willing to get intimate with the opposite sex.

In this chapter, we discuss the many elements of attraction—most of which are beyond even the most reasonable person's control. Remember those hormones we highlighted in chapter 2? Well, your sex drive is at their mercy. They're responsible for those lustful feelings when you crossed paths with the hottie in Lycra bike shorts . . . or the babe in the miniskirt waiting in line for the pay phone . . . or the sexy accountant who's auditing your department. Our brain is what separates man from beast—or at least most men. Societal expectations, the environment in which we were raised, and our awareness of sexually transmitted diseases (and other lifestyle challenges) enable us to rise above the oftentimes intense urge to jump each other's bones on the spot.

We have dating and mating rituals that set the tone for human relationships.

Aside from covering these issues, which lead up to sexual relationships, we'll also get down to the nitty gritty, discussing the specifics of sex—from foreplay and the most common intercourse positions to trendy, more adventuresome sex. And because an awesome orgasm is what we all hope to achieve from this info, we cap off chapter 4 with tips on how to build a better one.

Let's start with lust.

When You're in Lust

According to Theresa Crenshaw, M.D., "Lust is a chemically, hormonally, emotionally driven desire for raw sex," and testosterone is at the heart of it. We know from chapter 2 that testosterone is the primary male hormone that drives a man's libido and sends him cruising for orgasms. "It's the young Marlon Brando—sexual, sensual, alluring, dark, with a dangerous undertone," Crenshaw says. "Testosterone makes you want to pursue sex, initiate, dominate." And, men have 20 to 40 times more testosterone than women, which is one reason that male and female sex drives are so different.

What happens to a guy during lust? Usually a

Lust, Love, and Sex

fantasy revs up the desire for sex, kicking hormones into gear. "He'd like to have an orgasm, and he's looking for someone to cooperate," Crenshaw says. "As a last resort, he'll take care of himself."

What's Love Got to Do with It?

Love, like lust, is also hormonally driven, says Crenshaw. The mix of seratonin, testosterone, dopamine, and so on circulating in your body at any given time determines your physical and emotional responses. As some hormones surge, others decrease, affecting your feelings, thoughts, and behavior.

"Your various hormones, each with unique features to contribute, get in bed with you, too," Crenshaw says. "In a way, it's as if there were a corporate decision going on, with each chemical casting its vote."

Though Crenshaw acknowledges the impact of hormones on love, she admits it's a mystery why one special person knocks our socks off and we melt in a shimmery rush of emotions, excitement, and longing. "Logic and reason dissolve like smoke, and you can think of nothing else," Crenshaw says. "Your love becomes the atmosphere. You breathe it wherever you are. We try to explain it with a favorite feature or quality, but that's just our mind's way of trying to make sense of something that isn't supposed to make sense. It ignores the fact that other people with the same qualities don't leave us fighting for breath."

Perhaps it's the high levels of testosterone in men that make lust their driving force, while women, who have a considerably lower level of the hormone, are more likely to seek love first. But nature also plays a force, according to Patti Britton, Ph.D. "Women are raised to think of love and sex as inseparable, whereas boys are encouraged to follow their urges."

In fact, it's this dichotomy that led Michael Castleman, author of *Sexual Solutions for Men and the Women Who Love Them*, to dub love and lust "the yin and yang of male-female human relationships.

"Men identify with lust—raw sexual desire independent of the person's identity, the 'I want sex now!' urge. Woman identify with love—the deep feeling of profound connection with another human being."

Sexologists sometimes say that men love in order to have sex, while women have sex in order to love. Many men say that good sex leads to a good relationship, while women say the reverse, says Castleman, a former sex counselor who used to contribute to the *Playboy Advisor*. "They're two sides of the same coin—linked, but very different. Therein lies a great deal of the torment of men and women."

> "Men identify with lust—raw sexual desire independent of the person's identity, the 'I want sex now!' urge. Woman identify with love—the deep feeling of profound connection with another human being."
> —Michael Castleman, author of *Sexual Solutions for Men and the Women Who Love Them*

Men often feel guilty about their preoccupation with sex. Women aggravate that guilt with putdowns such as "Men are animals" and "Men have only one thing on their minds." Nonsense, says Castleman: "Men have two things on their minds. One of them is basketball."

Seriously, if you think about sex all the time, you're normal. According to a Kinsey Institute report on sexuality, men between age 15 and 50 think about sex every five to ten minutes. "It may not be admirable, but it's normal and not pathological," Castleman says.

"As you get more life experience, you learn to control or civilize your lustful feelings," says Isadora Alman, a syndicated sex and relationships advice columnist and board-certified sexologist. "You can't jump everyone you're attracted to. Choices have to be made with heart and head, even though the groin yells the loudest."

> "According to a Kinsey Institute report on sexuality, men between age 15 and 50 think about sex every five to ten minutes."

Why we're attracted to unattainable lust objects and indifferent to the people pining for us is a mystery. Alman pictures a pantheon of gods and goddesses playing a game by pointing one person at another to see what happens. "Whoever designed all this has a really quirky sense of humor," she says. "When lust hits, how strongly it hits, how inconveniently it hits is almost always a surprise."

Lust Is Easy. Love Is Tough.

"When Mom said that the way to a man's heart was through his stomach, she was about four inches too high," says John Gray, relationship guru and author of several books, including *Men Are from Mars, Women Are from Venus* and *Mars and Venus on a Date*.

Love and Lust and Everything in Between: Celebrities Talk About Affairs of the Heart— and Points Further South

Famous people are different from you and me; they get asked a lot more questions about their personal business. We sent writer Michael Szymanski to ask them their very personal opinions about love, lust, and the hardships of being rich, famous, and attractive. Here are some of the responses he gathered:

Drew Barrymore: "The best thing anyone can give a girl is a tattoo somewhere on his body with the girl's name on it. Boyfriends will come and go, but we know we'll always have each other."

Marisa Tomei: "I hate to admit it, but I don't believe that there's only one person out there for me. I think there are many different people you can love at different times in your life."

Sandra Bullock: "In my life, I've had a really-like-you-a-lot, lustful thing at first sight, but never a love at first sight. I'm a pretty hard sell. You have to send up flares and stand in front of me with a sandwich board before I'll realize you're attracted to me."

Jacqueline Bissett: "Romance is something very elusive. You have to trick yourself into it."

According to Gray, we might as well be from different planets given the way men and women think, act, interpret, and communicate. The lust and love differences between men and women, as in most other realms, are stark.

Sexual pleasure is a different experience for men and women, says Gray: "Men are like blowtorches; women are like ovens." For a man, sexual pleasure is a release of tension—but for a woman, it's the gradual buildup of tension and desire. A man doesn't need much help getting aroused; he needs help releasing. A woman needs help building up her arousal. "In a sense, he is trying to empty out while she is seeking to be filled up," Gray says.

Sexual arousal lets men connect and open up to love, and receiving love helps women feel sexual passion, Gray maintains. Though women think men only want sex, the truth is that men want love as much as women do. "It is through sex that a man's heart opens, allowing him to experience both his loving feelings and his hunger for love as well," he says. "Just as a woman needs love to open up to sex, a man needs sexual arousal to open up to love."

The goal is to find a partner who will support your emotional, mental, and spiritual needs as well: a soul mate. If it's just sex, a man will lose interest as soon as that immediate passion is satisfied, and the relationship won't last or grow. "Physical attraction can be sustained for a lifetime only when it springs from chemistry of the mind, heart, and soul as well," Gray says.

"Desire is wanting what you don't have; love is wanting what you have," he asserts, adding that that's the main difference between lust and love. Lust is easy. Love is tough. Anyone can be hot for the alluring body of a stranger. The real challenge is to continue feeling passionate desire for a woman after you get to know her by transforming physical desire into love. Says Gray: "This is what separates the men from the boys. Our challenge is to connect the sexual energy with your heart and your mind. That's what makes us a whole being."

It's All in the Response

Though men and women may seek out sexual partners for vastly different reasons, we both want the same thing in the end—mutual satisfaction. And a connection is important. Where men are concerned, it doesn't always have to be deep and meaningful . . . and it definitely doesn't have to last forever. But guys aren't as self-absorbed and selfish in the sack as the media likes to suggest. Witness: For the book, *Sex: A User's Manual*, four thousand men were asked to select the least pleasant element of a sexual encounter from the following five choices:

- guilt feelings
- odors and discharges
- foreplay
- a demanding woman
- an unresponsive woman

If guys fit that "Wham, Bam, Thank You Ma'am" mold, the answer would have been "foreplay" or "a demanding woman." It would mean they'd have to work harder. But the top pick was item number five—59 percent of the respondents chose "an unresponsive woman." In other words, guys don't like a cold fish.

Just ask Bernie Zilbergeld, Ph.D., author of *The New Male Sexuality: The Truth About Men, Sex and Pleasure.* "Men these days—and this is a reasonably consistent finding on my part—want partners to be turned on and responsive; they want them to participate in lovemaking and to get something out of it. That's the big change in male sexuality during the last 20 or 30 years," reports this Oakland, California–based therapist.

"It used to be that sex was something men took from women. Women were not expected to be particularly responsive," Zilbergeld says. "When I was in high school (in the late fifties), guys were satisfied with anything (they could get). The woman could lie there, she could cry, she could read a magazine—the only thing that mattered was that she let the man have sex. But during the past few decades, men—normal men—have increasingly begun to view sex as something conducted between equals."

On this score, Martin, a 38-year-old production-crew chief at a major Hollywood studio, considers himself a lucky man. Married nearly three years to Heather, Martin claims that the sexual rapport that exists between them continues to improve with time.

He explains: "When we make love—and sometimes it's not about love but simply a matter of grunt-variety sex—Heather is not afraid to move, to make noises, to moan, to ask for whatever it is she needs. I've been with women who barely made a peep, and that never turned me on to the extent that I get turned on by Heather's participation. That turns me on like nothing else."

By contrast, Justin's relationship with his girlfriend appears to be on shaky ground, precisely because "I rarely know whether Christa's turned on or not," he says. The couple (he's 30, she's 28) have dated exclusively for months, but Justin says the lack of response from his partner during sex has markedly diminished the pleasurable sexual tension he feels during lovemaking. According to Zilbergeld, "When this lack of responsiveness occurs in a relationship, the man tends to

Molly Ringwald: "I find it really romantic when a guy pushes hard for me, when he doesn't give up. I don't like guys who are pushy, just someone who will hang in there."

Martin Short: "I remember my first kiss. She walked away."

Tracy Ullman: "Lust is mystery. My husband gets me these little teddy bears and tries to be mysterious, saying it's from a secret admirer or some such nonsense, but he has the worst handwriting in the world, so I can always tell it's him. He has a favorite card with two teddy bears looking out to the ocean, and I keep saying, 'Not those damn bears again,' because it makes me feel so middle-aged."

Sharon Stone: "I was aware of my first sexual stirrings when I watched old movies. I remember it well. I dreamed about men when I was watching the screen. I dreamed of being swept away by Rock Hudson."

Bonnie Hunt: "I fell in love every time some guy spoke to me when I was in Italy. Like any married housewife who visits, you're flattered and tempted, but you just don't do anything about it."

Meg Ryan: "Women love to feel erotic and sensual, and so do men, but it's often overlooked. We all want to lose ourselves in the idea of romance as much as possible. It's the stuff for movies, something we have high dopey hopes about."

Sandra Bernhard: "You know it's lust when you satisfy all your real needs. It's when you need nothing else, except the feeling of it."

Matthew Modine: "You know it when it feels right, when it's clean. Lust is not something that is smutty. Lust is not something that is dirty, but is pure. You feel good in your gut. It's wrong to make it sleazy."

> "It appears that today's normal, healthy male increasingly prefers a partner who participates in sex on an equal footing."

Jason Priestley: "I know right away when it's lust. I mean, guys know. It's immediate. It's purely physical."

Ashley Judd: "[Lust is] when you don't have to change who you are."

Mike Myers: "I'm a lover of lust. Lust and love will never die. I do things for my wife to show her I care, like quitting smoking or something big like that."

Jennifer Jason Leigh: "Lust and passion must have a certain truth. Passion is a kind of love to feel in a physical way, to keep it private in real life."

feel rejected, to get upset with his partner, to eventually start criticizing her. Without a responsive partner, the sex act becomes a matter of servicing."

Marilyn Lawrence, a Los Angeles therapist and a founding fellow of the American Academy of Clinical Sexologists, agrees with Zilbergeld's assessment. "What that 59 percent means to me, and what my practice bears out, is that nobody wants to be alone in this thing we call sex," Lawrence says. "And it goes back to something that has to do with performance—as much as I hate to use that word. The only way to know that what you're doing is pleasurable is to receive a response from your partner. Sex is not conducted in a vacuum. Response is feedback; it signals that someone is appreciating your ministrations and effort. It answers the question: Are we feeling this thing together?"

"The basic reality is that the ego is part and parcel of sexuality," says Ann LaManna, a marriage and family counselor in Los Angeles. "One of the ways in which a man can feel validated for being who he is as a man is to know that the woman wants him sexually, that she responds to him. A man's sexual pleasure does not depend solely on physical release; more than ever before, therapists find there's a strong psychological component to a man's sexual pleasure as well, and that part needs to believe the woman wants him.

"When a man has a partner who participates with him in sex, there is a buildup of sexual tension that works well for both," she continues. "Having a responsive partner, therefore, serves the positive side of the ego in the mutual-sex equation, and that makes him feel connected to his partner in a most intimate way."

A further insight can be gained from the study cited earlier. While nearly two-thirds of the men surveyed preferred a responsive woman in bed, a mere 6 percent indicated that their greatest turnoff was a demanding woman. It appears that today's normal, healthy male increasingly prefers a partner who participates in sex on an equal footing. Unlike his predecessors, he no longer treats her as merely a receptacle. He wants a partner who brings her fair share to the picnic.

Credit feminism, which champions a woman's right to sexual pleasure, for at least part of this transformation of the male sexual dynamic. As a result of this movement, men's sexual priorities and attitudes have continued to shift.

For example, "The business about the virgin bride is pretty much myth today," says Ted McIlvenna, Ph.D., president of the San Francisco–based Institute for Advanced Study of Human Sexuality. "While men (may have) believed that their goal was to find a woman in whom they could awaken sexual desire, the real reason was that they were afraid of being compared sexually with other men. It was largely a performance issue.

"Especially since the birth of feminism, however, men have found that the performance burden in such a situation is simply too great. So what they have increasingly done over the past few decades is seek out women who are sexually responsive rather than those who merely take care of men's needs. Men have discovered that sex becomes a lot easier, much more satisfying and meaningful if the burden of performance is removed."

Phallic Fiction and the Burden of Performance

From grade school to the grave, men seem to be more governed by myths about sexuality than they are by the facts. Avodah K. Offit, Ph.D., a psychiatrist and sex therapist based in New York City, has worked with men for years to wrest reality from the web of sexual fiction. Offit selected ten myths that are particularly prevalent among men, and then refuted each. Here are her comments:

1. **A man should be ready, willing, and able to have sex at all times.** Men impose enormous physical demands upon themselves—unrealistic demands. Frankly, I think there's something wrong with a man who can have sex with anyone at any time—and this is true for men from 18 to 80. It's not only a physical impossibility, but a gross neglect of self-interest, self-awareness, and self-respect. You may simply be too tired, too angry, or just plain disinterested. The penis is a good barometer of your mood—if you're not in the mood for sex, don't expect your penis to respond at the drop of a skirt.

2. **The longer a man lasts during intercourse, the more pleasure a woman feels.** There's an erroneous notion that a man is supposed to keep pumping away for hours on end. He's not supposed to have an orgasm—or so the myth goes—until the woman is thoroughly exhausted. This is nonsense. Most women are not looking for endurance champions; they prefer to go up and down in excitement—taking periodic breaks before getting back into the hot-and-heavy sex. Of course, having the gift of longevity is no great liability, but it's not exactly what most women are after.

3. **A man should be blessed with the power of achieving instant erection.** Some women take it as a blow to their egos if you're not instantly erect in their presence. This problem rests with the woman, not the man. A woman's self-esteem must be pretty low if

William Hurt: "It's more than any moral judgment, it's not being judged. When you're loved, it's good for us as human beings."

Samuel L. Jackson: "I'd like to do a romance, just to do more than what I did with Geena Davis [in *The Long Kiss Goodnight*]. That was hard because her husband was directing it. On one hand I was kind of anticipating one thing, but then when we actually started to do it, it was bizarre because she was doing it and he was giving her instructions the whole time. She actually slipped me the tongue. He was telling her to do it, so there was nothing sensuous about that."

Robin Wright: "You simply know it. You know when you feel loved, and some people can get damaged by it."

Brad Pitt: "There's nothing that is as passionate as when you are at the end of each other's rope, like [when mountain climbing for his role in *Seven Years in Tibet*]. It is such an amazing feeling. You feel most alive when you're closest to death."

The Land of the Lust: Men Fitness' Lust Survey

The results are in, and the findings are indisputable: The *Men's Fitness* reader is a pretty horny guy. In order to truly understand the lustful nature of the human male, we conducted the first-ever *Men's Fitness* Lust Survey. We wanted to see what made your wheels turn, and, boy, did you ever tell us: We got 1,392 responses. From what we now know, the average *Men's Fitness* reader thinks about sex a few times a day, most often thinks about women he has seen but not met, is most aroused by a shapely butt, is more turned on by a nice smile and personality than intelligence, and, by a narrow margin, prefers the unattainable woman to one who's available to him. The stats:

How often do you feel sexual attraction?
A few times a day: 63%
Once an hour: 28%
Once a day: 5%
Less than once a day: 4%

Toward whom do you most often feel these attractions?
Someone seen but never met: 42%
Regular partner: 27%
Casual acquaintance: 27%
Close friend: 25%
Celebrity: 4%

(Many respondents selected more than one.)

Which body parts arouse you sexually?
Butt: 71%
Legs: 65%
Breasts: 52%
Eyes: 42%
Waist: 37%
Hair: 26%
Feet: 13%

(Most respondents selected more than one, obviously. Some selected everything. Others wrote in body parts like neck, shoulders, arms, eyebrows, hands, skin tone, genitalia, etc. A few decided that "waist" wasn't sufficient, and wrote in "stomach" or "abs." Finally, one wrote, "Nose—yes, the things you can do!" No, we can't imagine what.)

What other qualities cause you to feel sexually attracted?
Personality: 63%
Smile: 51%
Intelligence: 33%
Unattainability: 17%
Availability: 14%

(Again, most respondents selected more than one if they selected anything in this category, and many wrote in some interesting additions to the list: self-confidence, independence, voice, smell, laugh, sense of humor, personal style, ambition, talent, hobbies. One guy added "snobbishness" and "maturity"—an interesting combo. Other readers got almost poetic: "gentle shyness," wrote one, while another submitted "natural, innocent sensuality.")

That brings us to the first of the two fill-in-the-blank categories:

Which famous person arouses in you the most lustful feelings?
As many of us suspected, the most pneumatically enhanced sex symbols received the most votes. Cut-and-paste Barbie doll Pamela Anderson Lee got 61 votes, while bazooka-breasted Demi Moore scored 45. Jenny McCarthy tallied 41, and the woman who replaced her on *Singled Out,* Carmen Electra, received 36. Megamodels also scored in the survey: Cindy Crawford got 30 votes; Tyra Banks, 26; and Kathy Ireland, 14.

Strong finishers in the movie-star category include hot-cha-cha Salma Hayek (25 votes), nice-nice Sandra Bullock (22), Jennifer Aniston (21), bad girl Sharon Stone (19), Meg Ryan (16), Jennifer Love Hewitt and Teri Hatcher (15), Nicole Kidman (13), Courteney Cox (9), Sarah Michelle Gellar and Mira Sorvino (7), and Julia Louis-Dreyfus (4).

Our readers didn't discriminate by age or even mortality. Deborah Kerr, who once had *An Affair to Remember* with Cary Grant, got a vote, while Marilyn Monroe grabbed five—one of whom checked "unattainability" as a quality that makes him feel sexually attracted to a woman. Sixties icons Raquel Welch and

Ann-Margret got a total of 13 votes (11 for Raquel).

Among singers, country star Shania Twain got 20 votes to Madonna's 17 and Toni Braxton's 11. Belly-baring Mariah Carey, who seems to work the sex-symbol thing harder than anyone these days, got 8. Jewel and Janet 6.

Our gay readers also weighed in. Again, we didn't recognize many of the names (Blade Thompson got two votes), but the clear-cut favorites were Brad Pitt (14 votes) and Tom Cruise (8).

The Top Ten
Pamela Anderson Lee: 61
Demi Moore: 45
Jenny McCarthy: 41
Carmen Electra: 36
Cindy Crawford: 30
Tyra Banks: 26
Salma Hayek: 25
Sandra Bullock: 22
Jennifer Aniston: 21
Shania Twain: 20

What's the craziest thing you've ever done because of a sexual attraction?

The second write-in question drew the craziest responses, many of which, unfortunately, revolved around onanism. We'll spare you those, but here's a sampling of some of the more amusing ones:

"Walked four blocks at two in the morning, in a full leg cast and crutches, to meet a girl I was attracted to."

"Asked a girl who was carrying someone else's child to marry me. Luckily, she said no."

"Flew three thousand miles five times this year to pursue someone who did not know of my intentions . . . and I'm married!"

"While working out at my gym, I went upstairs to work abdominals for the sole purpose of checking out a girl. I must have done a thousand crunches. My stomach hurt for weeks."

"I kissed a guy to win over a girl I was attracted to [who] was known for being turned on by two men kissing."

Now they get a little more aggressive:

"I once dressed as a woman to see a girl in the nude."

"Chased a woman down in the pouring rain. She was riding a bicycle. I had a warm, dry car. It worked!"

"Xeroxed my schlong and mailed it."

"Spray-painted a message on the road in front of her house."

"Got drunk, took off all my clothes, and went to her sorority house to serenade her. P.S.: Don't try it. I got arrested by campus police."

"Oh, just your good old-fashioned stalking. No big whoop."

"Broke into her house."

Returning to nonfelonious acts:

"Introduced an older woman to my mother as a 'teacher' (this was when I was in high school). I said she was going to help with my 'assignments.' I had to explain student-teacher passions later when Mom caught us 'studying.'"

"Did an engine tune-up wearing only a coverall unzipped to the hairline so she could get a good look. It worked!"

"Got married!" (Several also said "proposed marriage.")

"Proposed to a go-go dancer, sober."

she is dependent on your instant erection for her own ego gratification. Many men need time to relax before getting an erection. Don't rush it. As long as you get one eventually, everything should be okay.

4. **A small penis is less satisfying to a woman than a large one is.** This falls under the heading of personal choice. It's really a matter of fit. Vaginas come in different shapes and sizes, and, of course, penises vary in length and width. In general, an average-sized penis—one that can fit comfortably in most women—will do the trick.

5. **You can use willpower to prevent a premature ejaculation from occurring.** This phallic fallacy is one of the more destructive. Delaying orgasm is more of a stop-start process than a matter of control. And don't try to distract yourself with thoughts of baseball and the stock market; instead, just stop what you're doing that has you so excited. (Check our advice in chapter 7 for tips and tricks regarding staying power and premature ejaculation.)

6. **An endless array of positions will improve your sex life.** And I suppose drinking a different fruit juice every morning will improve the quality of your breakfast! Most couples have a repertoire of two or three bread-and-butter positions, and that's fine. It's fun to experiment, but you don't have to go swinging from the chandeliers to enjoy a satisfying sex life and a meaningful relationship.

7. **Familiarity is the death of desire.** Most men are looking for a partner who's warm, loving, and caring. The more you love and trust your partner—traits that go with a long-term relationship—the better the sex will be.

8. **A man must be rigidly erect to excite a woman.** Like it or not, you're going to lose your full erection from time to time during sex. Masters and Johnson revealed that a man may lose his peak erection as often as four times during intercourse. Many women are aware that this happens and actually enjoy the sensation; soft erections offer a gentle feeling that's very stimulating. The notion that you must be completely hard all the time during intercourse is just plain false.

9. **Impotence can be overcome by taking charge of your penis.** The men who are the least potent are the ones who insist on controlling every single aspect of their lives. I treat a lot of macho types—business executives, officers in the military, star athletes—who insist on

taking charge of their penis, rather than just going with the flow. The most potent men are the least hung up on being compelled to perform. Stop trying so hard and you'll get better results.

10. **An erection means you must have sex right away.** Your hard penis may not signal that you're ready to jump into bed with the woman down the hall. Erections come and go; just because you have one doesn't mean you must act on it immediately. Enjoy the feeling, but don't put pressure on yourself to do something about it right away.

Foreplay—It's Not Golf, but It Can Help Your Stroke

Now that you're hip to all the myths related to your own performance, you can lighten up and enjoy sex along with your partner. Since we know that you do indeed want her to enjoy herself, we can tell you straight up that foreplay is going to be the best way to make that happen. Yes, there once was a time when a man's definition of foreplay was undoing his zipper. And sensitive foreplay meant not holding her head down.

But in these enlightened times, foreplay covers a broad spectrum of activities leading to sexual intercourse . . . and sometimes, it takes the place of the ol' in-out-in-out itself. Indeed, foreplay is often more than physical activities . . . remember, in its strictest definition, it's a prelude to intercourse. That means everything is fair game. Like a call at the office, describing what's going to happen tonight. Or a playful description of last night's tryst written on your bathroom mirror. In essence, foreplay can be sights, sounds, or thoughts of activities to spark the idea of sex. By building anticipation, you're engaged in foreplay.

The prototypical romantic dinner is foreplay of sorts, with each party wondering what dessert will be served up after . . . well, dessert. Foreplay is all about setting the stage, creating a mood. Those candles during dinner? They're helping create the receptiveness toward a night of passion . . . or raw sex. The champagne? Popping its cork can help you pop yours.

Dinner parties can also be a part of foreplay. Next time you and your significant other go to a crowded dinner party, do this: As you sit down to the first course, lean over to your mate and quietly whisper something suggestive, something sexy. Maybe how you can't wait to get home .with her. Maybe a detail of what you'd like to do with her afterwards. How radiant and sexy she looks.

> "A variation [of foreplay] from China is called the spring butterfly, where you substitute a paintbrush for your fingertips, making the brush skip and dance across your partner's skin, as would a butterfly in a field."

For the rest of the evening, she'll be anxious. Mill about. Talk with friends. Every so often, look across the room to your mate and give her The Look. You know what we mean. It builds anticipation and a sense of urgency. That's foreplay.

You can always try new approaches to touching, like gently stroking feathers, or sensual materials such as silk scarves, over your bodies. That's foreplay, too. Joel D. Block, Ph.D., suggests another idea he calls Spiders' Legs in his book *Secrets of Better Sex*. Have your partner close her eyes. Then use only your fingertips to occasionally touch her hair or skin. A variation from China is called the spring butterfly, where you substitute a paintbrush for your fingertips, making the brush skip and dance across your partner's skin, as would a butterfly in a field.

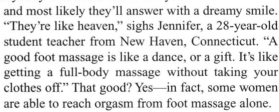

". . . some women are able to reach orgasm from foot massage alone."

Want to try something really sensual? Bow down before your partner . . . and perform . . . a foot massage.

Foot Massage—Therein Lies the Rub

A foot massage, hand to foot, intimate and sensual, is one of life's true luxuries. Ask anybody who's had one to tell you what it feels like

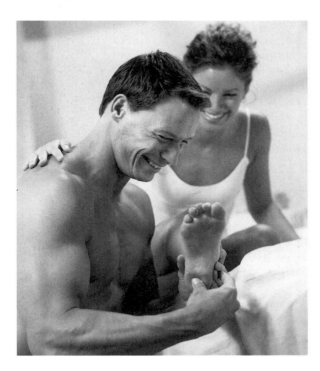

and most likely they'll answer with a dreamy smile. "They're like heaven," sighs Jennifer, a 28-year-old student teacher from New Haven, Connecticut. "A good foot massage is like a dance, or a gift. It's like getting a full-body massage without taking your clothes off." That good? Yes—in fact, some women are able to reach orgasm from foot massage alone.

Aside from their powerful sensuality, there are physiological reasons why foot massages feel so great. "We don't realize how much pressure we put on our feet and what kind of tensions they're under throughout the day from just standing or walking," says massage therapist Lee Direen, director of the North Star Bodywork Therapeutic Massage Center in San Francisco. "The feet bear the body's full weight."

But a massage can relieve more than just physical stress. The skin's surface contains neural receptors that affect heart rate, blood, and hormone flow. Pleasurably stimulating these receptors releases endorphins—natural painkillers that are structurally similar to morphine—which also triggers a sense of well-being. A school of therapy known as reflexology is based on stimulating pressure points in the hands and feet that are believed to be linked to all the body's organs and systems. And, while professional foot massages are exquisite, you needn't be a pro to give someone you're close to a taste of such bliss. Here are some guidelines for making a lover feel really good.

Make sure the room is warm enough—there's nothing like a chill in the air to cool things down. Consider candles and soft music. Turn off the phone. An ideal time for a foot massage is after a bath or shower and just before bed. The lucky recipient should lie faceup and slightly higher than you on a bed, in a soft chair, or in a nest of cushy pillows while you kneel on the floor. Support both feet just above your thighs. Stay comfortable—don't hunch over. You may find it easier to work on the soles of the feet—the primary focus of a good massage—with the massagee lying facedown and slightly lower than you.

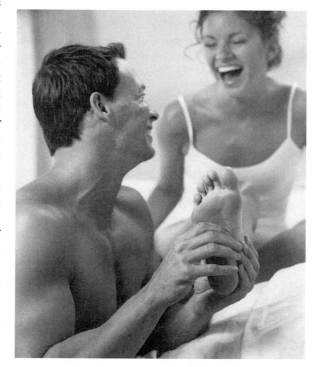

"First of all, let go of the idea of giving a professional massage," Direen says. "Ask your partner when it feels good and when it doesn't. Many people are afraid to either give or take feedback." But one of the pleasures of a massage for both people is tuning into the other person's body and its responses—knowledge that's beneficial in all sorts of circumstances. "Massages have to do with pleasure, but also with communication and a sort of energy connection," Direen says.

The key is to maintain constant contact between hand and foot, supporting and massaging one foot at a time with both hands. Use the contours of your hands to brush along and press into the contours of your partner's feet, generally using a solid, deep pressure and always paying attention to the foot's structure. Some things to watch out for while doing this:

Don't tickle. Using a single finger or your fingernails invites squirming. Use at least two fingers and the larger surfaces of your hand:

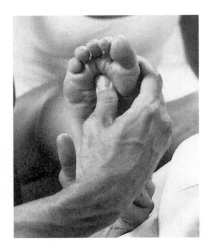

heel, palm, and knuckles. Thumbs are good, but try not to rely too much on them. A range of different touches makes for a more toe-curling massage.

Go easy. The skin is thinner at the top of the foot over the arch, with a network of tendons and muscles lying relatively exposed just below. Light pressure over this area—a cupped palm or a brush of the fingers—is about all you should use. If an area seems unusually tender, avoid it. If a certain motion hurts either you or your partner, stop it.

Careful with the toes. Fingers between the toes give an intense sensation that's either heaven or hell (the effect is even stronger if you're using oil or lotion). "People either love it or they'll say, 'Honey, that is so gross,'" Direen says.

Using thumbs, knuckles, or several fingers, apply pressure to the ball of the foot, kneading lightly while holding the top of the foot with your fingers or other hand. Press more firmly on the soles of the feet, where the skin is thickest, and less firmly on the tops, where the skin is thinner. Use all the surfaces of your hand to stroke your partner's foot. Try sandwiching a foot with your fingers and drawing them along the length of the foot. Then do it again while turning your hands slightly for a different sensation. Be creative here.

The body supports most of its weight on the arches and the area from the ball of the foot to the big toe, and these areas will appreciate a little extra attention. With one hand on top of the foot, roll the knuckles of your other hand into the ball, then up to the arch and heel. Gently wiggle the foot at the ankle and toe joints, and pull the foot gently toward you to help relieve the tension that accumulates.

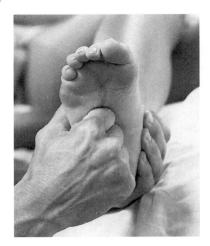

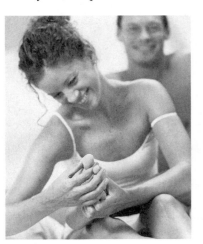

Starting at the base of each toe, apply firm pressure to several spots as you work your way to the ends. Also try kneading the toes all at once with the knuckles of one hand, supporting the foot with the other. Do unto one foot what you do unto the other—symmetry helps make the massage more familiar and soothing. Having the area around the ankle caressed is almost as much fun as having an earlobe nibbled or a shoulder nipped lightly. Spend some time on the ankles themselves, then work your way up the calves, higher if that's the way your encounter is headed.

The Story of O

While foreplay is the key to arousal, it's also an opportunity for her to enjoy multiple orgasms before you even begin intercourse. So let's talk about the female orgasm. Her movements, pulsations, and moans may be mysteries to you. Which shudders signify pleasure and which ones discomfort or dissatisfaction?

Actually, male and female orgasms feel very similar. Says Kenneth Reamy, M.D., professor of gynecology and psychiatry at West Virginia University Health Sciences Center, "Written descriptions of orgasms by men and women are indistinguishable."

Here's what is different: Many women take longer to become aroused and climax than men do, but they also rate higher in the variety of orgasms they experience.

Like most men, some women have one intense explosion, after which a second orgasm may be unlikely. Others will climax, then experience a slight drop and subsequent rise in arousal, often followed by another orgasm. Still others may have one "big" orgasm, followed by a succession of smaller ones—kind of a ripple effect.

Multiple orgasms are a huge source of fascination for men. While many women do have the capacity for them, they shouldn't be the goal of lovemaking; any pressure by either party is self-defeating. According to Lonnie Barbach, Ph.D., a sex therapist, psychologist, and author, "A single, terrific climax is perfectly satisfying for most women." Barbach describes a female client who claimed to have had 100 orgasms in 15 minutes using a vibrator, but says that person's experience isn't necessarily better than that of the woman who has one intense orgasm.

The Big Bang

Are orgasms essential to women's enjoyment of sex? Generally speaking, yes. The twist is, they don't necessarily expect it to happen during intercourse. In fact, about half of American women don't climax consistently or easily that way. Some 25 percent say they've never even had a coital orgasm. That doesn't mean they don't get a kick out of vaginal sex; most sex therapists agree that women find intercourse pleasurable whether they climax during the act or not.

But the orgasm should fit into a woman's sex life somewhere, and that's where the clitoris comes in. According to The Kinsey Institute New Report on Sex, 75 percent of women require some kind of clitoral stimulation in order to climax. Before and/or during intercourse, it's the key to female orgasm. (Though intercourse alone generally doesn't provide direct stimulation of the clitoris, there are coital positions and techniques that lend themselves to increased clitoral contact; more on these later.)

As noted in chapter 2, the clitoris is located where the labia minora—inner folds of the vagina—join on top of the vaginal opening.

(Take note: the labia minora are also sexually sensitive and swell with blood when a woman is excited.) For most women, the clitoris is by far the most sexually sensitive part of the genitals. It's also the only human organ whose sole function is sexual sensation—the clitoris contains specialized nerve endings so it gets erect when a woman is aroused. In fact, the clitoris is very much like a small penis. According to adult film star Nina Hartley, in her video *Nina Hartley's Guide to Better Cunnilingus*, the clitoris resembles a penis, in that it has a shaft, a glans—or head—and a clitoral hood, like the hood of an uncircumcised penis. "All the nerves you have in a penis are scrunched down into a small piece of real estate called the clitoris," she says.

"While many women do have the capacity for [multiple orgasms], they shouldn't be the goal of lovemaking; any pressure by either party is self-defeating."

The clitoris is not to be mistaken with the Grafenberg spot. The "G-spot," according to some sex researchers, is a dime-sized area on the vagina's front wall that's very sensitive to sexual stimulation. While there is still no conclusive evidence that it exists, some women report that the area is stimulated by penile thrusting, which can trigger orgasm. In chapter 2, we give tips on trying to find the G-spot. Don't feel you've failed if you can't locate it. Most couples we know are still searching. That's half the fun.

". . . most sex therapists agree that women find intercourse pleasurable whether they climax during the act or not."

The Sound and the Fury

Some women climax noisily—panting, moaning, yelling; others are virtually silent. Some women thrash around; others barely move at all. But physiologically the process is the same: As orgasm nears, breathing becomes more rapid, muscles tense, and the vaginal opening narrows, gripping the penis more tightly (a sensation the man may or may not feel). With orgasm, a series of muscular contractions, lasting several seconds, occurs in the vaginal, uterine, and anal areas.

"According to The Kinsey Institute New Report on Sex, 75 percent of women require some kind of clitoral stimulation in order to climax. Before and/or during intercourse, it's the key to female orgasm."

"There's a whole range of female orgasmic response," says Carol Ellison, Ph.D., a clinical psychologist. "Sometimes a woman's muscular contractions and her whole orgasm are very powerful and intense. Other times, orgasm is just a gentle wave of release."

Women can and do fake orgasms. It's interesting to note, however, that women in long-term relationships are less likely to do so, according to Ellison. The reasons? First of all, women tend to feel more comfortable with longtime lovers. In addition, if they're having difficulty achieving orgasms, they may be more likely to address the problem with a trusted partner.

If you think your partner isn't having orgasms, talk to her about it (though not while you're making love). In fact, it's best to discuss sex on neutral ground—not the bedroom. The best approach, Barbach says, is the caring and direct one. For instance: "What do you like and not like about our sex life? Are you having orgasms? Is there something I can do to make our sex life better?"

The Clitoris: How To Push Her Buttons

If she masturbates, that's good for her. And for you. David Hurlbert, a marital and sex therapist at the Adult and Adolescent Counseling Center in Belton, Texas, found that women who masturbated on a regular basis had orgasms through a variety of sexual acts with partners (intercourse, oral sex, manual stimulation), while the vast majority of women who didn't masturbate could only climax with their partners during oral sex. In addition, if she knows how to pleasure herself, she can more easily guide you toward her pleasure zones.

Sexbit 7

Watching most women laugh at the diner scene in *When Harry Met Sally* is evidence enough that most chicks have faked a guy out at some point or another. So here's some ammo—four ways to tell is she's fakin' the Big O:

She's a drama queen in bed. Don't get us wrong. You may be a stallion in the sack. However, if she's loud enough to wake the neighbors with her "Oh, Oh, Ohs," then she's probably putting on a performance. Which doesn't mean you should quiet her down, says Barbara Keesling, Ph.D. and author of *Super Sexual Orgasm*. "She may be exciting herself with her sound effects." And maybe the neighbors, too.

Her alabaster skin remains that shade. Blood flow increases at the moment of orgasm, causing a flush to develop on a woman's cheeks and chest. If her skin isn't at least a little bit rosy after she collapses in ecstasy, she's probably ain't all that ecstatic.

You don't feel the grip. A woman's vagina contracts every 0.8 seconds during orgasm. If you don't feel a clench, clench, clench as she shouts, "I'm coming!" the "O" isn't for real.

She looks straight as an arrow. A woman's sympathetic nervous system is also activated at orgasm, causing her pupils to dilate. In other words, if she's gotten off, she should look like she's been smoking something funny—but sans the bloodshot eyes.

So let her responses guide you. It's usually best to talk about love-making preferences, turn-ons, and other sexual "positives" in bed, but save discussions about sexual difficulties and turn-offs for later. Keeping in mind that each woman has her individual sexual preferences, here are a couple of general tips.

"Go easy on the clitoris; it's highly sensitive. Start out gently, touching only lightly and sporadically and gradually building up pressure as she becomes more aroused."

Go easy on the clitoris; it's highly sensitive. Start out gently, touching only lightly and sporadically and gradually building up pressure as she becomes more aroused. "For most women, indirect stimulation is perfectly adequate because [the clitoris] is so sensitive," Hartley says. "A couple layers of skin [on the hood] won't get in the way. I know guys like to pull things back and begin poking at it like a button, but the clitoris is not a doorbell. Every time you pull or pinch or tug another part of the pussy, the clitoris feels it. It's that sensitive."

Instead of immediate direct contact, Hartley suggests massaging the areas adjacent to the clitoris, such as the vestibule directly beneath it, as well as stroking the shaft with your fingers. First, position your index and middle fingers to either side of the clitoral hood. Then, slowly spread your fingers to a "V" shape, gently massaging the shaft in an up-and-down movement. By building the speed and intensity, you'll be able to read your partner's expressions, varying your movements until you reach a rhythm that's ideal.

Hartley also suggests pulling the clitoris slightly off the pubic bone for enhanced arousal. First, position your fingers at the base of the clitoris. Then gently pull the folds of the labia away from your partner's body, at a 90 degree angle. As the skin pulls away, the tension will pull the clitoral hood back, revealing the clitoris. By massaging the labia in such a fashion, you'll be using the clitoral hood as a means of friction. Since most women don't naturally tug at their labia this way, it also provides a unique sensation. Still, gentleness is a watchword. Read your partner's expressions and talk through what you're doing—as you do it.

After mastering the gentle pulls, tugs, massages, and ministrations, move toward oral stimulation. Hartley suggests using your tongue and lips on *all* areas of the vagina, not just the clitoris. As you move slowly upward toward the clitoris, remember the sensitivity issue. Oftentimes, gentle licking above and around the glans is enough to make a woman orgasmic. Or, vary the amount of time spent directly on the clitoris, building sexual tension and anticipation as a means of arousal. Just be gentle.

"Another mistake eager lovers make is trying to introduce a finger into the vagina before it's ready," Hartley says. "Some women take a little longer to get ready . . . hurried intercourse can feel very rude and intrusive. So some women feel it's a violation. If you're going to be a sensitive lover, you need to take your time."

Again, Hartley suggests looking for visual and verbal cues before doing something that may be viewed as intrusive. Then, and only then, should you attempt to insert a finger into the vagina. Even so, move slowly—a knuckle at a time. And contrary to all those backseat fumblings when you were 16, women don't typically like rapid-fire finger thrusting. You may want to slowly massage the vagina in a circular fashion, moving your finger around the rim of the vagina.

"As she approaches orgasm," Barbach says, "it's useful for her partner to keep on doing whatever he's doing and maintain a steady rhythm. This isn't the time to vary the pace, pressure, or activity." More rapid breathing, increased muscle tension throughout her body, and a tendency to focus on herself rather than you are all signs that she's about to climax.

Positions and Possibilities

In the sixties, every groovy cat had a copy of the Kama Sutra on his cinder-block-and-pine bookshelf. Thousands of positions! Mystical teachings! Twenty-hour sex sessions! Spiritual enlightenment at the tip of your dick! Far out, man!

Truth was, all those copies of the Kama Sutra just collected dust. We, as a nation, don't get into too much exotica . . . and holding the same position for twelve hours to receive Manna from heaven? Forget it.

Still, there is something to be said for variety . . . it's the spice of life and it can spice up your bedroom antics. After all, your partner will tire of the ol' in-out if it's just the ol' in-out.

> " . . . there are as many different [sex] positions as there are different shapes and sizes of breast and penises . . . the possibilities are infinite."

Just remember: There are as many different positions as there are different shapes and sizes of breast and penises . . . the possibilities are infinite. But as we've mentioned before, go with what's comfortable to you and your lover. Sex shouldn't be a sordid game of Twister—left

The Birds and the Bees

We're infinitely more logical and civilized in our mating behavior than other denizens of the animal kingdom. Consider these creatures' unusual sex rituals:

- The male weaverbird builds a nest and hangs upside down from the bottom of it, flapping his wings to attract the female. She inspects and picks at the nest for up to ten minutes before deciding whether to stay or go try someone else's nest.

- A scorpionfly female only mates when a male brings her a tasty gift, which she eats while they mate. If she finishes eating before he's done, she throws him off. Since it takes the male 20 minutes to deposit his sperm, he becomes adept at bringing morsels that take 20 minutes to eat so he can complete the act. If any food is left when he's done, they fight over the leftovers.

- Male lovebugs wait and fight for a chance with a fertile female. The male who gets to her first doesn't let go, having continuous sex with her for up to three days. By the time the honeymoon ends, she's ready to deposit her eggs, so he is assured they're his.

- The male pied flycatcher woos a female and mates. After the female starts incubating the eggs he's confident are his, he dashes off to find another mate. Then he returns to female No. 1, devoting most of his time to feeding her chicks, and delivering only half as much food to female No. 2's chicks, who are more likely to die or be smaller. Researchers theorize that female No. 2 doesn't know about the existence of No. 1 until it's too late. Males also try to slip in with females already mated to others and impregnate them so other males unknowingly feed the marauder male's chicks.

- A male rat ejaculates twice as much sperm when he knows the female he is mating with has been near another male recently. (Similarly, men whose wives have been with them all day ejaculate much smaller amounts than men whose wives have been absent.)

- Ever wonder why female spiders and mantises eat their mates? The male's chances of mating at all in a lifetime are so low that when he gets lucky, he gives it his all—literally. His instinct is to produce as many offspring as possible, and if he can provide the female extra calories and protein, she'll have more and healthier eggs. So she eats him while they mate. Distracted by fresh food, she lets him (the parts of him that are left) copulate longer. Sex to die for . . .

hand red, right leg green. And it shouldn't be an act requiring Olympian strength and agility. After all, it would be pretty embarrassing calling the paramedics to uncouple a couple in the throes of back spasms. Be sensible. Explore. But do what feels best—for both of you.

Following are a handful of positions—each designed for maximum enjoyment, without requiring a learner's permit.

Missionary Position

It's the most common position, the stuff of Hollywood movies—a woman lying on a satin-sheeted bed, her man on top, staring soulfully into her eyes. Then . . . the scene cuts away to both of them side by side smoking cigarettes. Here's what you missed:

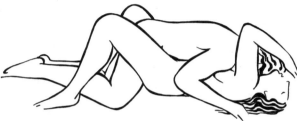

The woman lies face up, with her legs spread and a slight bend at the knees. The man rests between her legs, supporting himself with his arms. This allows for a steady rhythm.

To get deeper penetration and longer thrusting, bring your partner's knees up. This creates a more natural pathway and provides more stimulation for both you and her.

Or try this alternative to the missionary position: Instead of having your partner spread her legs, have her bring her thighs together. This time, mount from on top, instead of in between. That way, there'll be more clitoral stimulation, as well as friction for your John Thomas. Using this position, you'll experience more intense—and possibly quicker—orgasms. And your mate may just have her first orgasm via intercourse.

The Wraparound

Want to send your lover into orbit? Take the pillow from the headboard and prop it under her rump the next time you're in the missionary position. Then she can bring her legs up and wrap them around your waist. By bringing her pelvis higher than her upper torso, you're also aligning her body so her clitoris and G-spot get incredible stimulation.

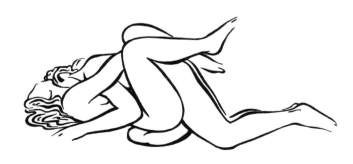

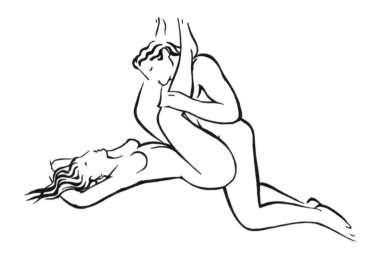

Getting a Leg Up . . . or Two

A variation of the Wraparound: Pull your partner's legs up—slowly, now—over your shoulders. This affords you the deepest penetration of all the prone positions, while still allowing balance and control. Or try just putting one leg up—this allows both of you easy access to each other's genitalia for fondling and stroking.

Sidewinder

Start with the previous position—both legs up over your shoulders. Then bring one leg down. Good. Now take the other leg and cross it over your chest, turning your partner in that direction until she's on her side. You may have to reposition so you straddle her "down" leg. Hold onto the leg you just brought down for support. This position is exceptionally effective in that it offers more friction during penetration.

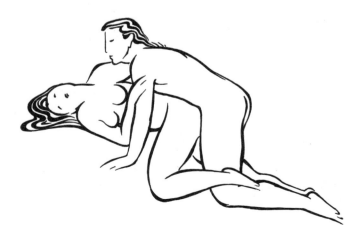

Rear Entry

Call it doggie style, if you will. Just don't spring it on your partner without warning, or you'll be in the doghouse. This position requires communication and a leap of faith, since your lover won't easily see what you're doing.

Typically, the woman gets on her knees with her partner behind her. By positioning himself between her legs, the man can place his hands on her buttocks to support himself as he thrusts. This position also allows the man to reach around and stimulate the clitoris with his hand.

Try this variation: Assume the position. Then slowly lean back, pulling your partner back, until you're resting on your calves.

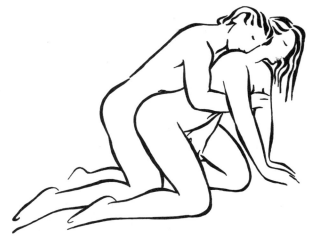

This allows your partner to control the rhythm and thrusting, since she can move back and forth as she "rides" you.

Or try this: Instead of having your partner get on her hands and knees, have her lie flat. This position provides more friction and contact with the G-spot.

Spooning

Think of it as rear entry. Except you're lying down. On your side. This position is ideal for clitoral stimulation, since you can reach over and fondle your lover.

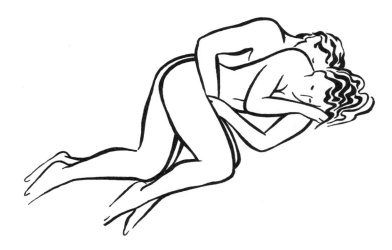

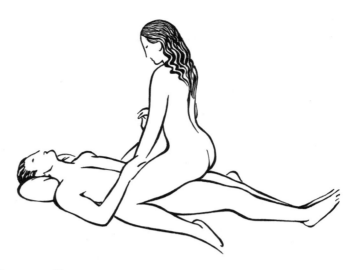

Woman on Top

Or, in truck driver parlance: Havin' her do all th' work. In this position, the woman is really in control. By straddling the man, who is lying flat, the woman can thrust and grind, creating the tempo and rhythm.

As a variation, try the woman-on-top position—backwards. In this case, your lover will straddle you, but face your feet. The angle is different, causing more friction and more clitoral stimulation. And, this allows you to provide anal stimulation . . . if she's up for it.

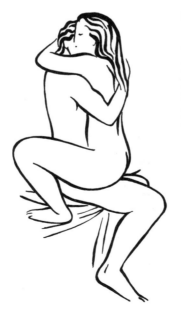

Sitting Down

In this position, you sit in a chair or the on the edge of the bed as your partner straddles you. She can either rest on her knees, or squat, providing more leverage. As an alternative, try reversing her position so she's facing away from you. This way, you can easily stimulate her clitoris with your hand.

Standing Up

Try the basic rear entry position—but this time, stand up. It's best if your partner has something to lean against, such as a bed or counter. And if you're a tall guy, hunker down a bit.

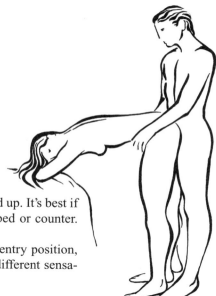

Try it a few different ways. As in the standard rear entry position, having your partner keep her thighs together creates a different sensation than when her legs are spread.

Coital Alignment Technique (CAT)

This new twist on the missionary position requires you to rest your body against hers, positioning yourself far forward between her legs so the shaft of your penis presses against her clitoral area. With this technique, instead of thrusting, the two of you move your pelvises together in short, rocking motions. By keeping your lower body in constant contact with her clitoris, you'll greatly improve her chances of achieving orgasm. It may not be the actual intercourse that does it for her (remember most women don't get off that way), but believe us when we say that she won't give a hoot how it happens. And neither should you.

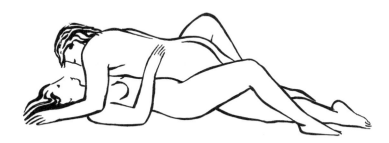

Want something exotic? First, make sure you've got that paramedic number handy. Then, try the Wraparound, except this time stand tall, lifting your partner as she supports herself with her arms around your neck. As you lower her onto your, um, manhood, she should wrap her legs around your waist. In this position, you'll be doing all the work, cradling her buttocks and lifting her up and down. Good balance is a must, as is a strong back and neck. Some weight training may be in order before you try this one.

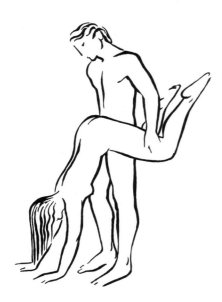

More Exotica

While you've got that paramedic number out, try this: **The Wheel-barrow,** a variation of a rear entry standing position. Except in this case, your partner bends over, puts her hands on the ground, and you lift her up by the thighs. (This can also be done in a sitting position.) Not for the faint of heart. Or weak of wrists.

Then there's a variation on the rear-entry-lying-down position, **Feet First.** In this position, you climb on top of your partner, backwards. You'll face her feet and enter her—slowly—backwards as you stretch your legs out until your weight is on your hands.

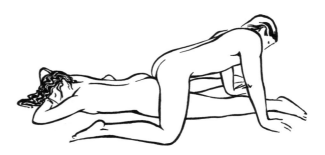

Or try **Thigh High:** Lie down. Bring your knees to your chest. Have your lover then straddle you while facing away from you, essentially sitting on your thighs. Hold onto your partner's waist to balance her. Then use those hamstrings to create the tempo.

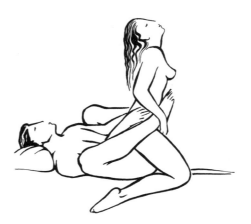

This just touches the surface of all the positions out there just waiting for you. Just remember: Talk everything through—before, during, and after you do it. After all, talk is sexy. Calling the paramedics isn't.

Bums the Word

Your gut reaction may be to quickly flip past this section. After all, people tend to think of anal sex in one of two ways: as a taboo—a hush-hush, dirty kind of sex favored only by perverts. Or as wishful thinking—something they're never going to get in this lifetime, so why waste a moment even considering it.

Well, as far as taboos are concerned, it's true. Anal sex is definitely something good girls and boys don't talk about. But that doesn't mean they're not doing it—about 30 percent of all heterosexual couples have tried anal intercourse, according to Tristan Taormino, author of *The Ultimate Guide to Anal Sex for Women*. She equates it to oral sex. As early as a decade ago, people wouldn't openly discuss fellatio or cunnilingus; these were the great secrets of the sexually enlightened. Now oral sex is considered a natural part of foreplay, with some couples even preferring it to intercourse. Women crave it. Men crave it. And no one is considered "nasty" for saying so.

> "Anal sex is definitely something good girls and boys don't talk about. But that doesn't mean they're not doing it—about 30 percent of all heterosexual couples have tried anal intercourse . . . "

Taormino, a self-proclaimed "ass aficionado," hopes anal play eventually achieves the same acceptance as oral sex. "Once people get past their hang-ups, they'll realize what a pleasurable part of the body the anus is."

Obstacle Central Part One

Foremost among those hang-ups is the fear of pain on the receiving end. Let's face it, the anus is a tight orifice. A bowel movement can hurt—never mind the insertion of a penis the size of a Polska kielbasa.

This is where the mind/body connection can help. To enjoy anal play, both partners need to be ready psychologically. It's not something you can fake and pressure won't work. As Nina Hartley says in her video guide to anal sex, "No one knows a lie like the anus. . . . You must, must do this because you want to do this."

Once that's established, partners need to talk about their concerns and comfort levels. "Get your feelings on the table. Set reasonable goals," says Taormino. "And start slow.

"If a woman feels safe and absolutely in control, she'll be better able to relax," she explains. "And relaxation is essential."

So is lubrication. "Spit is not going to do it," says Taormino, adding that guys need to get over the notion that if a woman is not getting properly aroused, she needs extra lube. "The anus does not produce its own natural lubricant, so it's essential that you use plenty of the manufactured stuff."

Make sure the lube is a water-based type, so it doesn't interfere with the protective capabilities of a condom. Experts agree, a condom should always be worn during anal intercourse, with only one exception: if you're in a monogamous relationship, and both partners have tested negative for all sexually transmitted diseases.

Once your partner is sufficiently relaxed and lubed, you can start exploring . . . again, slowly. Start by gently touching or licking the area around the anus. It's packed with nerve endings, so penetration isn't necessary to elicit a wonderful response. If your partner is comfortable and at ease, try inserting a finger—one joint at a time.

Toys, such as anal beads and butt plugs, are a natural progression. Though we talk about them in detail in the next chapter, our best advice where the bum is concerned is to start small and work your way up. Some individuals like a full feeling; others the in-out motion of intercourse. Experiment with a variety to see what is most pleasurable for you.

Once you're ready to make the transition to anal intercourse, keep in mind the delicacy of the area and proceed with caution. "Start by massaging the buttocks and inner thighs," writes Taormino. "Work your way around the anal area with your fingers, your mouth, or a vibrator. The more you stimulate the entire area the more the blood rushes there. You can combine anal stimulation with stimulation of the clitoris or vagina to get the entire genital region engorged and excited."

Never poke the anus, advises Taormino. Instead, gently caress it. "You'll know your partner is ready to move forward because she'll tell you so. If she says stop, do it. It's in your best interest to move at her pace. If you hurry—and it hurts—it may never happen again."

Here's a final tip to make the initial penetration less problematic. What often causes discomfort for your partner is the fact that you must insert your penis against the grain of the sphincter muscle. The more pressure you apply—especially the first time—the more the muscle will tighten reflexively. We suggest that your partner breathe deeply and naturally . . . holding her breath in anticipation may cause the muscle to tighten. Then tell her, gently, to push outwardly with the muscle. Once your glans has passed the sphincter portal, give your partner a chance to get acclimated to the sensations. Hold still briefly and enjoy the feeling before pushing in deeper.

Obstacle Central Part Two

Once women realize how much pleasure can be derived from anal eroticism, chances are good that they're going to want to reciprocate. This is where a second major anal sex hang-up comes into play. Many guys consider their own anus off-limits. "I know it sounds goofy," says Dan, a 38-year-old businessman. "But in the back of my mind, I'm thinking, only homosexuals do that."

Interestingly, during her research, Taormino discovered that while 50 to 60 percent of gay men have tried anal intercourse, only 30 percent of them enjoy it regularly. "People need to realize that the object of their desire won't change if they try something new. Gay men give each other blow jobs; that hasn't stopped heterosexual men from enjoying them, too."

Besides, she reminds us, anal play doesn't have to involve penetration. "If a man is uncomfortable with the thought of something being inserted into his butt, it's his prerogative. Comfort and trust must go both ways."

She points out, though, that many men can have much more intense orgasms through anal massage. Because it's in close proximity to the prostate, the male equivalent to the G-spot, a gentle massage is sometimes all it takes.

Obstacle Central Part Three

Another reason some couples are reluctant to explore anal eroticism is because they feel it's unclean. "It doesn't seem sanitary to put your penis in contact with fecal matter," says Darrell, a 27-year-old Michigan postal worker.

The fact is, there is only a small amount of fecal matter in the anal and rectal canals, says Taormino. It's stored in the bowel and only passes through on its way out of the body. Though some people like to take a bath or shower before sex, it's not necessary. Likewise, some people like to have an enema before anal sex, but this is also unnecessary. "Enemas deplete the rectum of natural mucus, which can aid in lubrication," she says. Of course, if having one helps you scale a mental hurdle, just remember to do it several hours before sex. That way the mucus will be replenished.

Obstacle Central Part Four

If you're worried that sticking something—anything—up your lover's bum will cause it to malfunction, don't. "It's a total myth that anal sex causes hemorrhoids or anal incontinence," say Taormino. In fact, most anal problems are caused by tension. "We store a lot of anxiety in our butts," she says. "Learning to relax that part of our anatomy has actually proven helpful. It makes for a healthier butt."

Tantric Sex, or . . . And Now for Something Completely Different

Although Tantric sex has been practiced for ages, it is one of the more significant sexual trends of our times. The good news is, you don't have to be acrobatic or even flexible to enjoy it. The bad news is, you have to have sex for a few hours.

Okay, so there isn't any bad news. But you do have to keep an open mind, because Tantric sex tends to sound like a bunch of New Age hoo-ha to the unenlightened. An ancient Hindu practice that links sexuality and spirituality, Tantra involves meditation, yoga, and breathing rituals designed to prolong lovemaking and lead to "full-body" orgasms (rather than the mere genital ones most of us know). It's through these orgasms that you and your partner can "ride the wave of bliss" toward oneness with God . . . the Goddess . . . or your higher power of choice.

Singles and couples of all ages and ethnic groups have been flocking to Tantra workshops here and abroad. Some of these how-to sessions are fairly tame, teaching techniques that couples can practice behind closed doors. Others are more intimate, with couples getting naked and "discovering God" in groups. And, of course, there's plenty of celebrity hype. Woody Harrelson and Sting are outspoken Tantra devotees, as are Jill Eikenberry and Michael Tucker, the real-life couple who played married legal-eagles Ann Kelsey and Stuart Markowitz on the TV show *L.A. Law*. Eikenberry and Tucker turned Tantric following her battle with breast cancer. For them, as well as many others, Tantra teaches far more than great sex; it's considered a path toward healing, a way to purge painful memories and hang-ups in order to connect with a partner on a deeper level.

Joseph Brown understands the deep connections that come with learning Tantra. A 44-year-old divorced father of two, Brown generally "avoids self-help workshops and pooh-poohs most New Age stuff." But two and a half years ago, he met girlfriend True Fellows through the personal ads and "we hit it off immediately," he says. On a camping trip, the couple made love for the first time and Brown, like most sexually satisfied men, ejaculated within 30 minutes. "I thought it was great," he said, "but True said 'You're going to have to learn to control that.'" Turns out, Brown's new girlfriend was a tantrika (a Tantra instructor) who had been studying sexuality for more than 25 years.

Fellows suggested they take a weekend Tantra workshop together, so Brown could learn ejaculatory control (a major focus for men) and so they could grow closer as a couple. "I led a pretty sheltered life and tend to be inhibited," Brown said, "but I trusted True and wanted to enhance our relationship."

Their workshop, one of the tamer types, ran from Saturday morning through Sunday afternoon. It began with brief introductions and moved right into emotional release work. According to Brown, these exercises in breathing and undulation (wavelike body movements) are designed to "help eliminate negative feelings, which keep you from truly connecting with your partner.

"I'm not the kind of guy who gets carried away by emotions, but I was pretty blown away by the experience. All the hurts from my divorce came back. I cried like I hadn't cried before. It was really good for me."

Next, couples were acquainted with the Tantra hug, a simple yoga technique in which the woman sits in the man's lap, and both remain still for about an hour. (Sorry, no snoozing allowed.) Dancing followed—but we're not talking the Macarena. "Tantra dancing is more like flowing body movements, a way to loosen up," says Brown. "It sounds silly, but you just give in to the moment like everyone else. No one is singled out or embarrassed."

After couples were sufficiently loose, the Sensuous Feast commenced. In all the variations of Tantra, food and feeding are key to enhancing sexuality. Finger foods—everything from pate to whipped cream—are placed before participants, who are encouraged to feed their partners sensuously. "It was fun," said Brown. "True and I smooched in-between bites. I put whipped cream on her tummy and licked it off. It was a lot of feeling, smelling, and touching."

At this point in the festivities, couples were asked to dress in their god and goddess costumes. "It could be a G-string or boxer shorts. Maybe a toga or lingerie for the women. Basically, it's whatever makes you feel sexy yet comfortable," says Brown.

More breathing exercises followed, with women focusing on methods of relaxing and men concentrating on ways to control ejaculation. "I used to think about baseball," jokes Brown, "but that takes you away from your lover. Tantra teaches you ways to remain connected."

One such way is the Cobra, a breathing technique which Brown describe this way: "You inhale deeply, clenching your pubococcygeus muscles [also called PC muscles; see chapter 7] and touching your chin to your chest. After holding that position for a moment, you breathe out in a hiss, raising your head and relaxing your PC muscles." Brown, who can now stop the inevitable with a mere tensing of the body, says the Cobra is the best place to start. "It helped loosen my erection, then I'd wait a minute and start making love again. Orgasms are a lot more intense."

So here's the big question: Why would a guy want to hold out for hours while his multiorgasmic woman enjoys all the fun? Because men who are into Tantra claim that it provides them with a wave of orgasms, too. "They're different than ejaculatory orgasms," Brown says, "they're like shivers that run up and down your body. They feel damn good. Even when I don't ejaculate at all, I'm never dissatisfied."

In fact, Brown says Tantra has improved his sex life and his relationship with Fellows, just as she promised. "For me, it's been a way of connecting sex with love. I've learned to be more romantic and to communicate, which is one of the toughest barriers. I'm also more open-minded and curious about other forms of sexuality."

Building Yourself a Better Orgasm

Want to improve something that's already a mind-blowing experience?

Building a more intense and longer orgasm isn't all that different from building a more fit and appealing body: You team up strategies, mental and physical, and end up with the desired result.

Sounds easy? It can be. But, paradoxically, not if you try too hard. Approaching orgasms like a competitive sport will sabotage your best efforts. Instead, take a laid-back approach, using these tips simply to feel more pleasure. Bigger and better orgasms will naturally follow.

Please note: if you're concerned about premature ejaculation—the act of having an orgasm too soon—check out our section on impotence in chapter 7 for specific tips on prolonging your sexual activity.

Untie Your Tongue

Most anxiety about sex stems from the belief that it's something you do without discussion. This assumes we're all sexual mind readers. Well, we flunked Sexual Mind Reading 101, and it's likely everyone you know has, too.

Talking about sex is difficult because it involves revealing our most private feelings. However, trust is a key factor in any personal relationship, and that's especially true when you're getting naked with another person—literally and verbally. People tend to have better sex with people they know and understand. Optimal sex means being able to deliver the bad news. If you're bored, physically uncomfortable, experiencing pain, or simply want a change of position or action, say so. No bonus points will be awarded for tolerating misery or tedium.

Take Your Time

Some men make the mistake of going straight for the finish as soon as they have an erection. They succumb to what may be an evolutionary urge to spread their DNA as quickly and as often as possible. If this is your usual pattern, try taking a detour—the longer, the better. An erection results from a circulatory traffic jam in the penis—more blood is taking the on-ramp than the exit. The pulsations of an orgasm feel great in part because they begin normalizing the volume of blood in the penis. The longer the buildup, the more blood to evacuate, the greater the pleasure.

To stretch things out, use the "balk method." That means going into the windup but not throwing the pitch. Approach the point of no return (referred to by therapists as ejaculatory inevitability), but stop just before you hit it. Let the urge to come die down by backing off on the stimulation or stopping it altogether. Then start up again, amplifying your arousal level and heart rate. Stop yet again when you begin approaching orgasm.

To do this, take some time alone to determine where the edge of your orgasm is, the place just before the point of no return. Play that edge with your partner. Pay close attention to your sensations. You'll climax longer and more intensely.

And what about masturbation? How many people don't dare share one of the most intimate sexual acts of all? True, it's

> "... trust is a key factor in any personal relationship, and that's especially true when you're getting naked with another person—literally and verbally."

also near the top of the list of activities many consider taboo. But watching others give themselves sexual pleasure can be a very arousing sight. Couples who share masturbation well into the relationship can also expand their ever-increasing knowledge of who their partner really is (translation: build intimacy), and that's what makes sex hot.

Adjust Your Mind

Don't obsess about what each sigh and wince means. It's impossible to do, and besides, if you try, you won't feel the great things that just began two groans ago.

And stay calm if things don't go as expected. Keep in mind that an entire relationship seldom revolves around one sexual experience. And if it does, doesn't that say a lot about your bedmate or about you if you're the hasty judge?

> "Don't obsess about what each sigh and wince means. It's impossible to do, and besides, if you try, you won't feel the great things that just began two groans ago."

Get Wet

It takes only ten seconds to demonstrate that lubricants enhance lovemaking, according to Michael Castleman in his booklet "The Slippery Secret of Sensational Sex." Here's how:

- Close your mouth and dry your lips.
- Run a finger lightly over them. Pay attention to how it feels.
- Now, lick your lips.
- With your lips moist, run the same finger over them. Again, focus on how it feels.

What feels more sensual? The moist lips, of course. The body provides several natural lubricants—saliva, vaginal secretions, and Cowper's gland secretions from your urethra—but all of these evaporate quickly because they're more watery than slippery. Water-soluble lubricants such as K-Y jelly, Ortho jelly, Probe, Slippery Stuff, Enhance,

PrePair, and Astroglide have staying power and are revivable with saliva or water (say from a spray mister at bedside) if they begin to lose moisture. Additional lubricant makes exploring those new territories more pleasurable, and it's virtually essential for experiments with sex toys.

Celebrate the Moment

Another way to intensify orgasm is to approach sex as a special occasion. Don't just add it to the list of things you do before going to sleep—wash face, brush teeth, have sex. Make love only when you've built up some desire for your partner (or would really like to). Also, learn the difference between horniness and "skin hunger." One is about genuine sexual arousal; the other is when you just want contact with another warm body and might really benefit more from a massage or snuggle.

Push Past Your Standard M.O.

Many men have found that they can build up to better orgasms when they incorporate overlooked and unexplored body parts and behaviors in their sexual repertoire. That means stretching the boundaries of what you've done before: Build muscle. Strengthen your PC muscle. The PC wraps around the base of the penis and the anus like a figure-eight, and reflexively contracts during orgasm, providing much of an orgasm's pleasurable sensations. A stronger muscle will contract harder and create a more intense orgasm, especially when combined with the "balk method."

To strengthen the PC, try Kegel exercises. Kegels consist of the same muscle action you use when you stop the flow of urine mid-stream, only you don't have to be peeing to do a Kegel: Perform that same squeeze action, holding the contraction for a slow count of three. Do this for about two minutes, three times a day. You should notice a difference in about two weeks.

A word of caution here. If you've never done Kegels before, you may feel tenderness in the area a day or two after you've launched into an exercise regimen. Don't worry. The slight discomfort is generally normal. Take a day off, giving the muscle time to flush out the lactic acid—that's what causing that slight ache—then return to the program. Eventually, you'll feel no discomfort. Instead, you'll notice a newfound sense of strength in the area. It's unlikely your unit will have the power of a catapult, but there should be a significant difference in your ability to delay orgasm.

Aim High

Lots of guys think nipple stimulation is just for women. Wrong again. Sex researcher Alfred Kinsey speculated that as many males as females may have sexually sensitive nipples. He even found a few men who could reach orgasm through nipple stimulation alone.

Aim Low

There's no need to be embarrassed: Incredibly sensitive nerve endings reside outside and just inside the anus and can create powerful pleasure when stroked with a well-lubricated finger. Moreover, the hidden part of the penis extends almost all the way back to the anal sphincter, which contracts forcefully during orgasms. Why stoically ignore a body part that's so clearly connected to sexual ecstasy? (More on this in chapter 5.)

> "Incredibly sensitive nerve endings reside outside and just inside the anus and can create powerful pleasure when stroked with a well-lubricated finger."

Hit the Volume

Most men won't hesitate to huff and puff and grunt when working out or playing a sport. But it's usually women who make real noise in the bedroom, taking their orgasms to a higher level. Why should they have all the fun? Experiment with the way you breathe during sex, working your way up to moaning a little as well. In fact, if you inhale and exhale deeply or moan and groan, your enthusiasm will probably turn your partner on more as well.

Order Extras

People aren't always comfortable with "extras" such as sex toys and unusual settings, but that doesn't mean they should be avoided completely. (Check our sex-toy test drive in chapter 5 for more information on a variety of possibilities.) A manageable amount of anxiety is one of the key ingredients to ever-improving sex. But if you're adamant in your belief that anything beyond the bodies involved is unnatural, then eliminate the sex toys. However, don't exclude sights, sounds, smells, and tastes as different types of "extras."

Make a Pact

Consider making this agreement with your partner: "I will do sexual things for you and with you for as long as I want to. If I am bored, uncomfortable, experiencing pain, or simply want to suggest a change, you can count on me to let you know. In other words, I won't do anything I don't want to do. If you'll make the same agreement, neither of us will need to second-guess what the other is feeling. Then we can relax and really enjoy the sex we're having."

Making an agreement like this permits people to luxuriate in their pleasure and enjoy their growing arousal. It's particularly useful for men with unreliable erections because they can stop worrying about their partner and simply enjoy their own pleasure. Anything that stops fruitless attempts at sexual mind reading can only boost the experience.

Open Your Eyes and Ears

Don't restrict your visual stimulation to videos and magazines; look at the person who turns you on. Be a voyeur, savoring what's happening to both you and your lover's body. For a really exciting ride, try keeping your eyes open the whole time. That way, you can teach your partner how to enhance your orgasms. Figure out what your hot buttons are and share your knowledge. Don't expect your lover to automatically know. Turn-ons can include oral sex, lingerie or other sexy clothing,

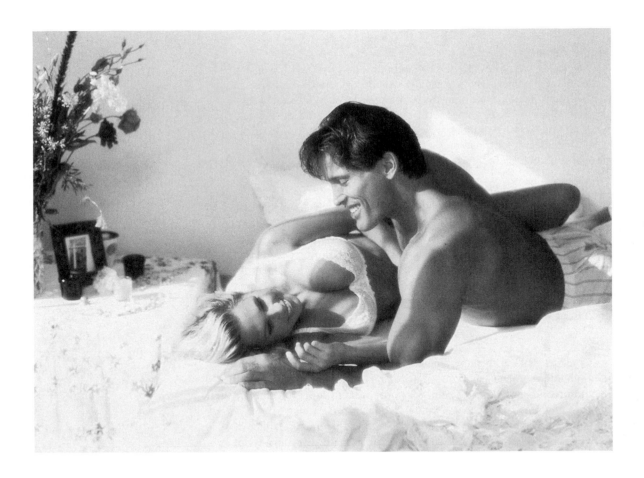

and having sex in "naughty" places. Get the full impact that playing out fantasies (both in your mind and in reality) can offer. Teach your lover how to take you over and rev you up.

Forget Winning a Medal

Stop thinking about your performance. Better yet, drop the word "perform" from your sexual vocabulary altogether. Take the focus off your penis and explore some of these new territories. Figuring out how to feel good, not trying to be good, is the necessary ingredient for a better orgasm.

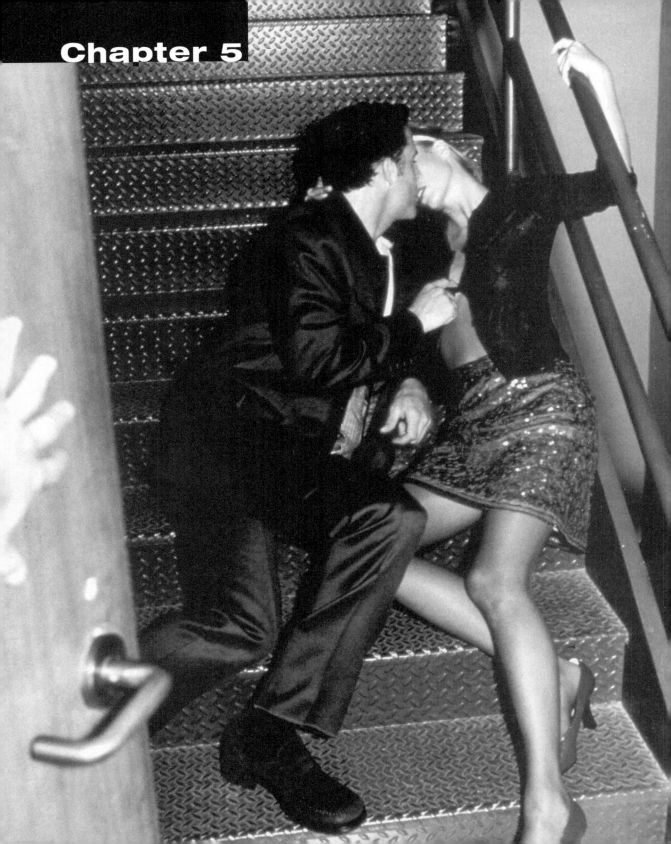

Chapter 5

We like to equate sex with athletes. You've got the squeaky clean, mainstream, Tiger Woods kind, and the over-the-top, extreme, Dennis Rodman kind. Though The Worm's choices may seem perfectly normal to him, to many, they're odd . . . bizarre . . . kinky, even.

The same can be said for pleasures of the flesh. The Woods kind of guy wouldn't dare be flogged by some Amazon in leather. Though their fantasies might swing in that direction, they'd never act on them—perhaps out of guilt or simply for fear of getting caught.

Well, here's a news flash: There are plenty of folks who couldn't care less if people learn of their wild sexploits. In fact, they take great pride in their open-mindedness and freedom. "Sex is supposed to be fun," says Damon, a 37-year-old real estate executive from southern California who dabbles in bondage. "We need to get over our hang-ups. There's a rainbow of flavors out there, but most people limit themselves to vanilla because it's the acceptable thing to do."

Well, if you're interested in what that rainbow consists of, here's what's happening several degrees left of the mainstream.

Porn Again

Your girlfriend is furious with you. She has just found your stash of old Victoria's Secret catalogs, which she'd thought were her catalogs, and which it's obvious you're keeping for purposes other than mail-ordering her an Olga's demicup underwire bra and matching tap pants. Or she's found your collection of British nanny-spanking photos, or your videos of lesbian convicts in bondage.

Why, she asks, do you need that stuff? Isn't she enough for you? Which is, of course, to miss the point entirely. She may or may not be enough for you, but having a collection of photographs of young ladies wearing bras and panties or tied with wrist-and-ankle restraints or standing in a field buck naked has nothing whatsoever to do with meaningful relationships. If love is never having to say you're sorry, a collection of porn is never having to say anything at all.

Many women claim they're not turned on by watching some anonymous hunk rip off a woman's skivvies. But they do get excited by an incredibly romantic guy in an incredibly romantic setting doing incredibly romantic things like sipping champagne in front of a roaring fireplace and saying she's the most amazing woman he's ever met. That, of course, is followed by dancing the tango and then ripping off

The Wilder Ride

Five Things to Say When Your Girlfriend Discovers Your Porn Stash

1. "Ahhh, I'm glad you found those. I was saving them to show you because the girl in those photographs looks a little bit like you, except that her thighs aren't as slim as yours."
2. "Oh, that's the research material the *Atlantic Monthly* sent me for an article they want me to write."
3. "I thought these sleazy examples of decadent sexist erotica would amuse you."
4. "I've assembled this material for us to review together so that it might lend variety to our long-term, monogamous, and otherwise incredibly fulfilling romantic relationship."
5. "It's not mine."

their skivvies. Most guys are turned on by just the thought of ripping off someone's skivvies.

Most women say they're simply not wired the way men are, that only men are aroused by purely visual stimuli. Most women, that is, besides the Vegas showgirls we once hung out with, whose take on the whole thing was rather like men's. They told us they're always checking out men's buns, sizing up men's bundles, having fantasies of anonymous sex, leering at porn videos, comparing notes with their showgirl friends about their lovers' prowess in bed and the size of their lovers' dicks and, in general, doing all the things that most women blame men for and claim not to understand.

What does this suggest? To us it says that women's attitudes toward pornography and sexual experimentation have more to do with permission and exposure than they'd like to admit. Among the closed society of the Vegas showgirls we met, there's permission to view pornography—or, for that matter, to do just about anything they want, as long as they show up for work on time. Although we're admittedly working from what scientists call "anecdotal evidence," we have to conclude that men and women may be more similar than we think.

Girls Peek Too

Though women may not admit it openly, a recent survey of 500 video stores found that female patrons have a say in at least 25 percent of all adult-video rentals. Journalist Sallie Tisdale wrote this in *Harper's* magazine: "I was interested in the discomfort pornography brings up, both for others and for myself, but no matter what else I could say about it, I had to admit that I found a lot of pornography exciting."

Women write porn, too. Best-selling author Anne Rice writes sadomasochistic fairy tales like *The Claiming of Sleeping Beauty* under the name A. N. Roquelar. Author Laurie Sue Brockway writes particularly graphic erotic fiction under the name Charlotte Rose. "One reason I write so graphically," Brockway says, "is because a lot of women don't know where everything is, what the clitoris is, how to have orgasms, how to pleasure themselves."

So porn can be useful as a how-to guide for the sexually unsophisticated. It can also provide fresh bedroom scenarios or lend variety to long-term monogamous relationships.

"Though women may not admit it openly, a recent survey of 500 video stores found that female patrons have a say in at least 25 percent of all adult-video rentals."

So the next time your girlfriend comes across your *Naughty Nurses Meet the Spanking Surgeon* video, why not suggest she join you in a stimulating and educational screening?

Wild—It's All Relative

Vanilla sex is clearly not the favored flavor among *Men's Fitness* readers. Here's the breakdown of their responses to our survey question: "Which of the following have you done?"

Used pornography to enhance sex	56.0%
Shared fantasies with a partner	53.6%
Used sex toys	45.6%
Had sex with someone much older than myself	36.9%
Been unfaithful when involved in a committed relationship	36.4%
Engaged in phone sex	34.2%

(Source: Taken from the *Men's Fitness* Sex Survey of readers, 1998)

Chick Porn Flicks

Better yet, save the Naughty Nurses for your own private moments and let her ease her way into adult entertainment with a more female-friendly porn flick. Candida Royalle, a former adult film star who now produces and directs her own features for her company, Femme Productions, acknowledges that many X-rated movies are sex-heavy and plot thin. As in real life, women need romance, says Royalle, "they don't want cheap and tawdry. A word commonly used to describe my films is 'class.'"

We previewed a selection of Royalle movies—*The Bridal Shower, One Size Fits All, My Surrender,* and *The Gift*—and noticed her "female-friendly" style immediately. A real woman, for example, probably wouldn't be too pleased if you ejaculated all over her face. In fact, she'd probably deck you—hard—if you did. So there are no facial "cum shots" in films created under the Femme Productions banner. Men either ejaculate inside their partner, or at a tasteful distance.

Women in Royalle's films also appear to be enjoying themselves. By contrast, the actresses in *Sorority Sex Kittens 3* might as well have been filling out their income taxes for all the enthusiasm they showed their masculine costars. (They did, however, seem to perk up during the all-girl sorority-initiation orgy scene.) Which brings us to another differentiation: Female-friendly porn flicks don't have girl-girl sex scenes for the hell of it. "Some women aren't turned on by watching two women pleasure each other,"

Next time you rent a porno flick to watch with your partner, think Candida Royalle. The former adult film star is now a director and producer of X-rated movies created for couples—with a special sensitivity to female characters. They have plots, hunky guys, lots of foreplay, and are absolutely cum-shot free.

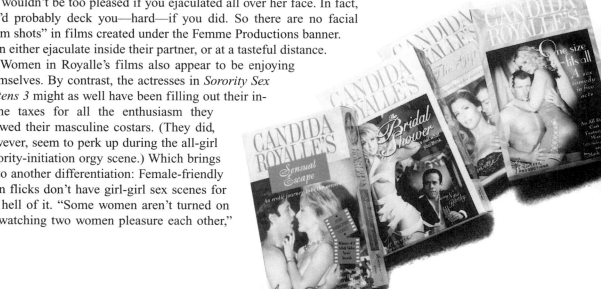

Porn: As She Likes It

Knowing that most people don't like to linger too long in the "adult films" room of their local video store, we asked Candida Royalle, producer and director of Femme Productions, to offer advice on how to choose titles both you and your partner will enjoy. "The number one way to pick is director, director, director," she says. Directors are known for having particular styles; those who have a loyal female following include Royalle, Cameron Grant, Andrew Blake, Paul Thomas, Veronica Hart, Jane Hamilton, Nina Hartley, and the husband and wife team of Missy and Michael. Dim the lights and pass the . . . vibrator.

says Royalle, "so we don't include this type of sex unless it has a plot connection."

And yes, her movies do have plots. One of our favorites, *One Size Fits All,* is a clever story that centers on a dress that seems to have erotic karma. Each woman who wears it (and there are about five throughout the one-hour film), enjoys a sexual encounter of romance-novel proportions. "It's all about fantasy," says Royalle, "I create sensual stories that appeal to a wide variety of tastes and preferences."

The women in Royalle's films seem more real, too. Instead of the typical porn star—a bleached-blonde Barbie on silicon overload—there's a mix of voluptuous blondes, brunettes, and redheads with beautifully flawed bodies. Their breasts have that telltale droop of authenticity, their hips are soft and round, their thighs a bit fleshy. "I think its more interesting and sexy to see women who haven't been overly altered," says Royalle, adding that it also helps female viewers feel less intimidated.

And the last—but perhaps most important—element of a female-friendly adult film are male costars who actually look good. Don't get us wrong. Ron Jeremy—a.k.a. The Hedgehog—is probably really nice. But then so is Nell Carter and we doubt you'd want to watch her make the beast with two backs. There are plenty of serious hunks in the adult film world. Look for names like Mark Davis, T. T. Boy, and Peter North. She'll like their looks. Take our word for it.

Do-It-Yourself Porno

Perhaps you and your significant other are bold enough to film your own erotic adventures. Our best advice is to get a good camcorder, a tripod, and a safe.

Choosing a camcorder can be a daunting task, considering the variety of options available. Compact VHS models, for example, record on miniature cassettes that fit into a gizmo that can be inserted into a standard VCR. The resolution of C-VHS recordings is the weakest of the tape formats. Eight-millimeter is better and Hi-8 millimeter is the best. Unless you have an 8-millimeter deck to play back your footage, you'll have to hook your camcorder up to the TV for playback. Sony incorporates a feature called LaserLink into its higher-end Handycams, which allows you to beam your videos to the television via infrared technology. (Cool!) Or you can watch your work on the tiny LCD screens featured in the newest camcorders from Sony, Panasonic, RCA, JVC, and Sharp.

If you have a really big budget—and want a picture so clear you can see the dimples on your lover's butt—opt for a digital camcorder. These $2,000-plus models can be connected to your computer for editing and some include digital snapshot functions that allow you to take still photographs.

Obviously, the tripod is a way to position the camcorder and forget it's there. After all, it's a lot easier to romp while your hands are free. It's just tougher to get the close-up shots.

And finally—and, most importantly, in our opinion—is a safe, or at least a safe place to store your home videos. You don't want any friends to find them. You don't want your niece or nosy neighbors to find them. You don't want your *Adventures of Pirate Pete* tape getting mixed up with your Blockbuster rentals. And you don't want the housekeeper to find them and sell them on the Internet à la Tommy and Pamela Lee—or maybe you do.

"If you have a really big budget—and want a picture so clear you can see the dimples on your lover's butt—opt for a digital camcorder."

The Buzz on Sex Toys

If you're like most Americans , your first sex toy was probably a vibrator or some metal-studded cock ring you received as a joke at a bachelor or bachelorette party. You may have chuckled—and blushed—along with the crowd, then tossed the "gag gift" in a bag with the rest of your marital booty. After all, good girls and boys don't use those nasty things.

Hah!

You'd be surprised to learn how many of your closest friends keep a closet stash of vibrators, dildos, and other sexual esoterica. Sales of these adult playthings have shot up 45 percent in the past three years, according to the International Academy of Sex Researchers. But you don't have to take their word for it. Pay a visit to Cupid's Treasures in Chicago, The Pleasure Chest in New York, Chicago, or Los Angeles, or Good Vibrations in San Francisco, and watch the traffic come through—business-

"Sales of [sex toys] have shot up 45 percent in the past three years, according to the International Academy of Sex Researchers."

women, construction workers, doctors, housewives. The new sex-toy retail outlets are boutiques, not shadowy adult bookstores. And some mail-order catalogs, such as the one put out by Good Vibrations, are about as wholesome as Victoria's Secret. The fact is: toys can add variety and adventure to your sex life. And they can be damn fun.

To get an idea of what's out there, and to put some of the most popular items to the test, we decided to take a trip to Cupid's Treasures, the largest adult-toy store in Chicago. There, we're greeted by Heather, a funky twentysomething urbanite with a vast knowledge of the products. Our mission, we tell her: Choose a variety of items for men and women to be evaluated by a group of eager friends. We explain that our volunteers are fairly adventuresome, but that we prefer to stick with some of the more mainstream stuff.

"Easy enough," she says, "let's start with the ladies."

Girls Just Want to Have Fun

Topping the list of popular female sex toys is the phallic-style vibrator—and Cupid's Treasures has walls of them. Heather points out that the store sells three types, all battery operated, which are generally referred to as Bullets, Vinyls, and Jellies. Most have adjustable speeds, with lengths varying from a few inches (great for travel) to more than a foot (Yikes!), and diameters to suit all tastes—from as thin as a finger to as thick as the fat end of a baseball bat.

Bullets are made of hard plastic and come in a wide range of colors, including metallic silver, "the most popular," Heather says. Vinyls are made of a flesh-toned vinyl ("for greater realism"). And Jellies are made of a soft, gelatinous rubber. Choosing among the three is a matter of preference. "It really depends on how much vibration you like," she explains. "The Bullets can be pretty intense—especially for direct clitoral stimulation. Personally, I prefer the Jelly type. They have the same type of motors, but the material tends to diffuse the vibration. Plus they're more comfortable to insert."

There's also greater variation in the Jelly category, Heather says, directing us to a section of blue, pink, orange, and glow-in-the-dark vibrators. She takes one, called the Jelly Delight, out of its packaging to "give us a feel." It seems slightly slimy at first, kind of like a stiffer version of Gak, that kid's stuff from Nickelodeon. But after a few good squeezes, we understand why many individuals might prefer this pliable material to the Bullet's industrial plastic.

And talk about creative design. There are Jelly vibrators that resemble a penis—complete with veins, scrotum, and glans. We notice a ribbed model that got considerably larger from tip to base. There are Jelly vibrators that can function in water and some that can actually be filled with warm water for "an especially cozy feel." Even more unique is a "dual vibrator." Designed specifically for insertion, this type combines a swiveling shaft with an extra appendage—so to speak—on the front for stimulating the clitoris. We can't help but laugh at some of these offerings. A dark green, textured model called the Alligator, for example, has a scary little gator whose tail flicks at the clitoris. And another has a teddy bear that performs the same trick with his tongue. (According *The New Good Vibrations Guide to Sex*, this type of vibrator hails from Japan, where it's illegal to make sex toys that resemble genitals. Hence, the accommodating fauna.)

We also chuckle as Heather points out a jumbo Jelly vibrator called the Earthquake. Assuming it's something most couples need to work up to, we decide to ease our pals into the wonderful world of sex toys with the Buzz, a fire-engine red Bullet by Private; the Jelly Fantasy Waterproof (ideal for the shower or Jacuzzi); and the Dragon Lady, a lilac-colored (and scented) dual vibrator with a rotating shaft filled with pearls and a little purple tongue that has no animal resemblance.

Another popular toy for women is the hands-free vibrator. This garter-belt style device is designed to be worn during intercourse to provide nonstop clitoral stimulation. The actual vibrator portion is positioned directly over the clitoris and labia and has varying speeds, generally adjustable via an attached remote control.

There's lots of variety here, too. One of the most well-known hands-free vibrators is the pink plastic Venus Butterfly. And a newer type called the Hummingbird looks like the frisky feathered friend it's

The Hitachi Magic Wand is a vibrator that defies categorization. Actually, it's technically not a vibrator, but a massage tool. But its legion of devoted fans knows that's just semantics. Called the "Cadillac of Vibrators" by women in the know, this plug-in device has a tennis ball–sized head that buzzes intensely—so much so that it causes blissful orgasm by just coming close to the clitoris. It's priced at $40.00 in the Good Vibrations catalog. Get your girlfriend one. She'll love you for it. In fact, she may drop you for it. Just kidding.

named after. Be forewarned: Customers often complain that many of the models are weak and tend to have flimsy straps that do a poor job of keeping the vibrators in place. Heather says Cupid's Treasures has received great feedback on the Onyx Climaxer, so we toss one into our basket.

"A dark green, textured [vibrator] called the Alligator . . . has a scary little gator whose tail flicks at the clitoris. And another has a teddy bear that performs the same trick with his tongue."

A third type of vibrator (notice the trend here) is a capsule-shaped kind that can be rubbed gently over the clitoris or inserted into the vagina. Some are covered in soft rubber, other are made of the same hard plastic as the Bullet vibrator. Most are controlled by a battery pack attached to the capsule via a long cord. For pure fun, we choose the only cordless model. Called The Egg, it's the hard plastic variety similar in size and shape to a small Grade A egg—with a high-tech spin. It's operated by a remote control. The idea is for one partner to insert the egg in the vagina while the other secretively commands it from across the room. Imagine the party possibilities here.

Moving on, Heather directs us to the section of anal stimulation devices. From chapter 4, you know that the anus and rectum are loaded with nerve endings, making "the backdoor" a highly sexual spot. And men have an added benefit: Anal penetration can stimulate the prostate, which often results in incredibly intense orgasms.

Still, the majority of Americans consider anal sex taboo. Because of homosexual connotations, many guys cringe at the thought of deriving pleasure from their anus. And the fear of pain keeps many couples from even considering incorporating it into their lovemaking. That's fine. Pressure should never be placed on either partner to do something with which he or she is uncomfortable. However, if you're feeling relaxed—and are willing to experiment with anal play—toys are a great place to start. Be sure to have plenty of lubricant on hand, and never insert a toy into the vagina after it's been near the anus without washing it first or covering it with a condom. We strongly recommend that non-monogamous couples cover all shared sexual devices.

That said, we agree to include a couple of anal toys in the test. "Butt beads are definitely a good place to start," Heather says. These successions of beads, often connected by nylon string, are inserted into the anus (or vagina) and pulled out during climax as a way to intensify orgasm. "Some people prefer that they be removed quickly; others like it done slow and steady. It's really a matter of personal taste," she says.

Heather points to a display of red, yellow, black, and glow-in-the-dark beads. Most people start out with the tiniest (about the size of a garbonzo bean) and work up to jawbreaker sized, she says, adding that there are much larger (billiard-sized) balls, but "the general public wouldn't be interested in them." No doubt. When we pick up a pair that vibrates for added stimulation, she cautions us. "Notice the rough seams and how the beads are attached together with rubber-coated wiring. That makes me nervous," she says. "You want to look for toys that aren't abrasive."

Good point. We put them back and instead choose Butt Buddy's, an 11-inch long strand of gelatinous balls with segments that graduate in size from 1 to 1½ inches. We also toss Anna Malle's PowerBalls into our basket for a more seasoned friend. This string of five 2½-inch beads is dipped in black latex. Inside each of the beads is a smaller bead; the extra heft reportedly enhances the experience.

Butt plugs are another option Heather recommends. Again, these vary in size and are designed to be inserted into the anus to intensify orgasm during oral or vaginal sex. Some are made of hard plastic, some vinyl, and some soft rubber. We go for the latter, selecting a product called Dynamic Duo, which consists of a jelly-coated egg and anal plug. Both vibrate (at multiple speeds) when connected to a battery pack remote control. The anal plug is T-shaped to follow the natural curve of the rectum.

Boy Toys

Although all of the items we chose for women can also be used by men, there are some toys designed primarily for male pleasure. Take cock rings. Typically made of rubber, silicone, or leather, these toys fit snugly around the base of the penis, restricting blood flow and causing a buildup of pressure that some men find extremely pleasurable. This restriction of blood flow can also help prolong an erection and even make it firmer—a bonus for both partners.

Gay men tend to prefer the leather-studded rings, according to Heather, whereas straight guys go for the silicone or rubber types. These come in varying degrees of thickness and stretchability. Some have nubby extensions, which can be positioned near your partner's clitoris. And many come with vibrating eggs that can be attached to the base

". . . there are also dildos in lovely jewel tones, dildos that look so real we wondered if they were warm to the touch. Dildos that are smooth and dildos that are ribbed for extra pleasure. There are even dildos based on the penises of famous porn stars."

of the ring to heighten pleasure. We choose three different types. The first, Sean Michael's Love Ring, is a basic rubber cock ring (endorsed by the adult-film stud) with beads at the base for loosening or tightening the tension. The second, a more adventurous device, is the Tuscan, a jelly model with a tongue extension for massaging the clitoris and an anal stimulator (similar to the Butt Buddy) attached via a nylon cord.

The cord is long enough to allow the stimulator to be inserted in either partners' sphincter. And last, but not least, there's the Super Stretchy Cock-Ring, a silicon model with a vibrating egg for added sensation.

Penis sleeves are also hot sellers. Made of stretchable rubber or silicone, they're also designed to fit around the shaft of the penis in an effort to restrict blood flow. Most have a nubby side that can be worn inward to enhance your pleasure or outward for hers. (Some people put sleeves on hard plastic vibrators to make them more texturally interesting.) At first glance, the sleeves look painful—almost bristle brush–like. But Heather lets us touch a few to convince us they're essential for our test.

> "Penis sleeves are hot sellers. Made of stretchable rubber or silicone, they're also designed to fit around the shaft of the penis in an effort to restrict blood flow."

She's right. We choose a collection called the Super Stretch Stimulator Sleeves, which includes seven sleeves that stretch up to eight inches in diameter. Each has a different bumpy texture.

And finally, because not all heterosexual guys are closed-minded to the idea of anal stimulation, we felt it important to include a butt toy for boys. Before you say, "no way," keep in mind that you don't have to be penetrated to enjoy the sensation. Having your partner gently massage the toy around that nerve-packed area, or the area between the scrotum and anus, can produce intense pleasure.

The ideal—nonthreatening—tool for doing that is the Anal E-Z Bend Vibe. This finger-width toy has a six-inch-long shaft with "vertebrae" inside that allow you to bend the toy into a variety of positions. A vibrating egg at the base delivers multispeed action. And a special polymer coating becomes extra slippery when slathered with a good water-soluble lubricant.

Cleanliness Is Next to Godliness

Okay, so the Puritans weren't thinking of sex toys when they came up with that statement. But you definitely want to keep your toys germ-free. According to Ann Semans, co-owner of Good Vibrations, it's a pretty easy task. "Any antibacterial soap will do. You can also wipe them clean with a cloth moistened with alcohol, or use a product specifically designed to clean sex toys called ForPlay Toy Cleaner." And if you use vibrator sleeves, pop them in the dishwasher. Just remember to take them out before the housekeeper arrives.

But There's More

The toys we tested are among Cupid's Treasures most popular items. But Heather reminded us that there are lots of other options: "People tend to come in here and buy a vibrator, come back later and get a string of beads, and then keep returning for increasingly exotic stuff."

Handcuffs and leather restraints are high on the list of hot-selling exotica, according to Heather. So are strap-on dildos. The former doesn't phase us. Plenty of people fantasize about being tied up and pleasured. But we're definitely surprised to learn that half of the buyers of dildos and harnesses are gay and the other half are straight. "It's another way to play out fantasies," says Heather. "Many heterosexual men, particularly those in high-power, high-stress positions, enjoy having a woman take control."

Try It, You'll Like It . . . Maybe

Special thanks to our enthusiastic panel of reviewers. But then, what are friends for if you can't get them to test your sex toys? Here are the verdicts. We recommend a good supply of rechargeable batteries.

Toy:	The Gist:	He Said:	She Said:
Buzz (by Private, $9.00) *For Her*	This bullet-style vibrator is long (about seven inches) and made of smooth, hard plastic. Its intensity can be adjusted by twisting the base, which stores two D batteries.	This is your basic vibrator. Nothing fancy. Nothing that will threaten your manhood.	It was kinda loud . . . but then so am I. At full throttle, I reached orgasm in a matter of seconds. Nonthreatening? If you say so.
Jelly Fantasy Waterproof (by Pipedream Products, $13.00) Superior Alternative: The Aquasagger ($30.00 waterproof vibrator from Good Vibrations).	A bright pink vibrator made of gelatinous rubber, the Jelly Fantasy is meant for use in the shower or bath, but could also be used on the breach or in a rainstorm, if that's how your get your kicks. It's adjustable at the base and runs on two AA batteries.	This is one fat, wobbly vibrator. 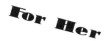	I love the idea of taking a vibrator in the shower, but this one is weak. So it's frustrating—and really unsatisfying. I'd say save your money.
Dragon Lady (by Doc Johnson, $60.00)	A dual-vibrator, the Dragon Lady has a shaft (for insertion) and a small appendage (for clitoral stimulation), both of which are coated in a translucent violet-colored rubber. The shaft is filled with pearls and rotates at varying speed both clockwise and counter-clockwise while the appendage vibrates slowly or rapidly in synch.	It twists, it turns, it spins, and buzzes. How can I compete with that?	You can't. 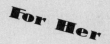
Onyx Climaxer (by California Exotic Novelties, $40.00)	This black hands-free vibrator is worn like a garter belt and is operated via an attached remote control. A tiny vibrator covered in soft rubber fits directly over the clitoris. Tiny rubber nubs enhance clitoral stimulation.	It looked sexy and she could wear it during intercourse. I liked that. *For Her*	Yes, it does look sexy. But I didn't climax. This vibrator might work for some women, but I need something with a little more oomph.

Toy:	The Gist:	He Said:	She Said:
The Egg (by California Exotic Novelties, $120.00) *For Her*	A small egg-shaped vibrator with a tamponlike string is inserted into the vagina. Either the wearer or a friend can control the vibration via remote control from up to 20 feet away.	I really liked the idea of having a secret little sex session in the middle of a party . . . you know, keeping the power switch in my pocket and watching my wife's reaction across the room as she trying to concentrate on conversations. Except . . .	Except the minute you turned it on, it sounded like an electric razor went off in my pants. Man, was that ever embarrassing. I had to go to the guest bathroom and take it out. Come to think about it, there's something weird about putting something inside you that has batteries. I mean, batteries are even hazardous to landfills.
Butt Buddy (by Adam & Eve, $17.00) *For Her*	These yellow jelly butt balls get slightly larger from tip to top. Designed to be pulled out slowly as you orgasm to increase the intensity.	They seemed like the perfect texture, really soft . . . like they couldn't hurt anyone. Except it was so soft that it bent every which-way.	That was a problem. We had to stop and start and stop and start, because this thing wasn't rigid enough. It really broke the mood.
Love Jel-Lees Dynamic Duo (by T.L.C., $30.00)	This vibrating combo includes a blue jelly butt plug with a T-shape to fit into the rectum and a green jelly covered egg, both operated by a plug-in remote control.	This was a lot of fun. We don't get much into anal sex, but this plug thing was really soft so we tried it. *For Her*	I was a little hesitant at first. And it took some time to slowly get into it. But the plug was incredible—especially the vibration. The egg was a little weird, but it was a fun change of pace to our usual foreplay.
Sean Michaels Love Ring (by Adam & Eve, $7.00) *For Him*	This soft red rubber cock ring has beads on the top and bottom so it can be adjusted to fit penises of various sizes.	At first, I felt a little funny. Foolish, like I was dressing up while being undressed. But when you tighten the ring, you can really feel that the blood flow is constricted. And it made my penis bigger.	It did look a little funny. I mean, he looked like some kind of porno stud. It did make his penis seem harder, though.
Anal E-Z Bend Wand (Adam & Eve, $20.00)	A remote-controlled purple bendable buddy, the finger-width Anal E-Z Wand is flexible and conforms to a variety shapes. An attached variable speed vibrator is included for further stimulation.	It looks like E.T.'s finger. I really wasn't comfortable with it. *For Him*	I thought it would add a nuance to our lovemaking, but it was almost as if he was dreading it. Why are men so weird about anal sex . . . unless they're doing it to you?

Toy:	The Gist:	He Said:	She Said:
Anna Malle's PowerBalls (by California Exotic Novelties, $20)	Anal beads for the enlightened, Anna Malle's PowerBalls is a string of five, two-and-a-half-inch beads covered in latex. Each bead contains a smaller bead for extra weight—and orgasmic boost. *For Her*	They looked pretty ominous . . . like something Darth Vader would use. But we've done this before so we went slow and tried it.	There are two basic problems with beads. Usually, they're made out of plastic, so there's always a little ridge on each one. And the string that attaches them together . . . sometimes you can feel that when you're pulling the beads out. It's an uncomfortable little feeling in the midst of a great rush. But these beads were great. The whole thing is covered in latex: the beads, the string, everything. So once you put lube on them, they're slick and slippery. I had a wild orgasm with these.
Tuscan (by Wildfire, $20.00)	Another variation of the cock ring, but this one is made of fuchsia rubber with an attached anal plug and a tongue that stimulates the clitoris during intercourse.	This thing was like some outer space gizmo. We really had to navigate to make it work right. *For Him*	It may be something you use every once in a while, but it took a lot of the spontaneity out of sex, because we had to really guide it in.
Super Stretchy Cock Ring (by Pipedream Products, $17.00)	A cock ring with a bonus: a vibrator egg that attaches to the base and is operated via a wired remote control.	It was pretty wild . . . even though I had to hold onto this remote control thing. The tightness made my penis really big and the vibrating really set me off.	He said it really felt good. It didn't do anything for me . . . but was it supposed to? *For Him*
Super Stretch Stimulator Sleeves (by Doc Johnson, $20.00) *For Him*	Made of miracle polymers, these sleeves fit over the penis to offer constriction and come in a variety of shapes "for her pleasure."	This seemed more like a novelty. The sleeves were tight, so they did their job, but the little nubs kind of flattened out once I stretched them out.	I don't care what he says . . . it felt great. The best was when he didn't penetrate me but rubbed his shaft over my clitoris. Those nubs were really stimulating.

If the idea of visiting an adult toy or video store turns your face a vibrant shade of red, you're probably an ideal catalog or Internet shopper. Here are several of the best direct-mail alternatives. Keep in mind that with the exception of Good Vibrations and Femme Productions, all may sell your name and address to other adult vendors. To avoid this, insist that your information not be sold.

Adam & Eve
Toys, videos, and lingerie
800-765-ADAM
www.aeonline.com

Adam and Gillian's Sensual Whips
   and Toys
Fetish toys
516-842-1711

Blowfish
Toys, books, and videos
415-864-0880
www.blowfish.com

Condomania
Safer sex supplies and novelty toys
800-926-6366
www.condomania.com

Eve's Garden
Women-oriented toys, books, and
   videos
800-848-3837
www.evesgarden.com

We're even more shocked by the range of dildos available. Yes, there are tiny ones and huge ones. But there are also dildos in lovely jewel tones, dildos that look so real we wondered if they were warm to the touch. Dildos that are smooth and dildos that are ribbed for extra pleasure. There are even dildos based on the penises of famous porn stars. If your significant other fantasizes about John Holmes, try strapping on his likeness. Never mind that he died of AIDS. That dude was scary big. We guarantee, with one look at your John Holmes she'll never be curious—or interested—in porn-star proportions again.

Speaking of sex toys molded in the image of porn stars, guys can fly solo with a vaginal simulator (a.k.a. Personal Pussy). Now we're not here to pass judgment. "Whatever floats your boat" is our motto. However, we can't help but wonder what kind of guy would enjoy having sex with the vinyl vagina of Kobi Tai, Christy Canyon, or Jenna Jameson. Guess it's as close to being "with" a star as some men will get.

Likewise, we wonder about those blow-up dolls. Cupid's Treasures sold the standard, plastic model with the caroler's mouth. But there's a newer, twenty-first-century version called the Real Doll that's been receiving lots of attention thanks to coverage on the *Howard Stern* show. In short, the Real Doll is a woman made of a silicone material that feels eerily close to human skin—and it can be made to order, with blonde, red, or brown hair; dark or light skin; blue, green, or brown eyes; a slender or voluptuous build. Heck, you can even choose her nail polish color. The Real Doll ranges in price from about $3,000 to more than $5,000—depending upon the number of usable orifices. No, you can't return her. Mike Saenz, national sales representative, tells us a chatty Real Doll is in the works. We can only guess what she'll say.

For women with deep pockets, there's a $1,400 sex device called the Sybian that looks like a smaller, stationary version of that mechanical bucking bronco in the movie *Urban Cowboy*. It's designed to be straddled (like a horse) and has a probe that vibrates and rotates at speeds that are controlled by two little knobs on the Sybian's front. To make the device more comfortable, the probe is covered with rubber phalluses, which vary in length and thickness from finger-sized to average-guy sized. This vibrator-on-steroids comes with it's own little nightstand/storage case; however, for the price, we'd expect something with a little more panache. And we're sorry, we can't vouch for its effectiveness. We received it in the mail and watched the instructional video. One look at that writhing phallus was all it took for us to seal up the box and send it back to the manufacturer. Sorry, but that looked a little too aggressive for us.

"We can't help but wonder what kind of guy would enjoy having sex with the vinyl vagina of Kobi Tai, Christy Canyon, or Jenna Jameson."

Exploring Fantasyland

If you're guilt-tripping over a fantasy involving the blonde accountant down the hall, get over it. Or better yet, enjoy it. According to Patti Britton, Ph.D., a San Francisco–based sex therapist, sexual fantasies are a perfectly normal—and healthy—form of expression.

Clinically speaking, Britton describes a sexual fantasy as a picture that you hold about an erotic object or an erotic act—visual imagery that's sexually arousing. But a fantasy can also consist of a longing that has a sexual charge to it. "For example, if remembering an encounter with an old girlfriend gets you excited, it's a fantasy," she says.

When working with clients to enhance their imaginative abilities, Britton likes to discuss the four elements of sex: "the Mental realm; the Emotional realm; the Body—and I mean the whole body, not just the genitals—and the Energy or Spiritual realm."

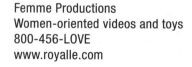

Although fantasy can be triggered by any of these four realms, it tends to play out most dominantly in the Mental realm, through imagination and the senses. "The nose—or the olfactory system—can be sparked by the scent of old lover's perfume," she explains. "When you breathe in the aroma, it can trigger your rewind button and cause you to fantasize about that person or various aspects of the relationship."

Although everyone is capable of fantasizing, many people aren't in touch with that aspect of their sexuality, according to Britton. Either they're not exactly sure what they find arousing or they have hang-ups or inhibitions that keep them from exploring this aspect of their sexuality. Women in particular tend to be less prone to fantasizing.

"They aren't encouraged to embrace their sexuality, much less fantasize about sex—unless there's a romantic aspect to it," she says.

About ten years ago, for her book *Swept Away*, author Carol Kassel conducted a monumental study that attempted to define the different things that make males and females tick. What she learned was that boys give love to get sex, and girls give sex to get love. "It has a lot to do with the wiring of our society," Britton explains. "Girls today may have more permission to explore their sexuality, but there's still a great difference in the way it's nurtured. Boys are encouraged to express their sexual prowess, whereas girls have to have that love connection before they can feel their sexuality and power."

Consequently, men tend to enjoy richer fantasy lives. According to Britton, one of the primary reasons women experience a lack of sexual

Femme Productions
Women-oriented videos and toys
800-456-LOVE
www.royalle.com

Good Vibrations
Toys and videos
800-289-8423
www.goodvibe.com

House of Whacks
Latex fashions and fetish toys
773-SM1-6969
www.whacks.com

desire "is because their well is dry." She likens it to going to a well for water and finding it empty. "You need to keep the well filled with material—books, magazines, video tapes, etc.—in order to keep the fantasy, lust, and intrigue going."

Men seem to have an easier time keeping their well at least wet, says Britton.

At the most basic level, fantasizing can increase or sustain arousal, Britton says. But it also can add an element of play that keeps a relationship from getting stale. We are, after all, human animals who have sexual parts and sexual energy that can't be shut off. Although we can—and often do—try to suppress it, our sexual energy is an essential component of who we are. "It's a lot healthier to find ways—like fantasizing—to enjoy our sexuality," says Britton, "than to attempt to stifle it."

> "Longing for a three-way may primarily be a guy thing, but when women take the lead and act on this desire, it's the guys who are often left feeling vulnerable or jealous."

The Dark Side

Exploring fantasy can backfire, though. As Britton explains: "Sometimes when people are engaged in sexual sharing—through foreplay, intercourse, or any of the other ways their bodies can merge—they're fantasizing, yet unaware of it. For example, a man might be wondering 'Oh my God, is she going to think I'm good enough?' or a woman might be thinking 'Where's he going to put his hand now? I wish he'd touch me there.'"

Both are forms of fantasy that take you out of the moment, she says. By leaving the here and now of lovemaking, it can cause anxiety or concern about sexual performance or the relationship.

For the most part, Britton believes fantasies enhance sexuality, but there are two types that can be damaging. The first involves fantasies that go outside the relationship (i.e., cheating, threesomes, or group sex).

Although she acknowledges that it's not uncommon to have sexual encounters with multiple partners simultaneously ("many people swear by it"), acting on this fantasy means taking a big leap—one that's best taken slowly.

Interestingly, studies have found that easing into this scene is as crucial for men as it is for women. Longing for a three-way may primarily be a guy thing—"there's a lot of bravado in male fantasizing," says Britton—but when women take the lead and act on this desire, it's the guys who are often left feeling vulnerable or jealous.

The other dangerous fantasies are ones involving physical pain. These days, an increasing number of people are experimenting with bondage and S/M. Although these lifestyles can offer exquisite pleasure for those truly experienced in them, they can also lead to serious injuries if you don't know what you're doing. "People who don't learn the rules—and play by them—are putting themselves and their partners in danger both physically and emotionally," Britton says.

Again, this is an area in which "easing in" is essential. Start by reading the section in this chapter titled Whip It, Whip It Good. Then pick up a few good books and videotapes. And if, after experimenting, it doesn't seem like your thing, it may not be your relationship either. A guy who wrote to Britton said he really wanted to tie up his girlfriend, but she wasn't into it. He stated, "I keep thinking about it, and obsessing about it. She'll do it, but it doesn't turn her on, and I need to see her turned on."

Her response? "I told him they might not be right for each other. You can't force someone to share your erotic fantasies."

Gender Bending

Everything about men and women differ—including their preferred fantasies. As we already mentioned, men tend to be more visually oriented. Looking at the anatomical parts of a female, either in person or in magazines, books, or videos, tends to get a guy going. Women are more relationship-oriented. Love and romance are their passions.

Whatever your pleasure, Britton assures us that fantasy is 100 percent safe and 100 percent natural—but it does not necessarily lead to interaction. It does generate erotic energy, though, and that energy is a wonderful gift that can be brought into the bedroom of a significant other.

Interestingly, Britton doesn't always advocate sharing fantasies. "They often have more charge when they're kept private," she says. "If you let your partner in on your fantasy, and it's one that helps you reach orgasm or maintain an erection, the fantasy may no longer work."

Reality Check

How can you tell if your fantasy life is interfering with reality? According to Britton, if the fantasy is bordering on obsession—if you can't think of anything else—you may need help. It's not natural, for example, to be heavily dependent on pornographic material in order to pleasure yourself or receive pleasure. Likewise, you shouldn't *have* to conjure up images of Pamela Lee in order to have sex with your girlfriend.

Most Common Fantasies and What They Say About You

Men:

I fantasize about . . .	Says . . .
. . . having sex with two women.	. . . you're an acculturated American male—John Q. Normal.
. . . tying my girlfriend up.	. . . you're a Don Juan Good Boy. You want to totally pleasure your lover with no resistance.
. . . anal play.	. . . you want to explore "the forbidden," "the nasty," "the taboo." (Though many people enjoy anal sex, it has a far-from-the-mainstream rep.)
. . . cheating on my girlfriend/wife.	. . . your current relationship may be in the dumper. It's time to rediscover your sexual spark or cut loose.
. . . watching other people have sex.	. . . you like things safe and easy. Voyeurism is a turn-on that doesn't require performance. You're off the hook.

Women:

I fantasize about . . .	Says . . .
. . . being taken.	. . . you want to let go of yourself and your inhibitions. It's not about violence, but about letting someone else take charge of your sexuality so you don't have to be responsible.
. . . my boyfriend falling desperately in love with me.	. . . you're an acculturated female—Joan Q. Normal. It's how girls are raised: love begets lust.
. . . having sex in public places.	. . . you need some excitement in your life. You want to live on the edge. The fear of getting caught is the aphrodisiac here.
. . . being desired by many men.	. . . you need a self-esteem booster. There's no better ego trip than being wanted by the masses.
. . . tying up my boyfriend/husband.	. . . you want to do the dominatrix thing, to take control of the sexual relationship.

There are ways of desensitizing, refocusing, and reprogramming your fantasies, so that the lure of the flesh, or the sound of breathing, or the scent of your partner can become more compelling than the longing to look at the silicone breasts of your favorite actress or porn star. This is where a professional can help.

On the flip side, if you haven't tapped your fantasy potential, there are some ways to jump-start your imagination. Play some games. Tell each other sexy stories. Watch videos together. Try on costumes and role-play. Buy her lingerie from Victoria's Secret. Explore some of the foreplay advice offered in chapter 4. Experiment with toys and lubes. Britton rec-

"If [your] fantasy is bordering on obsession—if you can't think of anything else—you may need help."

ommends Hot Stuff, a fruity-tasting lotion that you can blow on to generate heat. "And ask her how it feels. That's what fantasy is all about—getting out of the mechanics and monotony of sex and reaching another level," says Britton.

One Ringy Dingy

Alexander Graham Bell would just shake his head in bemusement. The telephone—his invention, his life's work—being used for sexual gratification. Indeed, phone sex is giving new meaning to "reach out and touch someone." And it's big business—a billion-dollar industry that's growing bigger every day.

It's no wonder, what with AIDS and other STDs. Phone sex is the ultimate in safe sex. If it's done by a couple, both parties (a party line, anyone?) get off; if a man calls a commercial phone sex service, he has a guilt-free release. (These 1–900 services most often advertise in the back of men's magazines and on late-night television.)

Commercial services offer a variety of fantasies, with a bevy of different voices on the other end of the line. Want a sultry-sounding Latina? Got her. Want a demure southern belle? Got her, too. In fact, most fantasies can be fulfilled at a charge-per-minute rate.

But since you are being charged anywhere from $2.00 to $5.00 per minute, you better get your money's worth. According to *The New Good Vibrations Guide to Sex*, men engaging commercial services for phone sex should keep this in mind: The gal on the other end of the line is talking on your dime, so you'd better take charge and direct the conversation. Steer it by talking through what—and who—you want and state exactly what kind of role-play you're looking for. That way, the operator isn't spending ten minutes discerning what rocks your world. Ten minutes at $5.00 a minute before the good stuff even starts? Now *that* would be a bad connection. And remember, phone sex may be fun to try on occasion, but to rely on it to get sexual release may signal serious problems.

With that said, if you just want to engage in a little long-distance romance with your loved one, here's some tips: Get in the right mood by suggesting the tele-encounter earlier in the day. That way, when you call back, your partner is already flush with anticipation.

Then, set the appropriate stage. Good phone sex doesn't dive immediately into the nitty gritty. Paint an erotic picture with words. Talk about what you're wearing, the surroundings, how you're feeling, what you're not wearing.

Pick a comfortable part of your abode to engage in phone sex . . . clearly, you don't want to talk dirty near that sink full of dishes in the kitchen.

Above all, make sure you've got all your self-love accoutrements nearby: your lube, tissues, or towel. You don't want to break the erotic tension to run to the other room. And finally, give as good as you get. Remember, there's someone on the other end of the line.

It's Not the Bandwidth . . . It's the Length

Ah, the computer. The marvel of the modern age, the personal computer allows us unprecedented productivity. Advanced computational possibilities. Lightning fast communications. And the ability to download pictures of frisky college coeds ditching Psych 101 for an afternoon orgy.

Those Silicon Valley technoids probably never knew what all their round-the-clock efforts in developing computers would lead to: an explosion of cybersex, where a virtual reality created through hard drives, modems, and servers provide people with sexual—albeit, virtual—interactions. So now, a guy is as likely to be surfing the web—one hand on this mouse, the other on his, um, joystick—as he is recalculating spreadsheets for work.

Chatting It Up

Almost all online services offer chat rooms, virtual spaces where everyone who's logged on can type in messages—and see these messages posted onscreen—to an assembled horde. If you've ever visited a chat room on America Online, CompuServe, or through a smaller regional server, you know it can be a chaotic mess. For one thing, if it's a popular room, there are loads of people "chatting" (i.e., typing away), so messages enter a fast-moving slipstream onscreen. You may have just typed in a message to, say, BooBear, but in the time you took to key in that message, 50 others have popped onscreen. Then, BooBear has to sift through all the scattered messages to find the message you just posted.

Another problem: the screen names. Like BooBear. Screen names offer anonymity and give users a sense of adventure; users can make up a persona—or onscreen profile that's viewable by everyone online—and attach a name to that persona. That's the problem. BooBear's profile may say she's a 30-year-old divorcée from Little Rock who likes macramé and aerobics, but in truth it can be an 18-year-old boy from Tacoma who's a surf punk. And a punk in general.

> **"BooBear's profile may say she's a 30-year-old divorcée from Little Rock who likes macramé and aerobics, but in truth it can be a 18-year-old boy from Tacoma who's a surf punk. And a punk in general."**

Teens in chat rooms are another problem. Teens are at an awkward age, just discovering themselves sexually . . . so they sometimes don't know how to handle themselves. Fortunately, most chat rooms on commercial sites have an option for two people to establish a private chat. Here's how it works: In a general chat room, two people hit it off, among the clutter of dozens of other postings. One asks the other if he or she would like to "take a walk," which is cyberspeak for establishing a private chat. Sort of the equivalent to getting a motel room. If agreed upon, one party gets the system administrator to set up a separate "room" with access only to the two individuals. Then, the two can chat privately. And typically, private chat gets steamy pretty quick.

Because it's often anonymous, chat can take the form of keystroked phone sex: One person says something suggestive. The other responds. Before you know it, both are masturbating to the messages. And typographical errors increase, as each tries to maintain the flow of typed "conversation" with one hand:

Nightcrawlr: Ummm. What are you wearing?

DoonaD: Just a pair of white panties. Am I getting you hard?

Nightcrwlr: Rock hard.

DoonaD: I'm soooo wet. I've got to squeeze my niples and paly with myself . . .

Nightcrawlr: Im strorking my cck. babygve it to me now im gong to come yr so hot

Aside from cramped hands from typing and cramped hands from, well, you know, cybersex does allow people to meet and interact. It also can be a great door-opener for real contact, if that's what cybernauts choose. Because all the commercial services have rooms designed for specific interests (B/D, butch dykes, femmes, singles looking to swing, men looking for older women, etc.) you can pretty much cut to the chase. Imagine if you went to a singles bar and that woman you were eyeing had a sign above her head stating Likes It Doggie Style. That's what you get in the chat rooms. And if you find someone you like, you can attempt a real-life encounter.

> **"Imagine if you went to a singles bar and that woman you were eyeing had a sign above her head stating Likes It Doggie Style. That's what you get in the chat rooms."**

"Typically, I like to get out of the chat rooms as quickly as possible," says Jon, a twentysomething graphic designer. "I ask the woman during chat if I can send her direct, instant messages from my browser. If she says yes, I'll continue a conversation that way, to feel her out. Then, I suggest meeting someplace or I try to get her phone number." Does it work?

"More often than not, yeah," he says. "On the Internet, all things are equal. The way you look isn't the first thing a woman notices. . . . It's how witty you are, what kind of conversation you can come up with, what your hobbies and interests are. Try getting to that level of conversation at a bar. . . . If you're not Brad Pitt you get shot down pretty quick. But this way, women get to know you quickly and easily. And besides, there are so many horny teenagers online that a normal guy with a real job and a bit of politeness stands a great chance of meeting someone."

So, where to go? If you're looking for down and dirty sex talk, try an Internet Relay Chat (IRC) available through your browser and web service. Once you log onto your service, use your browser to access the sites (sometimes the command is simply typing in IRC). Then you'll see information on software and modem requirements. Once in the mix, you'll see a number of current

> **"If you're looking for down and dirty sex talk, try an Internet Relay Chat (IRC) available through your browser and web service."**

channels where all the talk is occurring. Type in the # sign and the name of your channel and you're there. Here's a partial listing of available channels (you can probably figure out the focus of each): #bdsm; #bisex; #teensex; #wildsex; #dirtysex; #desade; #30plus; #passion.

If you're looking for love in all the Net places, try www.match.com, a cyber-dating service. Or try www.cupidnet.com, which offers chat, events, and links to singles sites. And remember, all good things in moderation.

Workin' the Web

Okay. That's chat. Want to delve into uncensored free trade? Want amateur cheerleaders engaged in highly unusual splits? Or pictures of horny housewives? Want Quicktime movies of group sex you can watch from your computer? It's all there waiting for you on the World-wide Web.

There's a plethora of online services devoted to offering the finest in hard-core pornography—all for a monthly fee, of course. Once you subscribe, you can cruise the service's photo archive, where up to tens of thousands of explicit pictures are stored for you to view in all their high-resolution glory. X-rated chat rooms are available, as are video downloads of sex acts.

The services cater to different interests: older women, S/M, water sports, you name it. One thing to remember when exploring, though: it's illegal to possess photos of minors, even in electronic format. For this reason, so-called "teen" sites are usually comprised of photos of 18 and 19 year olds—still teens, but all legal. If you do run across real teen-sex photos and, say, bring in your hard drive for repairs, the technician will be able to retrieve your images. And alert the police. Your best bet: Don't even court the whim of an inkling of a notion of getting teen photos.

Another caution: Sex sites on the Web disappear on a regular basis—taking your credit card information with them. If you want to subscribe to a site, check it out by referencing other sites. For example, check out Persian Kitty at www.persiankitty.com, a compendium of free and pay-site links that is a kind of porn seal of approval. If a link gets onto Persian Kitty, it's legit. Persian Kitty also has links to the best homepages of aspiring adult video starlets and strippers, as well as free web sites featuring nude photos.

CU-See-Me Get Naked

Technology is such a beautiful thing. No sooner do we get video downloads of bored housewife hijinks than streaming video emerges. With a program called CU-See-Me, people can send quasi-real-time videos of themselves over the Internet. For pay services, this means subscribers can request a strip tease from a stable of beauties. Select a girl. Onscreen, the image appears. But if your modem is equipped with voice capabilities, your stripper will talk with you, asking your name, asking what you want her to do or take off. And you can talk back. At some sites, you can use this technology to direct two women as they have sex with each other: "Now lick her thigh . . . grab her butt and spread her legs . . ."

Sex on Disc

CD-ROMs store up to 650 megabytes of information—a vast, vast amount. So it was only a matter of time before enterprising pornographers used the storage capacity to their advantage, creating CD-ROM versions of their adult titles. Now, you can order adult releases directly

Cybersex: The Cheating Debate

Davis sounded frantic when he called. He'd discovered that his wife was spending her wee hours as a surfer girl on the Internet, sharing sexual intimacies with an array of cyber-suitors in one of those raunchy chat rooms.

"I feel like she's been having an affair," he said. "You know, cheating on me."

Is cybersex—sharing steamy chat with strangers over the Internet—really cheating? It's a tough call, since this area of sexual exploration is still so new. We decided to get feedback from a trio of women, who we'll call Fran, Mary Ellen, and Marie, and a couple of prominent men. Dennis Prager is a nationally known lecturer-philosopher-writer who hosts a popular daily talk show in Los Angeles on KABC-radio. And Leslie Pam, Ph.D., is a talk show host, psychologist, and marriage counselor; he's also cowriting a book on relationships. Here's what they said about cybersex:

Q: Is it cheating when someone in a monogamous relationship engages in "dirty talk" online with someone other than his or her partner?

Dennis Prager: Revealing fantasies or any other truly intimate part of one's life to a member of the opposite sex who's not one's partner can be a form of disloyalty. But like all sins, there are gradations. I have asked women on the air if they would prefer that their husbands had an anonymous one-night affair with a woman, or weekly lunches with a woman that involved no touching but during which he poured out his soul. The great majority voted for the one-night stand. The issue isn't just sexual. Therefore, "cheating" needs to be defined. If cheating refers only to sex, then verbal intercourse isn't cheating.

Leslie Pam: Cheating is anything you do secretly that, if your partner were doing it, you'd feel he or she was cheating. You apply the rule of "Do unto others . . . ": switch roles for a second to see how it makes you feel.

Marie: Absolutely, it would be cheating if my husband were spending time away from me, having a relationship with someone else when he should be having it with me.

I would ask, why is he doing that on the computer and not with me? Obviously, that kind of communication gets into very personal, private areas. Even though he doesn't see the person he's interacting with, it's still an intimate relationship.

Fran: I wouldn't consider it cheating, not unless you're going to file for divorce and seek partial custody of the children with your computer. Not unless there's a chance that you and the other person on the computer could become a couple. What's the difference between this and talking to someone on a 976 number? Or reading a romance novel or pornography? If it was something you were just curious about, I wouldn't think it was a violation. But if it was ongoing, that's indicative of something missing in the relationship; it means you're going to someone else to satisfy a sexual need.

Q: Would you prefer that your husband talk dirty with the same person night after night or with different people?

Fran: I'd be more concerned if you did it with the same person; that might indicate it's going to a different level.

Marie: I wouldn't want my husband to go outside our relationship for anything like that. It's one thing if, together, we share an erotic movie or magazine—but I don't even really know how I'd feel about that. Whether he comes back to me to talk about it or keeps it to himself, I would still find it offensive; it smells like a ménage á trois.

Mary Ellen: If he's engaging in a sexual activity on the computer or in any other form, that is cheating.

Whether you actually engage in physical activity is not the point.

Q: So if a guy has sexual fantasies about a woman other than his wife, is that cheating, too?

Mary Ellen: Yes. I'm coming from a Biblical base. In the New Testament, Jesus says that if you have lustful thoughts about someone other than your spouse, you've committed adultery in your heart.

Q: Does that extend to reading pornography as well?

Mary Ellen: Yes.

Leslie: What you want to avoid is putting a wedge between yourself and your partner. God knows, it's hard enough to stay connected to somebody in an intimate way. It's like disconnecting some part of you, as though you were a circuit board, and connecting that part to somebody else. That means a loss of energy to the relationship. But the secrecy is the cheating part.

Q: So if it's out in the open, it's not cheating?

Leslie: This is about being honest regarding your sexual needs. Obviously, you wouldn't be doing this if you were 100 percent sexually satisfied at home. A monogamous relationship is difficult in the best of circumstances, but maintaining honesty helps a lot. Honesty keeps you connected to the other person. Live long enough with someone, and biologically you get in tune with that person. Any deceptive behavior partially disconnects you from him or her.

Q: Do you make a distinction between what constitutes cheating for men and for women?

Leslie: The issue transcends gender. People who are into sex-chat rooms have built-in barriers: time, space, and anonymity. Most people don't want to break those barriers, which is why this is proliferating. It's safe. When you really think about it, you're actually having sex with your computer screen—with typed words. The mind does not distinguish between real or imagined. Like when you have a nightmare—it's just as real as if it were happening to you during the day. We fool ourselves that a flesh-and-blood person is more real than the person we imagine from the screen, but in fact, the brain doesn't see any difference.

Fran: I think it's the same for men and women, though I can't imagine as many women doing it as men.

Dennis: When a woman does that, it usually indicates a real discontent at home. This is not the way women are wired; talking about cunnilingus is not their thing. I would consider it a serious problem if (my partner) sought other men for titillation.

Q: When does someone cross the line from recreation to infidelity?

Dennis: When he gives his name.

on CD-ROM ... but who would want to? Even though you get unedited video releases, there are limitations, like only seeing a jagged image on a tenth of your computer monitor.

Our recommendation: You might want to try some adult titles that are truly interactive. There are titles in which the plot outcomes—and who has sex with whom—is determined by the choices you make onscreen through dialog boxes. Or try an adult CD-ROM game like *Rodney Rubber,* which makes you solve puzzles or correctly answer adult-oriented trivia before you can see a video clip. Best yet, these titles now have a "quick escape" key, which you can hit to change the salacious images onscreen to a timid-looking spreadsheet, good enough to fool the boss when he saunters into your office. (Be forewarned: This trick only works with CD-ROMs. Your company can obtain software to easily print out info about your Internet whereabouts.)

> "... these [CD-ROMs] now have a 'quick escape' key, which you can hit to change the salacious images onscreen to a timid-looking spreadsheet, good enough to fool the boss when he saunters into your office. "

Whip It, Whip It Good

Adding a playful little spank on the buttocks to foreplay from time to time is hardly scandalous. Likewise, restraining a partner to the bedposts with silk scarves or handcuffs—and doing with them what you please—is one of the most commonly acted upon fantasies.

There are those, however, who need to do these things—sometimes to the extreme—in order to get off. They would be devotees of B/D (bondage and discipline), D/S (dominance and submission) or S/M (sadism and masochism). All of these overlapping sexual practices involve the submission of one person to another. Of the three, S/M is the only one based on pain. By definition, sadists (named after the brutal Marquis de Sade) like to give it; masochists (named after novelist Leopold von Sacher-Masoch) like to receive it. There is a strict code of conduct among followers. Those in command stop instantly when their submissives indicate they've had enough or give a predetermined code word. Orgasm is often achieved without penetration; a few strategic flicks of a whip on the behind, chest, or between the legs is sometimes all it takes.

> "There are chicks in latex flogging guys in dog collars and leather pants. There are guys in dog collars and leather pants dripping hot wax on the chests of chicks wearing vinyl bustiers and panties ... "

And that may be precisely why BDSM (for short) is growing in popularity. No exchange of bodily fluids means no risk of contracting a deadly disease. Some are even calling it safe sex for the millennium. The mainstreaming of these once-considered perverted practices are evident on several fronts.

In the music world, Madonna hinted of things to come with her under-the-coffee-table book *Sex*. Though this black-and-white glimpse of BDSM pleasures caused a furor among middle Americans when it was published in the early nineties, it would raise but a few eyebrows today. After all, every parent's nightmare, Marilyn Manson, paraded around the stage of the MTV Video awards in bondage chaps—exposing his pasty (dare we say flabby) ass to the world. And sweety pie Janet Jackson—free from her family's bizarre clutches—showed her true colors. Posing for a *Vibe* magazine interview in a latex catsuit to hype her late 1997 release *The Velvet Rope*, she's alluded to her own preferences for edgy sex and has boasted of her high-tolerance threshold, saying "pushing the limits of pleasure is exciting."

Capitalizing on this apparent trend, nightclubs across the country are attracting huge crowds with sexy shows depicting bondage and light S/M. Black Market Chicago, a fetish shop that sells a wide range of BDSM fashions and gear, for example, hosts wild events at the city's hippest dance clubs—Crobar, The Dome Room, and The Exit. Patrons play dress-up for the night in next to nothing made of latex, vinyl, or leather. Whips, restraints, and other toys are available for purchase. Tattoo artists and body piercers are on the premises to decorate the daring (or drunk). And those who can last until midnight can catch The Rack. This traveling interactive bondage show has steamed up clubs from coast to coast and even worked up the crowds of Lollapalooza. At the centerpiece of the show is a towering pentagon-shaped "rack" made of wood with a variety of restraints. A troupe of S/M-trained actors initially entertain the audience with pyrotechnic S/M theatrics. There are chicks in latex flogging guys in dog collars and leather pants. There are guys in dog collars and leather pants dripping hot wax on the chests of chicks wearing vinyl bustiers and panties. There's a big guy (also in a dog collar and leather pants) who applies "electric shock measures" to another big guy using a battery charger with long steel shanks. You get the picture—pretty edgy stuff for most Americans.

Once the 20-minute show is over, the real fun begins. Voyeurs in the audience have the opportunity to come on stage to be watched, whipped, dripped, and flogged 'til last call.

Tony Duffy, owner of The Rack, calls these evenings out an "opportunity to dress up, get into these involved situations in public with other consenting adults, and have a really good time without endangering your life." (That battery charger looks at lot worse than it feels, he assures us.)

> "Posing for a *Vibe* magazine interview in a latex catsuit to hype her late 1997 release *The Velvet Rope,* [Janet Jackson has] alluded to her own preferences for edgy sex and has boasted of her high-tolerance threshold, saying 'pushing the limits of pleasure is exciting.'"

And this is just happening on the club scene. There's a New Jersey bed-and-breakfast equipped with its own private dungeon and an S/M-themed restaurant in New York called La Nouvelle Justine featuring waitstaff dressed in bondage garb and a menu that includes a service fee for those who prefer to "lap their linguine out of a dog bowl," as the *New York Post* put it.

Owner Hayne Jason, a former tax attorney, says he's amazed by the success of La Nouvelle Justine, a restaurant he opened because "it sounded like fun.

"I thought people might be horrified. But they flock," he said in an interview with the *Village Voice.*

And many of those who flock fit the BDSM profile: conservative types who need to relinquish control every now and then. "When we opened, I wasn't looking to have this Wall Street crowd," Jason says. "It was a big shock when men would call and book late-night reservations in tough-guy voices. I'd say, 'Sure, we're open late, no problem.' And they'd say, 'Good, because we wanna come after the hockey game.'"

Rules of the Game

Another explanation for the mainstreaming of kink, beyond its safe-sex appeal, is that BDSM allows willing couples to explore erotic alternatives without taking them too far. The strict code of conduct among BDSM practitioners has been communicated well by the individuals who are packaging it for pop culture. Safe, sane, and consensual. This motto sets limits on the play, allowing those who are taking the licking—be it verbal or physical—to stop when they're no longer having fun. To be more specific:

- All of those involved in the BDSM play must consent before any activity begins.

- Partners should discuss in advance which activities they find displeasing and agree not to participate in any of them.

- There should be an agreed-upon release word or signal that is honored instantly.

- Only knots that are easy to undo should be used. When handcuffs are used, the person in them should be released immediately upon asking.

- Breathing should never be restricted.

- No one should be left bound or tied without supervision.

S/M Lite: Adventures in Restraint and Pleasure

If you're intrigued by the prospect of BDSM play, but hate pain at any level, Frank, a 50-plus-year-old Dominant—or Dom—who goes by the name Trainer assures us, "it doesn't even have to enter the picture." This former cop-turned-carpet-salesmen is a kind of BDSM personal trainer, providing couples and groups with instruction in "restraint and pleasure," a variation of the practice that "doesn't leave marks."

"It's all about touch," Trainer says, inviting us to check out the tools of his trade in the "playroom" of his Oak Brook home. It was an offer we couldn't refuse. What would a Dom's private quarters look like and what toys would it reveal?

Proof that fantasy is often better than reality, it turns out Trainer's playroom is merely a bedroom in a rather standard suburban home. He grabs a special key off the top of the refrigerator. ("I keep the room locked cause I have a young daughter.") As he lets us in, we immediately stumble over a gynecological table. "Got it from a client who sells medical supplies," he tells us.

Moving along, we see whips and flogs scattered all over the carpeted floor. There's a scuffed-up rack shaped like a humongous "X" jammed into a corner and duffel bags brimming with vibrators strewn about. ("I get some pretty strange looks from airport security when I'm carrying these," he says with a wink.)

We smile as we navigate this sexual obstacle course, making our way to a wall on the right covered with more whips and flogs. Trainer takes down one that looks like a graduation tassel and brushes it along each of our forearms. We nod in agreement—it definitely has potential. So does the mink-lined paddle and a feathered flog Trainer takes to our necks in a figure-eight pattern. "I can turn a woman on with anything," he boasts, adding that he loves to show couples how to get creative at home with brushes, plants, household appliances, and the tool chest in the garage.

One of the coolest toys Trainer shares with us is a steel medical device that resembles a pizza cutter with tiny spikes on the outside of a wheel. At first glance, it looks rather torturous, but he tells us to close our eyes and then takes turns lightly running it along the back of our necks and forearms.

Tough Love: One Woman's Road to Dominance

We asked writer Ginger Darren to explore her wilder side by taking a sexuality course titled How To Be a Dominatrix—Love, Fun, or Profit. Here's her report:

Our instructor was growing impatient with her roomful of neophytes. We had asked our volunteer male enough probing questions about his childhood and why he liked being dominated by women. It was time for action. "Quit asking and tell him what you want him to do," the teacher said, dropping a black leather duffel bag on the floor.

"Take off your tie. Loosen that shirt collar," ordered Mistress Lorraine, an attractive brunette in her forties. She seemed to be the one woman in the class of about 15 who knew the ropes, so to speak. Daniel complied, eagerly.

That broke the ice. Acting on ensuing orders, Daniel shed his clothes item by item—three-piece suit, tailored shirt, conservative boxers—until only his pink satin bikinis remained. A Southern California newsletter publisher in his late twenties, Daniel seemed pleased with himself, as the circle of women around him expressed approval of his tall, well-muscled body.

Next, the instructor emptied the duffel bag's contents at our feet—ropes, paddles, dog collars, whips, chains, kitchen utensils. A woman

with obvious ranch experience quickly hog-tied our volunteer, detouring the rope around his genitals. Another snapped a dog collar on Daniel and placed the leash handle in his mouth. Soon after the blindfold went on, all eyes turned to me, the only person who hadn't joined in the free-for-all. Mistress Lorraine led the hobbled Daniel to kneel in front of me. I flinched seeing him so close up, bound and gagged, and wondered just how the hell I'd gotten into this situation.

My interest in being a dominatrix started as a prank pulled by my friend Kat, who lives in Washington, D.C. A new phone-dating service was just starting up there, and Kat talked me into leaving this message: "Hi, my name's Ginger. I'm a Southern belle gone bad. I like bad boys who know when they need to be punished. So leave me a message, and I'll call you back . . . if you're worthy."

The responses practically jammed the phone lines: more than 100 takers in five days. Most sounded like educated, "normal" guys—lawyers, accountants, congressional aides, military men.

Kenny: "I'd love to be your bad boy. Call me at work, but be discreet."

Gary: "I've been so naughty. I need to be disciplined."

Jan: "I'm usually on the other side of these things, but from the sound of your voice, I might be willing to switch for you."

Matt: "I've heard about the kind of thing you're talking about but never tried it. I'd love to know more."

Steve: "My wife is a wimp and lets me dominate her. Let's see what you can do."

Michael: "It sounds like you know what a man needs, what a man likes. I'd travel the earth to be wrapped around your pretty finger."

Based solely on my message and my Southern accent, these men were ready to do anything for me. My friend Larry, a veteran newspaper reporter and a D.C. resident himself, called the city a hotbed of S/M-bondage-dominatrix activity.

"Just think of all those power-mongers," he told me, "all those guys needing a brief, albeit controlled, release from all that control. Maybe even needing to have someone tell them they really are the unworthy dogs they suspect they might be."

It got me thinking. A few weeks before placing the message, I'd lost my job as a newspaper editor because of a repetitive-use injury. I didn't know if I'd be able to write again. New career options weighed heavily on my mind. So my ears perked up when my physical therapist told me about his friend, the professional dominatrix. "What does she do?" I asked. "It depends," he told me. "She plays tennis with one client every week, for instance. They play a fast, hard game. Pretty soon, the sweat makes his tennis whites cling to his body, revealing the black panties underneath."

"No whips? No sex?"

"Nope, for this guy, simple humiliation does the trick." It sounded like easy money.

A short time later, Ava Taurel, a professional dominatrix with a "role-play" agency in New York who'd come to town on a national lecture tour, was teaching a class on the topic at The Learning Annex. I signed up, thinking it might be the perfect career.

My first move: to relieve Daniel of the thick leather leash he held between his teeth. "Thank you, mistress," he said, working his jaw loose. So as not to appear a complete wimp, I picked up the metal ice tongs, clicked them a few times near his ear, then slid the ends over his chest to squeeze one nipple, then the other. I heard a soft gasp. Then, before I knew it, someone snuck up and took off his blindfold. Our faces were a foot apart. I froze in embarrassment. Many mortifying seconds later, somebody led him away.

After class, Daniel (who'd been recruited from the previous night's lecture on fantasies and fetishes)

confided that whips and flogging don't turn him on. His idea of submission is to please a woman by brushing her hair, rubbing her feet, whatever she wants.

"Sometimes I think that if I had a strong woman running my life, I'd be a bigger financial success," he said. With that, he gave me his business card. "I find you a sane, definitely attractive woman," he added, "and I'd love for you to put me over your knee." I muttered something like "thank you" (how should I respond to something like that?) and left.

My dreams that night were the most erotic I'd ever had—odd because the whole experience turned me off. I have no urge to whip men, and I've never been attracted to weak, passive guys who need me to run their lives. As for my career, I realized that I'd run out of steam real fast if I encountered many Daniels along the way.

Besides, I believe that once you open some doors, there's no turning back. Vanilla sex is fine by me—although now I understand how a little fantasy role-playing, some mink-lined wrist restraints, and a paddle or two can round out the experience. I haven't met a man yet who wouldn't give it a try.

That's something I never would have imagined before this experience. I know part of the attraction for men must be that they enjoy having someone else assume the burden of control. But, in larger part, I think, it stems from a point made by Ava during our course: "Men like a woman who

knows what she's worth, who will stand up for herself. Men will try to put a woman down, but if she doesn't allow it, it will stop. And he will respect her more."

My first-generation Italian mother, who wouldn't know a dominatrix from an aviatrix, said virtually the same thing to me in an unrelated conversation. It's tough for women like me, who are natural givers and romantic idealists, to accept such aphorisms. But sometimes that may just be the best thing to do: Get tough and give him a little reminder of why he should worship his woman as the goddess she is.

Wow! We would have never guessed that tiny pin pricks could feel so good. Trainer tells us some people like him to press harder, but the thing to remember when using of any of these toys is to determine how you can use them to please your partner of the moment. "Just because one woman liked me to run this little gizmo along her inner thigh, doesn't mean all women will. You need to talk lots in advance of any play to learn each other's pleasure/pain thresholds."

Before we leave, Trainer shows us some photos from a demonstration he gave at a swingers convention. He's wearing a black leather vest, leather pants. A hoop earring dangles from his left ear and his head is shaved completely. Quite a contrast to the harmless-looking bald fellow in street clothes who stands before us. "It's all about fantasy," Trainer says. "I dress the part and it works."

You bet. Mr. Clean with a whip.

One Man's Ceiling Is Another Man's Floor

It all depends on your perspective—the sex you think is normal is positively strange to the next guy. And we're not about to cast judgments. Except when a practice isn't mutually agreed upon. Then there's some damaging psychology at work with one or both partners—and that's wrong. Following is a glossary of the extraordinary, with help from Brenda Love's *Encyclopedia of Unusual Sex Practices*. Take a look through it . . . the cravings you thought made you seem strange may not be so strange after all.

Acrophilia Next time you're on a plane and the lady next to you grips the hand rest during ascent, consider this: She may not have a fear of flying, but rather may get aroused by heights. And that guy panting next to you at the Empire State Building observation deck? Well, he ain't panting because he walked all the way up there. Acrophilia also is attributed to that swingin' seventies pastime known as the Mile High Club, where randy passengers tried to get it on in airplane lavatories—lending a different twist to the motto "Fly United."

Acrotomophilia This is the act of fantasizing about sexual experiences with an amputee. Some acrotomophiliacs want their partners to bind their limbs. Now, that's not to be confused with an apotemnophiliac, which is a person who gets off at the thought of having a limb or another part of his body surgically removed. Nuff said.

Anasteemaphilia See that really, really short guy with that leggy, statuesque woman? That's anasteemaphilia at work: the act of finding a significant difference in physical height sexually arousing.

Arachnephilia Take a spider. Let it crawl on your partner's body during your foreplay session or intercourse. If she doesn't scream and leap off the bed, she's probably in this category and thinks spiders are a part of a great sex session.

Autoerotica asphyxia The only time you ever hear about practitioners of this act is when they go a bit too far—that's when the ambulance shows up with the body bag. Autoerotic asphyxia involves self-strangulation during masturbation. People who practice this think the sensation of near-suffocation heightens orgasm. Here, we will pass judgement—this is just too way out!

> "Safe, sane, and consensual. This motto sets limits on the [S/M] play, allowing those who are taking the licking—be it verbal or physical—to stop when they're no longer having fun."

Autonepiophilia Also known as infantilism, this is the ultimate in role-playing. Autonepiophilia involves having one party act and dress as an infant, while the other assumes the role of parent—diapering, feeding, rocking, and sometimes disciplining the "child."

Autopederasty This refers to the act of inserting your own semierect penis into your anus for sexual pleasure. If you can do this, you might also qualify for the circus.

Axillism An axillist isn't necessarily a lover of Guns 'n' Roses. He's a guy who is aroused by armpits . . . and would love nothing more than to engage in a bit of armpit sex, sliding his penis between his partner's clenched upper arm and torso.

Bestiality The act of making the beast with two backs with . . . um, a beast. Having intercourse with animals is often viewed by society as depraved. It certainly isn't healthy! And dare we say it? This type of thing ain't just horsin' around.

Blood sports This very risky practice involves bloodletting—shallow cuttings or scratching of a partner's body—as part of sex. It's risky because of STDs and the chance that the cut will get infected. Bloodletting and vampirism (drinking blood) are practiced at underground clubs in major metropolitan areas across the country.

> "Next time you're on a plane and the lady next to you grips the hand rest during ascent, consider this: She may not have a fear of flying, but rather may get aroused by heights."

Some cuttings are intricate; paper towels are left on the etchings to pick up residue blood. The towel is then peeled off and dries as an "art canvas" of sorts.

Choreophilia If you got all hot and bothered at the last scene of *Footloose* (break dancing, line dancing, ballroom dancing, and just-plain-dancing dancing in that grain-elevator-turned-senior-prom-hall), then choreophilia just may be your ticket. It's the act of getting aroused by dancing. And you know what the Baptists said dancing leads to.

Coprophilia The act of getting aroused by feces. We have absolutely no witty rejoinders here.

Dendrophilia "I think that I shall never see, a poem as lovely as a tree." And then he masturbates to it. A dendrophiliac loves the forest. Literally.

Felching The act of sucking ejaculate out of a partner's vagina or anus.

Frottage Rub up against someone on the train going to work this morning? It's called frottage, son. And it's usually against the law.

Homilophilia You know that guy in accounting who keeps volunteering for those presentations to the board of directors? He may not be such a brown-nose after all. He may be a homilophiliac—a guy who is sexually aroused by giving speeches . . . or listening to them.

Maieusiophilia This refers to men who are aroused at the sight of visibly pregnant women. And the act that gave us such stellar magazines as *Knocked Up and Milky*.

Mysophilia In the back of adult magazines—way back—you'll find ads from adult stars offering their soiled panties for sale. A mysophiliac wants 'em . . . or any type of soiled undergarment, be it a jock strap, a bra, panties, or what have you.

Nasophilia Nose sucking. There. We said it.

Oculolictus Eye licking. There. We said it.

Podophilia This refers to a love of feet: the shape, size, and overall look of them. It should be noted that a foot love isn't considered a fetish unless the person fixates on the feet and forsakes the rest of his partner's body during love play.

Pseudonecrophilia Pretending your partner is dead. Which is different from wishing your partner was dead, which happens with warring or divorcing couples.

Psychrocism This refers to the act of arousal in the freezing cold. So maybe those Polar Bear Club swimmers who dive into the lake on New Year's Day have something else in mind. Hmmm.

Pygophilia Into pygophilia? You're an ass man, plain and simple.

Pyrophilia Refers to someone who is aroused by fire.

Sacrofricosis This is the practice of cutting a hole in your pants pocket and playing a little pocket pool out in public places. Practitioners are highly aroused by the experience of secretly masturbating in such a manner.

Urophilia People who like urine water sports (their gratification comes from being urinated on or urinating on someone) are urophiliacs.

Xenophilia This refers to people who are only aroused by strangers. This is not to be confused with Weird Al Yankophilia, which refers to people aroused by strange singer/accordionists.

Public Play

Frank and Laurie (not their real names) were in the tiny broadcasting studio in New York where Laurie is a deejay and newscaster. While the tunes played, they'd been kissing and fooling around. As Laurie began to read the hourly news report, Frank slowly took down her jeans and then her panties and proceeded to perform rather spirited oral sex on her. Listeners attributed the quaver in Laurie's voice to emotion at the tragic news stories she was reporting. Laurie tells us it was the most exciting sex she's ever had.

Alan was having dinner with his fiancée, Jennifer, at an extremely posh French restaurant in Beverly Hills. As the sommelier uncorked a bottle of vintage montrachet, Jennifer slid her hand under the table-cloth and unzipped Alan's fly. The sommelier mistook Alan's facial expression and sharp intake of breath as he tasted the wine for dis-approval and swiftly whisked it from the table.

Making Safe Sex Sexier

In our age of AIDS, this kind of risky sex might make more sense than ever: Carnal activity in situations where discovery or miscalcula-tion might result in public humiliation, incarceration, physical damage to one's most tender parts, or worse. Of course, adventurous sex is dif-ficult today; picking up a stranger for an anonymous quickie must be classified not as risky sex but as Russian roulette. Many people who aren't suicidal are looking for ways to put back the excitement that's missing in bed, and risky sex seems a way to recapture that old rush. Are your fiancée's folks over for dinner? Why not go into the kitchen to assist her and slip a helpful hand into her undies? Did your wife talk you into accompanying her to the opera? Why not try to make her yell "Bravo!" at the end of the aria?

Why on earth would an otherwise sane person do such things? "Novelty and uncertainty are the two components of eroticism," ob-serves Alan, although he's not a professional psychotherapist. Bernard Berkowitz, who is one, explains it like this: "It's the excitement of get-ting away with the forbidden. So many of our early sexual experiences occur in parked cars or behind shrubbery in the park. It's a Pavlovian association of danger and potential embarrassment with the excitement and tension of sex."

New York psychiatrist Harvey Greenberg, M.D., has other explana-tions. "One is the infantile wish to look and be looked at, often when one or both parties are naked," he says. "That idea of showing off, of exhibitionism runs very deep in all of us. Another has to do with the incest taboo. In most Western countries, it's forbidden to have sex with a parent. And one of the things young people do when they have sur-reptitious sex is have it in their parent's bedroom."

Though the parental-bed thing can seem outrageous when you're a teen, it's tame compared to the risks some adults are willing to take. A writer we know admits to having had sex in public swimming pools, on

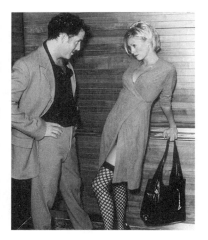

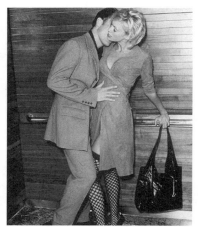

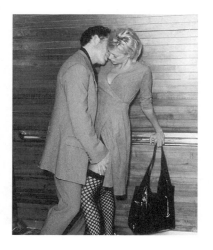

crowded beaches, standing on a bridge over the Hudson River, and on a public pathway at night in Westchester County. Friends of his have had sex in airliners, in advertising agencies, on roofs and fire escapes, in public stairwells, in the men's room of the posh New York Yacht Club, and on a religious retreat. Some of Greenberg's patients have done the nasty in elevators, on trains, on the lawn at garden parties in broad daylight, and in hospital beds.

People of both sexes have admitted to boffing their exes at their own weddings. Others have masturbated or performed oral sex on a partner while he or she was driving—surely one of the riskiest forms of risky sex. Greenberg assures me it's not teenagers, but adults—people in their forties and fifties—who do it most, especially if they've had unadventurous earlier lives.

Besides the possibility of getting caught, another huge attraction of risky sex is that it has to be done quickly, before being interrupted. In welcome contrast to the advice given in many sex manuals, which often make men feel hideously guilty if they don't spend a minimum of two hours in foreplay, risky sex demands that you get it over with as fast as possible or suffer serious consequences. It's license to have a quickie, without foreplay and without the deadly responsibility of simultaneous mutual orgasms. It also allows us to be naughty . . . to take dares, to refuse to be Goody Two-shoes, to shake our fists at authority. During the deed, and for hours afterwards, we feel vital and ready for anything. That's great sex.

The Swing Set

The suburban recipe is simple: cookie-cutter housing tracts, strip mall on every corner, and minivans full of soccer moms and their kids. But swingers' clubs? That kind of sleazy stuff is reserved for sin-soaked city folk, corrupt politicians, and sixties leftovers, right?

Not quite. Mate-sharing organizations are popping up in suburban communities all over the country. The 'burbs provide the perfect—discreet—environment for couples who, after tucking their toddlers into bed, prefer to seek entertainment within a grocery store's distance from home. And that "entertainment," according to couples who participate in the lifestyle, centers on socializing with other free-spirited adults and enjoying recreational sex—lots of it, with lots of different people.

Swingers believe in sharing. Their relationships, they say, are so honest that intimate experiences with others won't destroy their primary partnerships. Because the lifestyle seems so bizarre in the age of AIDS and political correctness, we wanted to find our what swinging in the twenty-first century is all about, so we sent our coauthors on a mission.

Rambling On

We place our first call to the North American Swing Club Association. Much to our surprise, a spokesperson for this governing body of swingers tells us that membership is greater than ever before. Hmmmmm. Could it be baby boomer boredom? Or perhaps a backlash to nagging right-wing conservatism? Whatever. Organizations such as Couples Choice, one of the Chicago area's more exclusive swinger's clubs, are thriving.

We call Couples Choice exclusive because its owners, Dave and Dawn, personally interview potential members. "Not all clubs do that," says Dave, a soft-spoken fiftysomething gent who's been part of the lifestyle for 20 years. "We do it to make sure all partners walk through the door with equal enthusiasm."

> **"A writer we know admits to having had sex in public swimming pools, on crowded beaches, standing on a bridge over the Hudson River, and on a public pathway at night in Westchester County. Friends of his have had sex in airliners, in advertising agencies, on roofs and fire escapes, in public stairwells, in the men's room of the posh New York Yacht Club, and on a religious retreat."**

Men usually make the first contact, says Dawn, Dave's wife and business partner of nine years. A petite ball of energy who's totally miffed by "straights" (that's swinger lingo for monogamous couples), Dawn says new members used to find out about the club primarily through word of mouth and ads in swingers magazines. But befitting today's times, the Internet now leads lots of people to their door.

And what a unique door it is. When we pull up to Couple's Choice, located in a suburb about 40 miles from the Windy City, our first thought is that it looks like a typical two-story home, but with a warehouse-style addition built onto the back to accommodate a business. In this

> **"Swingers believe in sharing. Their relationships, they say, are so honest that intimate experiences with others won't destroy their primary partnerships."**

case, the business is pleasure, which comes in the form of Saturday night, anything-goes parties that begin at 8:30 P.M. and often end after brunch the following morning. To get in, partners pay $45, which includes a buffet dinner for two. Because Couples Choice has no liquor license, its gatherings are BYOB. And, interestingly, unattached women can attend, but single guys aren't welcome. "They can't handle the scene and tend to get out of hand more easily," explains Dave.

As we enter the club, we can't help but chuckle to ourselves—it looks like your basic sports bar. There are football helmets hanging from the ceiling, photos of Indy race cars and other sports memorabilia on the wood-paneled walls, and dozens of tall, circular oak tables with barstools. There's even a dance floor at the far end of the room, complete with a disco ball, strobe lights, and a DJ booth.

Over the Rainbow

Then Dave directs us toward a doorway adjacent to music central. Passing through, we find ourselves in a cozy sitting room with a fireplace and an abundance of futonlike sofas. Following Dave up a staircase at the far end of the room, we realize instantly that we are not in Kansas anymore.

You see, Couples Choice is an on-premises swingers' club, meaning it offers multiple rooms and alcoves where members can share all manner of intimacies with one another. We make our way through several rooms with king-sized beds, an orgy room with seven beds lined up in a row, a room with a swinglike contraption suspended from the rafters, a loft-style room with stars painted on the ceiling, and, the most popular room of all, according to Dave, the bondage room. Here, members can play with a wide variety of gear while restrained to the wall, a bed, or a Grecian Bench, a device that resembles a saddle to which an adventurous soul gets strapped in on all fours. Because this room gets so crowded, Dave and Dawn have had to put a sign-up board on the door, limiting members' restraining and spanking time to half-hour intervals.

With that image of the facilities in mind, you're probably wondering about the members. Personally, we thought they'd be a mix of free-love throwbacks from the sixties and seventies and sleazy types who couldn't get it anywhere else. And there are some of each of these in the group, we're sure. But mostly, they're normal people. Really normal. "Our members are a combination of blue- and white-collar suburbanites," Dave says, "Ages range from 21 to over 60. You should come to a party sometime and meet them."

Sounded like an opportunity to us. So in the name of investigative journalism, we accepted Dave's offer to attend a Couple's Choice masquerade ball. When we arrive at 10:00 P.M. the party is jumping. Couples, dressed up in costumes, look like they're attending some ersatz Mardi Gras. There are several angels and devils, a couple of scantily clad construction workers, plenty of French maids, and lots of women in slinky lingerie—all competing in a costume contest that gets more risqué as the night wears on. Everyone appears to be having a ball, and one woman is having two of them as she kneels on the floor, unzips some guy's fly, and satisfies him to roaring crowd approval.

"Wild things happen at this club," says Nancy, a peppy, 41-year-old mother of two who started swinging with her husband, Steve, after 24 years of marriage. Like most of the couples we speak with, Nancy and

Steve say they got involved in the lifestyle as a way to spice up their marriage. "It's made me a more conscientious lover," says Steve, who admitted that prior to swinging he was the kind of husband who would satisfy himself, then roll over and catch some zzzzs. "Now, I know what it takes to pleasure a woman—because I've pleasured lots."

In fact, Steve and Nancy have been with 27 other couples in the three years since they adopted the lifestyle. Due to the sheer volume of sexual encounters, it's common among swingers to reserve something special just for their partners. For Steve and Nancy, that something is wearing a condom with everyone but each other. Yes, that sounds like it should be a given in the age of AIDS, but here it's not. Swingers are surprisingly nonchalant about sexually transmitted diseases. Although Dave and Dawn supply plenty of prophylactics in the club's eight bathrooms, Steve says he'd estimate that 80 percent of the members don't even use them.

"People are extremely courteous here," says Dick, a handsome 51-year-old who runs a construction company with his wife Susan. "They won't come to the club if they have so much as a runny nose."

Swing Appeal

But when chatting with Steve, we learn that couples don't have to be married to gain entrance to a party. "They just have to prove to Dave and Dawn that they're together," he says. In other words, just about any sweet talker can get in, which seems pretty risky to straights like us.

That's risky. There's also a weird part to this swinger scene—the practice of rinsing the genitals with mouthwash between sexual encounters. "We're a really well-groomed bunch," says Steve, adding that the mouthwash routine "keeps the ladies and men smelling and feeling fresh." (All we could think about was how much our gums burn after a quick gargle with Listerine. Yowch!)

But Steve seems to be right. The partygoers appear to be a clean bunch. Admittedly, many of them are attractive. Take the tiny, hard-bodied harem girl who approaches one of us. "Did you see *The Arrival,* that movie with Charlie Sheen?" she asks. "You look just like him . . . so handsome." She giggles, flips her long blond hair, and proceeds to rub her entire body up against both of us.

Or Steve, who had an uncanny resemblance to an old flame. He quickly becomes a de facto fashion adviser. "You," he says, pointing to one of us. "You need to wear tighter pants . . . show the ladies

> **"We make our way through several rooms with king-sized beds, an orgy room with seven beds lined up in a row, a room with a swinglike contraption suspended from the rafters, a loft-style room with stars painted on the ceiling, and, the most popular room of all . . . the bondage room."**

what you've got. And you . . . the denim shirt, skirt, and a leopard print scarf make you look prudish. Now, if you just wore the scarf alone . . . grrrr-yow!"

In a different setting, these exchanges wouldn't have bothered either of us. Lots of people have told John he resembles Heidi Fleiss's best customer. And Beth has had her fair share of suggestive remarks. But here, it confirmed what we already knew: Neither of us could ever swing. We're much too jealous.

Interestingly enough, swingers don't get jealous watching their partners have sex with other people; it's the little things that set them off. Carla, a 32-year-old brunette who looks like a former high school cheerleader, recalls her bout with the green-eyed monster. "After my husband and I had finished having sex with another couple, he let the woman give him a back massage. That was too personal."

> **"Everyone appears to be having a ball, and one woman is having two of them as she kneels on the floor, unzips some guy's fly, and satisfies him to roaring crowd approval."**

Nancy got equally ticked when Steve spent an entire evening talking to the same woman. "We told each other we'd move around, meet lots of people. He was way too focused on her for my comfort," she says.

Most of the couples we meet here work through these issues, saying it "makes their relationship stronger." But swinging isn't for everyone. Cynthia, a thirtysomething Chicagoan, says the lifestyle destroyed her marriage. "Watching your spouse have sex with other women ruins your intimacy as a couple," she says. "My husband and I don't even sleep in the same bed anymore."

Dawn would argue that Cynthia and her husband had problems before they began swinging. "The lifestyle only makes good relationships stronger. People tell us they come to our parties, have a great time, and go home and have the best sex ever," she says.

> **"There's also a weird part to this swinger scene—the practice of rinsing the genitals with mouthwash between sexual encounters."**

Dick agrees, saying that "a bad night here is better than a good night anywhere else."

But don't expect swingers to openly discuss their wild Saturday nights at the water cooler come Monday. "I'm paranoid about people finding out," admits Joseph, a corporate executive who bears a striking resemblance to Martin Scorsese, unibrow and all. Ironically, he and his wife, Mary, hit the swinging scene as a way to act out their fantasies. "We'd go to public places so we could get caught," Mary explains. "Then we heard about Dave and Dawn's. Everything here is public—and consensual."

Because of the stigma attached to swinging, Carla and her husband Don won't share details of their lifestyle with friends either. But they do have an inside joke: The license plate on their Corvette reads "Swingers."

"We tell everyone we're bigtime golfers," Don says with a laugh.

As for us? We're not converts; We're perfectly happy with our straight lifestyle. But we do have to admit, we were impressed by the group's openness and total lack of inhibition. In fact, we can't help but think that if our society weren't so repressed, we could all find a thoroughly happy medium—and be open about it.

Swing, baby.

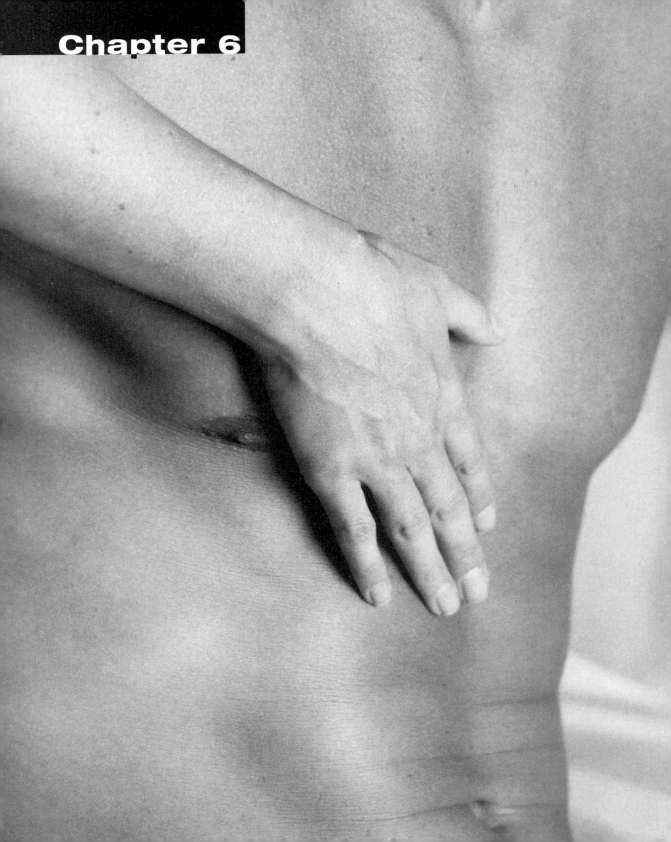

Chapter 6

According to conventional wisdom, a man's sex drive reaches its peak at around age 18. After 40, it really begins to dive—erections start petering out, so to speak. Or they get stuck at half-mast. This thinking contains a tiny germ of truth—yes, aging brings some sexual changes. But for most men, these changes are minor. The fact is, if you want a great love life at 45, 55, and beyond, you can have it.

To give you an idea of the impact aging has on your sexuality, we've created sexual profiles of both men and women in their twenties, thirties, forties, fifties, and beyond. Though physical changes that impact sexuality generally don't occur until both genders are well into their forties, there are psychological and lifestyle issues related to aging that may have a major impact on your sexual preferences and performance. We believe that awareness of these issues—both your own and your partner's—will enable you to tailor your sexual expectations to maximize your pleasure through the Golden Years and beyond.

The Twenties
What's Up with You

Good news. According to the Kinsey Institute, your sexuality doesn't peak at age 18—your sexual daydreaming does. That means in your twenties, that vision of Alyssa Milano slathered in whip cream will hit you every half-hour instead of every two minutes as it did when you were a teen. Which is good, because after college, you'll be embarking on the real world, where constant daydreaming can wreak havoc on life, love, and the pursuit of happiness. In other words—adulthood.

Yep. The world considers you a grown-up now and with that comes responsibility. Two years into this decade, most guys are either entrenched in a trade or graduating from college and grasping the first rung on that tall ladder to success. Believe it or not, your desire to get hootchie five nights a week will probably go from spot one on your list of priorities to somewhere at the bottom of the top ten, according to San Francisco–based sex therapist Patti Britton, Ph.D. "Guys this age expect to get their B.S., M.B.A., and Ph.D. by the time they're 24. There's no time for relationships, and even if a guy in his twenties would like to connect with a woman, he's exhausted from working day and night. The sheer pace of the twentysomething man's life leaves him with little stamina for sex."

That's the bad news. The good news is all your manly parts are still working full steam. The mere thought of that wildcat in whip cream will put you at full mast, so be careful. You'll also want to be careful of your sex partners. Studies indicate that 25 percent

Sexuality and Aging

Twenties:

Him: ". . . in your twenties, that vision of Alyssa Milano slathered in whip cream will hit you every half-hour instead of every two minutes as it did when you were a teen."

Her: "Though teenage girls often settle for less in the orgasm department, most women who've reached their mid-twenties have acquired enough knowledge to know that sexual satisfaction is a two-way street."

of men in their twenties have had intercourse with five to ten different women; 10 percent have been with 20 or more. If you're on the high end of that scale—gettin' jiggy with untold numbers of strange females—this would be a good time to review chapter 3 on Responsibility and Protection. Acquiring a nasty (possibly deadly) infection is one of the risks of nonmonogamous sex. So is an unplanned pregnancy. Unless you want to be an STD statistic—or a daddy—use a condom.

Ironically, television, magazines—the media in general—would have us believe that guys in their twenties are having the most sex. But volume is not one of your bragging rights. According to the University of Chicago's Sex in America study, young studs are getting it the least—unless they're in steady relationships. It all goes back to Britton's theory. Single guys fresh out of college are career-obsessed. To them, getting a promotion is more satisfying than having an orgasm. If you happen to be in a relationship, though, you're enjoying the best of both worlds.

Of course, the closer you and your partner get to that 30-year mark, the more you'll be hearing the "M" word—marriage—from your girlfriend, your buddies, her parents, your parents, the family dog. Well, maybe not from her parents, but pressure to tie the knot could weigh heavily on you from a variety of fronts. It's a natural progression. We meet, fall in love, marry, have children, etc., etc. Though we're the first to say knockin' boots is damn fun, sex is also about propagating the species. And in the U.S. of A., unless you're a celebrity (á la Madonna), getting hitched is still the common first step in the quest to create heirs.

Her Deal

Get ready to work a little harder, guys. Women in their twenties are becoming more aware of their sexuality and sexual preferences. That quick romp in the backseat of your parents' sedan will no longer cut it—especially if you're the only one enjoying a payoff.

Though teenage girls often settle for less in the orgasm department, most women who've reached their mid-twenties have acquired enough knowledge to know that sexual satisfaction is a two-way street. This bodes well for both genders, says Britton. "As women become more aware of their own pleasure, men become less self-focused. It's not about getting their rocks off any more. They become better lovers because they learn quickly: if they want to get off, they're going to have to get her off, too." (This isn't a huge surprise: 60.9 percent of the *Men's Fitness* readers surveyed felt bringing a woman to orgasm is a shared responsibility.)

The more sexually experienced a woman is, the more comfortable she'll be telling you exactly what she likes. However, in most cases, your list of sexual partners will outnumber hers, which means she may be aware of her preferences, but she still may have a tough time talking about them. Take your time. Make her comfortable. Ask her what feels good. You'll both end up having a grand time.

That's her sexual profile. Psychologically, the twentysomething woman is searching—seriously—for love. "For females, sex and love go hand in hand," according to Britton. "It's the way we're raised." Though women are no longer considered "old maids" if they're unmarried in their late twenties, they're getting as much pressure—perhaps more—than you are to take the plunge. After all, there's that thing called the biological clock. It usually starts ticking in the late twenties and doesn't stop until a woman fulfills her reproductive destiny, adopts a child, or enters menopause. We should point out that not all women desire children, but research indicates that the biological urge to reproduce is difficult for even the most independent females to ignore. "I was sure I never wanted kids," said Jenny, a 35-year-old Chicago writer. "Then I turned 28 and it was all I could think about. I'd see babies and get all mushy. I wanted one—bad!"

Jenny's clock was right on target. A woman has the best chance of conceiving a child in her twenties, with her fertility tapering off from the age of 35. Men, on the other hand, have no limit on the time frame in which they can father a child. (Witness actor Tony Randall, who became daddy to a second child at the ripe age of 78). Though this can create a bit of an imbalance between the genders, for the most part we seem to remain in sync. Career-driven couples are putting off marriage and families, but it's still happening primarily in late twenties and early thirties.

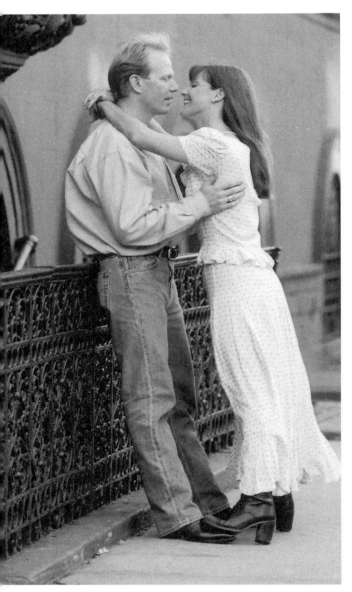

The Thirties
What's Up with You

Because many men in their thirties have a spouse or significant other, they at least have the opportunity to enjoy sex on a consistent basis. That old joke about a person's sex life heading downhill after marriage is just that—a joke. Men in their thirties claim to have more frequent sex than they did in their twenties—and it's better, too.

"By this decade of a man's life, he's either become a wonderful lover or is divorced," jokes Britton, who says men generally focus more on their partner's pleasure as they get older. "And, of course, pleasing her ends up pleasing him," she adds.

Speaking of being pleased, your equipment is still working well. It may take you slightly longer to get erect again after ejaculating than it did ten years ago—but not an amount of time that would put her to sleep. And the healthier you are, the better. At this stage of your life, poor eating habits and couch-potato tendencies not only impact your overall well-being, but begin to take their toll on your sexuality as well. As you'll read in the next chapter, that 16-ounce steak, baked-potato slathered in butter, and cigar-and-brandy chaser may satisfy the palate, but smoking, drinking, and a steady diet of fatty, high-cholesterol food is one of the quickest routes to impotence. The best way to ensure that your manliness remains manly for the long haul is to get fit and healthy—now.

Likewise, you need to learn to lighten up. Your continuing ascent up the corporate ladder has brought added responsibilities and headaches. They're working you like a dog for that growing paycheck, which mean lots of stress and little time to decompress.

If you're a family man, double the anxiety. You *need* your paycheck. To pay the mortgage. To cover the credit card bills. To save for college tuition. Instead of butting heads with the boss, you've learned to grit your teeth and present

Thirties:

Him: "That old joke about a person's sex life heading downhill after marriage is just that—a joke."

"Let's just say if you're too uptight, you probably ain't gettin' any. Anxiety can kill the libido."

". . . regularity in sexual activity, ejaculation, and orgasm, not only helps to keep your gear (particularly the prostate) in good shape, it also helps you retain your sexual capacity."

one hell of a convincing faux grin. Anything to avoid the unemployment line.

What does all of this have to do with sex? Let's just say if you're too uptight, you probably ain't gettin' any. Anxiety can kill the libido. You may worship your partner, but if you spend your day stressed and exhausted, you'll probably be happier collapsing in bed than using it for amorous purposes.

And that's where trouble can start. At this stage of your life, sex becomes necessary. Research has shown that the male and female sex organs can fail if they're not used for their intended purposes. Moreover, regularity in sexual activity, ejaculation, and orgasm, not only helps to keep your gear (particularly the prostate) in good shape, it also helps you retain your sexual capacity. Britton prescribes "an orgasm a day," though she says twice weekly will suffice. And the Big O doesn't have to result from intercourse. Oral sex and masturbation work just as effectively.

Her Deal

This is a big decade for women. As we mentioned in the section on the twenties, you'll notice the females in your life becoming increasingly assertive between the sheets. By now they're well aware of what bad sex is and many won't hesitate to let you know when your techniques qualify as such.

But don't sweat it. A little constructive criticism offers you an opportunity to share your preferences, too. As Britton points out, "One of the greatest sexual lubricants is talking about sex." And think of the benefits of a friskier partner: She may occasionally initiate action. According to our sex survey, more than 60 percent of you feel she should take the lead half of the time. Because women reach their sexual peak at 38, this may be the decade in which that wish comes true.

The Forties
What's Up with You

For many men, the forties marks the beginning of slight changes in sexual capacity. But slight is the operative word. Testosterone levels begin to decline gradually during this decade. Typically, it may take a bit longer to get aroused. Whereas in the past, you may have become erect by merely watching your partner undress, you may now need direct stimulation. And even with that stimulation, you may notice that your erection may not be as firm as it once was.

Our most important words of advice: Don't worry about it. If you've been enjoying a healthy sex life up until now, it will continue as long as you and your partner understand that the changes you're experiencing are physiological—and absolutely normal.

Yes, your lovemaking may take longer. But look on the bright side: Your lovemaking may take longer. Use this opportunity to rediscover the joy of foreplay and to enhance your intimacy as a couple. By exploring new and adventuresome ways to please each other, your relationship will continue to grow stronger.

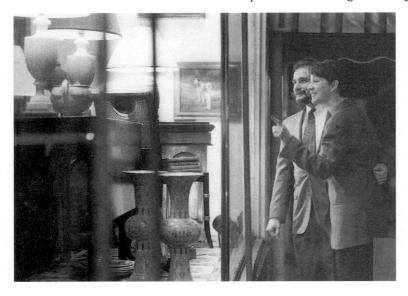

Start doubting yourself, however, and trouble will creep in. After a few failed attempts at lovemaking, it's not uncommon for some men to rechannel their sexual energy. Feeling inadequate, you may feel the urge to bury yourself in work, household projects, gardening . . . anything to keep from thinking about sex. Though these activities are clearly distractions, your partner may read them as disinterest—in other words, "He's more passionate about his azalea plants than me."

Direct that energy into improving your relationship—and

Forties:

Him: "If you've been enjoying a healthy sex life up until now, it will continue as long as you and your partner understand that the changes you're experiencing are physiological—and absolutely normal."

Her: ". . . women in their forties are healthier and more physically active then ever, which works well in the boudoir, as studies indicate that people's sexual enthusiasm is much higher when they feel good about themselves."

your health. Continue those healthy habits you started in your thirties—eat right, exercise, and limit the stress in your life. Your sex, psyche, and physicality will be much better for it.

Her Deal

There are three things that tend to have the greatest impact on a woman's sexuality during this decade—her body, children, and perimenopause (premenopause).

In terms of a woman's body, the visible signs of aging may become tougher for her to take. Though you may love the fine lines around her eyes and mouth, she may start sampling lotions and potions to get rid of them. But don't fret. Her concerns will have little bearing in the bedroom. Just as women tend to become more sexually confident as they get older, many women in committed relationships lose the hang-ups they've had regarding their bodies. That pocket of cellulite on her thighs may have sent her bolting for the light switch in her thirties, but it's a fact of life now.

Men's Sexual Frequency Through the Decades (%)

Age	Never	Few times a year	Few times a month	2–3 times a week	4+ times a week
18–24	15	21	24	28	12
25–29	7	15	31	36	11
30–39	8	15	37	33	6
40–49	9	18	40	27	6
50–59	11	22	43	20	3

Note: These results are based on the question: "How often have you had sex during the last 12 months?"
(Source: Sex in America survey, University of Chicago, 1994.)

Tips for a Healthier Penis

The Massachusetts Male Aging Study (MMAS), conducted on nearly 1,300 men between the ages of 40 and 70, found that 52 percent had some degree of erectile dysfunction.

However, if you fit this demographic, and can't perform sexually the way you like to, the MMAS research has an upside: erectile problems are preventable. Even if you have the risk conditions we mentioned—high blood pressure, heart disease, and diabetes—you can take these steps, which improve your overall health, and the long-term health of your penis.

- **Pop a rod.** The more erections you have, the more erections you're likely to have, as your penis will get the nutrient it needs most—oxygen. If your equipment is oxygen-deprived, permanent damage to blood vessels and muscles may occur. The end result: impotence. Again, it's the use-it-or-lose-it syndrome. Three erections a week and a couple of orgasms will give your penis the O_2 it needs.

- **Get some extra sleep.** An hour of extra Z-time a day will add up to extra energy . . . for work, play, and sex.

Of course, that doesn't mean she doesn't care about the way she looks and feels. On the contrary, women in their forties are healthier and more physically active then ever, which works well in the boudoir, as studies indicate that people's sexual enthusiasm is much higher when they feel good about themselves.

That enthusiasm may be coupled with motivation if she still wants to have children. Thanks to increasingly healthy lifestyles, and remarkable advances in reproductive medicine, more and more women are having children after hitting the 40-year mark.

Needless to say, the clock is loudly ticking at this point in her life, which means you may find yourself under extreme pressure to perform. Or you may find yourself at a fertility clinic trying to speed up the natural process. Either way, "trying" to have children can put serious stress on a relationship. Sex becomes scheduled and oftentimes clinical. If you're prepared for that—and for the potential disappointments (assisted reproduction has improved greatly, but it still offers no guarantees)—you can get through this final quest for kids with your commitment intact.

Finally, some women begin to experience perimenopause symptoms in their early to mid-forties. Hot flashes, night sweats, and irritability are just a few of the indicators that "the change" is around the corner. Though perimenopause doesn't have a direct impact on a woman's sexual capacity, she may not be "in the mood" as often due to hormonal fluctuations.

The Fifties
What's Up with You

Most of the physical changes we covered for the forties also apply to men in their fifties. A reduction in testosterone may inhibit your libido and your ability to achieve an erection. Plus there are medical conditions relative to aging, such as heart disease, high blood pressure, and arthritis, that may begin to interfere with your desire—and capacity—to make love.

The best thing you can do for yourself—and your sex life—is to nip your problems in the bud. Don't wait until they get out of hand, harming your health and your relationships. As you will discover later in this chapter, and in chapter 7, there are medical treatments for just about everything that may ail you.

Her Deal

While a man's body, and primary sex hormone (testosterone), change gradually throughout his forties and fifties, women experience dramatic physical changes during menopause. As we mentioned, this

Fifties:

Him: "The best thing you can do for yourself— and your sex life—is to nip your problems in the bud. Don't wait until they get out of hand, harming your health and your relationships."

Her: "Whereas a younger woman can become comfortably wet after 10 to 30 seconds of stimulation, a menopausal woman will take a few minutes—and then still may need additional lubrication."

phase of life, which marks the end of a woman's reproductive years, begins with common symptoms—hot flashes, night sweats, irritability, etc. By the time it's complete (the average age of menopause is 51), a woman will no longer menstruate and will have lowered levels of estrogen, progesterone, and testosterone that could have a major impact on her sexuality.

Lower levels of estrogen, in particular, can cause a woman to go through extreme discomfort at the time of menopause, according to Dr. Saul Rosenthal, author of *Sex Over 40*. "Symptoms can manifest themselves emotionally (in anxiety, irritability, insomnia, nervousness, or depression) and physically (with hot flashes, fatigue, and headaches)," he writes.

But this is only the tip of the iceberg. Because menopause results in a permanent decrease in estrogen, there are also long-term effects. By understanding the changes that take place in her body (as well as your own), you can adapt your lovemaking to ensure mutual comfort and satisfaction. Here is what Rosenthal says to be aware of:

- Her breasts may lose some elasticity and may not swell as much during arousal, but the nipples will continue to become hard, erect, and sensitive with stimulation.

- The clitoris will remain sensitive, but it may take somewhat longer to respond to stimulation.

- Though most women notice little if any change in their orgasms after menopause, laboratory measurements of uterine contractions during orgasm indicate that they may become slightly less powerful.

- The loss of estrogen after menopause frequently causes a condition called atrophic vaginitis. Her vaginal walls become thin, losing

- **Chill out.** Stress can interfere with many aspects of your life, including your ability to perform sexually.

- **Speak up.** If something is bugging you, get it out. The MMAS study shows that the men who were assertive and took control of situations were less likely to have erectile problems. Probably because they have less stress, which causes the hormones to go out of whack.

- **Eat your veggies and reduce fat.** We said it before, you'll derive all kinds of benefits from a diet rich in vitamins and low in fat. Aside from feeling great, you'll reduce your risk of heart disease and cancer, and your penis will be more likely to function at full capacity. Just be sure not to eliminate fat altogether. Super low-fat diets have proven to deplete testosterone levels—and we all know what that means.

- **Exercise.** You know this drill— getting in shape will give you more energy, improve your well-being, and add extra years to your life. Your penis will benefit from improved blood flow that results from a healthier heart.

their soft folds and the cushioning effect they previously had. This loss of elasticity may also cause the opening of the vagina to become more narrow. Without the elasticity, the vagina is unable to expand to accommodate the penis. The result: painful intercourse.

- A loss of vaginal lubrication compounds the previously mentioned problem. Whereas a younger woman can become comfortably wet after 10 to 30 seconds of stimulation, a menopausal woman will take a few minutes—and then still may need additional lubrication.

- Some women also report urinary symptoms, such as burning, after intercourse. Rosenthal says this is due to irritation of the urinary passage and bladder, "since they are no longer as well-cushioned or protected by the vaginal lining during intercourse."

- Some women also report painful uterine contractions during orgasm.

- Low levels of estrogen accelerate osteoporosis, a condition in which the bones throughout the body become thin and fragile. Low levels also accelerate heart disease and arteriosclerosis.

Keep in mind that many of the most serious conditions brought on by menopause can be treated with estrogen replacement therapy (ERT). Aside from arresting the immediate symptoms of menopause like hot flashes, ERT can also prevent other, long-term effects on the vagina and skeletal bones. Note: A link to uterine cancer in the mid-seventies caused many doctors to rethink estrogen replacement therapy. And there is still concern that it may increase the risk of breast cancer. But many physicians remain confident that it's the best way to prevent the long-term physical problems associated with menopause. A woman should consult with her doctor about the regime when she starts showing signs that the change has begun.

The Golden Years
What's Up with You . . . and Her

A survey of six thousand married couples over 60 showed that 55 percent made love one or more times a week. In addition, sexually active retirees rated themselves as happier with their love lives than 20-year-old single guys. And demographics work to the older man's sexual advantage. Statistically, women live longer than men. At age 65, there are 1.25 women for every man. By age 80, women outnumber men two to one. Stay healthy and sexually active long enough, and you'll live to see what the Beach Boys sang about in "Surf City"—two girls for every boy.

The Challenges of Aging

You've read our decade-by-decade account of the effects aging has on your hardware. Now we'd like to elaborate on five major life issues—namely, growing families, male menopause, changes in lovemaking, the empty nest, and age-related illness—that have been know to deflate even the heartiest sexual appetites. Read on.

#1   Kids: How to Have Them . . . and Still Have Sex

You can't open a newspaper, or turn on the television, without encountering stories of poverty, violence, and eco abuses throughout the world. It makes the choice not to have children seem very practical. And yet, Americans are in the midst of another baby boom. Our solid economy over the past several years is part of the reason. Never mind that there are scary things going on all over the planet—we're feeling optimistic about our own future and are having babies in droves.

If you've hit your thirties and are just contemplating children, then you know that your precious little "tax deduction" will actually impact seriously on your

> **"Never mind that there are scary things going on all over the planet—we're feeling optimistic about our own future and are having babies in droves."**

bottom line. As we mentioned earlier, the financial aspects of parenting often put serious pressure on both partners. Sometimes Mom has to work to help make ends meet. If she'd rather take care of Junior full time, it could mean plenty of weepy moments on the home front. If you'd like to tell your boss to shove his spreadsheets where the sun don't shine, the best you can do is bite your tongue or start to freshen up the résumé. After all, your beautiful bundle of joy must be fed.

All of this adds up to stress—and too much stress usually means too little sex. Couples with children need to work extra hard to keep family pressures out of the bedroom, according to Britton. Though it may sound silly, she says, that date-night becomes an essential means of ensuring that the spark in marriage remains strong.

Making Babies: The Natural Way

You both want children, so you have sex—lots of it. Two months into trying that little blue line appears on the pregnancy test strip. You're going to have a baby.

And you're lucky, because according to Sherman Silber, M.D., getting pregnant isn't easy. As he explains in *How to Get Pregnant with the New Technology*, with all other animals except humans, the desire for sex corresponds exactly to the moment a female is about to ovulate. "The human inclination to have sex at any time during the month or year is reproductively inefficient," he writes. "A period of fourteen days is required for a follicle to develop in a woman's ovary from day one of menstruation until the egg is sufficiently matured so that it is ready for ovulation. After ovulation , there is another fourteen-day period after the egg is fertilized (assuming sex has occurred at the right time), when the embryo grows and then implants in the uterus, or womb. If intercourse occurs sometime other than those few days around the time of ovulation, it is unlikely to lead to a pregnancy."

Determining exactly when a woman ovulates can be challenging—but it's one of the best ways to achieve a pregnancy. There are ovulation predictor kits on the market that help pinpoint this critical time. But most are pricey (between $20 and $100 per month) and come with no guarantees. The smarter option is for a woman to get to know her body. There is no better book on this subject than *Taking Charge of Your Fertility: The Definitive Guide to Natural Birth Control and Pregnancy Achievement* (by Toni Weschler; HarperPerennial, 1995). If you and your wife are serious about making a baby, this is the book to read, as it will teach both of you how to identify signs, such as changes in cervical mucus and basal body temperature, which signal the onset of ovulation. Other great reads on the subject include *How To Get Pregnant* (by Sherman J. Silber; Warner Books, 1991) and *Getting Pregnant: What Couples Need to Know Right Now* (by Neils H. Lauersen and Colette Bouchez; Fawcett Books, 1992).

> "... retire those snug Calvin Klein briefs for a while and, instead, wear boxers. Infertility specialists claim that the baggier alternative keeps the temperature of your testicles at a more appropriate level for sperm production."

To do your part, retire those snug Calvin Klein briefs for a while and, instead, wear boxers. Infertility specialists claim that the baggier alternative keeps the temperature of your testicles at a more appropriate level for sperm production.

Making Babies: The High-Tech Way

Most gynecologists recommend that you see a fertility specialist (or reproductive endocrinologist) if you've been trying to get pregnant for more than a year without success. Though 12 months can seem like an eternity once you decide to start a family, it actually takes an average of 7 months for healthy couples to conceive. When you think about it, reproduction is truly a miracle. Not only do your sex organs and hormones need to be in sync, there's that mere three- to four-day window of opportunity for the egg and sperm to meet. Even the slightest malfunction can cause infertility.

Fortunately, this is a diagnosis most couples can overcome, thanks to amazing advancements in reproductive medicine. But it's not easy.

Infertility treatment results in a lot of nail-biting and anxiety, as well as a fair share of physical and mental discomfort for both partners. Right from the start, your fertility specialist is likely to put you through a battery of tests.

Because 40 percent of infertility is related to low sperm counts and motility (the inability for the little guys to swim fast enough to fertilize the egg), you'll have to provide a sperm sample for a count. Many doctors provide cozy little rooms with a selection of X-rated flicks and skin mags to help speed up the monkey-spanking process. But don't be surprised if you find yourself in a cold bathroom stall with nothing more than tiled walls to arouse you. Fertility clinics are notoriously female-focused, so we suggest you arrive prepared—with your own stash of reading material or a wife who is willing to help out.

Of course, she's likely to experience an even heftier dose of poking, prodding, and yanking. Women must undergo several standard fertility tests before a diagnosis can be made. All are designed to ensure that her sex organs are functioning properly, and all involve considerably more discomfort than those cold tile walls. There is a procedure called a hysterosalpingogram, for example, in which a dye is injected into woman's cervix and observed via X-ray as it passes through her uterus and fallopian tubes. Cramping is common—and sometimes severe—for hours after the exam.

"With fertility drugs and procedures such as in vitro fertilization, not only is it possible for couples to have a family who could never conceive on their own; it gives women the opportunity to give birth well beyond their peak childbearing years."

If the tubes are obstructed (a common cause of infertility), the doctor will then prescribe a surgical procedure called a laporoscopy. Though it's performed on an outpatient basis, the surgery requires general anesthesia and results in at least a few days of bed rest.

The purpose of a laporoscopy is to provide the physician with a detailed, inside view of a woman's uterus, fallopian tubes, and ovaries. It also provides an opportunity for the doctor to correct mild blockage or scarring in the tubes. However, if serious problems are detected, a second surgery may be recommended.

This may sound like a lot to go through to have children. And couples who have "been there, done that" may agree. But assisted reproduction is truly remarkable. With fertility drugs and procedures such as in vitro fertilization, not only is it possible for couples to have a family who could never conceive on their own; it gives women the opportunity to give birth well beyond their peak childbearing years.

We should note that infertility treatment is not without its risks. Multiple births are on the rise due to the increased use of fertility drugs.

One of the more powerful pharmaceuticals, an injectable drug called Metrodin, was responsible for the Iowa septuplets, the seven babies born to Bobbi and Kenny McCaughey in late 1997. They were lucky. Though their children were born about six weeks early, they were relatively healthy. Most parents of multiples don't have such happy endings. The babies are born so early—with so many problems—many don't survive and those that do have long-term physical ailments.

For this reason, the ethics of infertility treatment has sparked great debate. While there is great sympathy for infertile couples, there are also valid concern regarding the ethics and risks of the today's more invasive procedures and experimental ones (such as human cloning).

Our advice to couples who find themselves knocking on an infertility specialist's door: Read up on treatments available, so there are no surprises. Some of the best books on the subject include:

- *In Pursuit of Fertility: A Fertility Expert Tells You How to Get Pregnant* (by Robert R. Franklin, Veasy C. Buttram, and Dorothy K. Brockman; Henry Holt, 1996)

- *Overcoming Infertility: A Compassionate Resource for Getting Pregnant* (by Robert Jansen; W. H. Freeman & Co., 1998)

- *The Couple's Guide to Fertility: Updated with the Newest Scientific Techniques to Help You Have a Baby* (by Marc Goldstein, Mark Fuerst, and Gary S. Berger; Main Street Books, 1995)

Children: The First Change of Life

Once that home pregnancy test strip turns blue, you'll be facing a whole new set of challenges. For the next nine months, sex will

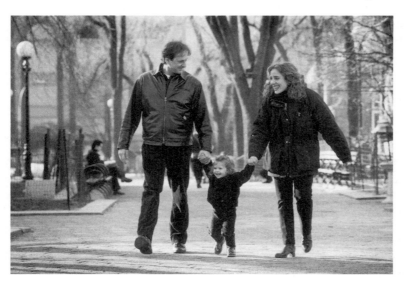

be vastly different. You and your partner may have all kinds of anxieties about "hurting" the baby. Don't worry. Unless your doctor tells you to avoid intercourse (which only happens if there is a threat of miscarriage), you can romp with abandon.

And don't worry . . . there is absolutely no chance Mr. Happy will come in contact with Junior. Likewise, there is no chance that Junior will be scarred for life by catching an early glimpse of Mr. Happy. In fact, the only thing you really need to worry about is satisfying your hungry partner. And we're not talkin' food cravings.

The hormonal surges of pregnancy cause many women who are otherwise quite passive in bed to become total wildcats. "Pregnancy made me hornier than I've ever been in my life," says Nancy, a 35-year-old mother of two from Chicago. "I couldn't keep my hands off my husband. He was exhausted."

Most OB/GYNs say it's safe to have sex up until the baby is delivered as long as the woman is comfortable. The key is to use positions, such as Woman on Top and Rear Entry that don't put pressure on her growing abdomen. Oral sex is okay, too. Just be careful not to blow air into her vagina. Doing so could force air into the bloodstream and cause an embolism (obstructing a blood vessel), which might prove deadly to both mother and child.

> "The hormonal surges of pregnancy cause many women who are otherwise quite passive in bed to become total wildcats."

That's the deal on sex during pregnancy. After the child is born there are other hurdles to cross. The first is getting past the vision of your partner giving birth. Most women will agree: About the only thing better than the presence of their partner in the delivery room is an epidural anesthetic placed strategically in their spine. If you're in the delivery room, you will immeasurably help her get through the agony of childbirth. The downside is that you may view her body—particularly her sexual organs—in an entirely different light.

"It's understandable that men change their view of the woman's sexual anatomy after pregnancy and childbirth," says Britton. "Fortunately, the image fades much more quickly than the average guy's sex drive. It's really much more difficult for a woman to rebuild her sexual image after having a baby. She may be carrying extra weight. If it was a difficult birth, sexual intercourse may be painful for months after the delivery. It will take a while for her to get back to where she was before motherhood."

Here again, making time for intimacy becomes critical in keeping your relationship going strong. It's very easy to go so gaga over your beautiful baby that you forget about each other. You'll want to work through the kinks of postpregnancy sex slowly and carefully, Britton advises, and definitely have a list of baby-sitters you can call when you need a night out alone. "This one-on-one time is essential," she says.

To put this new family life into perspective, we asked writer Kevin Cook to chronicle his experiences after the birth of his first child.

Tales From the Crib: One Man's Story

They warned us. Friends, relatives, even the UPS man nodded at my pregnant wife's belly and said, "Just wait. You'll never be the same after the baby comes."

"Right. That's the idea," my wife, Pamela, said. After all, Pamela and I had never imagined parenthood would be a mild diversion, like premium cable. We wanted a mission. We had already done the carefree thing, spending our twenties and early thirties exactly as we pleased, eating and drinking and smoking ourselves silly, blowing our money on plane tickets and champagne. But even the snappiest tune wears thin with repetition. At last we decided to beget with the program.

Another reason for action was Pamela's biological clock. It was melting. As she passed her 33rd birthday, still totless, her mood swings began showing up on radar. We pictured her ovaries glowing in the dark. "Seed me," she said.

Our final reason to spawn: death. Through some cosmic snafu, the general rule of mortality seems to apply to Pamela and me as well as to everyone else. We plan to file an appeal; the problem is jurisdiction. Meanwhile, we settled for entwining our DNA into something new, tethering ourselves to the future before our souls could slip away.

The Bentleys laughed at us. They said parenthood wouldn't make us immortal—it would make us boring.

The Bentleys, Penny and Jon, are our yuppie friends. She's a doctor; he's a chef. They are dinner-party animals. Childless by choice, prizing their carefreedom, they won't have kids because kids have stolen so many of their friends. "Poof. The baby comes and you vanish," Penny said.

"You unmake the scene," said Jon. "There's one final cell-phone transmission about little Tyler or Alison, 7 pounds 10 ounces. Then silence."

". . . parenthood wouldn't make us immortal—it would make us boring."

"Even if you pop up again a year or so later, it's not the same. All you'll talk about is spit-up, bowel movements . . ." We all laughed, looking at Pamela's stomach.

Up All Night Then Cal arrived, all wet and red with big, immortal eyes. He took over the house. His feeding schedule kept us awake almost the entire night. Pamela did all the hard work, but I, too, learned how quickly sleep deprivation can give you a window on psychosis—the grinning teddy bears and Raggedy Andys of the apocalypse.

We learned to sleep hard. It turns out a first-time parent can dream a night's worth in 15 minutes. I had Schwarzenegger dreams in which I defended the baby against evil armies of skeletons on Harleys. It was the first time I'd ever worn a bandoleer.

Of course, we had no time to return our friends' calls. Maybe tomorrow, or when Cal goes to kindergarten. Books and newspapers were off-limits; they used up precious sleep and/or burping time. Still, those early days brought valuable new knowledge. I learned why Kmart shoppers look that way: They all have young kids. Frantic efficiency experts like me, they wear the same clothes for days on end, and, man or woman, they don't have time to shave.

I became one of those shoppers you hate—the guy shifting his yelling infant from one shoulder to the other as he takes a full minute to dig through his pockets for his wallet at the cash register. I'll empty my pockets, spilling keys, pacifiers, change, nursing bottle, lint, a dead moth, and one tiny sock. But no wallet. My wallet is in a sandbox somewhere.

One day, walletless, I shoplifted diapers and kept waiting to hear sirens and police choppers. But that day, crime paid. A minute after our escape, Cal unleashed a quarter-pound steamer in his swiped dipe. Who says there's no adventure in this job?

An expert diaperist, I am a stool student. Nothing pleases Pamela and me like a firm, healthy log in Cal's diaper. We debrief each other on his dumps: "It was nice and smooth, tapered at the top, kind of like a Henry Moore," she says.

All Booked Up We plan to get back to the Bentleys. We must thank them for the silver Tiffany's spoon they sent baby Cal, though it came too late for him to be born with it in his mouth. Penny has left a few messages. She says we must dine ensemble. We will, but she's talking about Thursday, and we're thinking 2003.

They must think we're boring. But we think we've merely traded a couple years of party time for Cal time. And while it has been every bit the challenge the UPS man said it would be, there's at least as much good magic as bad sleep in the job.

Sometimes I miss debating books and plays and TV over fine wine with the Bentleys, but the crows Cal and I watch outside our house are cool. Crows are all Jack Nicholson. One will fluff himself up and caw tough, sidling over to a mockingbird's nest to maybe cop an egg. Then mockingbird dad starts dive-bombing him, and he flies off cussing. Cal and I can watch crows for hours.

Soap bubbles are hilarious. So are mirrors—step right up and see you! A trash truck, a helicopter, rain, ice, ants—all miracles.

Like all tykes, Cal loves early Elvis. We sing and dance to "All Shook Up," with its goofy country lyrics, and "Blue Suede Shoes." Yesterday we were showing off for the neighbors and I asked him who's the greatest singer in the world. I expected the cute answer "Elvis!" and got something better instead: "Daddy!" Now, you can knock me down, step on my face, slander my name all over the place, but that's mine forever. Roll over, Elvis, I'm the king around here.

Cal is three now. Pamela and I are seriously considering adult company again. After a long search involving local experts, the FBI, and

Interpol, we have found a baby-sitter we trust. We're dipping our toes in the party waters again. Pamela and I think we've beaten BPS—the dreaded Boring Parent Syndrome. In fact we're planning to host the Bentleys at our crib next week. There's only one thing we have to work out: What color wine goes with oatmeal?

#2   Male Menopause

It begins with the slightest twinge of self-doubt, then progresses to become an incessant tick-tock pounding away at your psyche: *life is passing me by, life is passing me by, life is passing me by.* That's not bad enough ... perhaps you've gained weight that only a year ago would have been erased in a few quick trips to the gym. Now, no amount of sweat makes a difference.

And sexually—sexually you have lost a step, so to speak. It may take longer to get aroused, or may require an undue amount of fantasizing. And once you get an erection, it may not be as rock-hard as it was when you tumbled in the backseat after Junior Prom. Worse yet, it may not stay as hard as long ... or you may sometimes have trouble even getting an erection.

Taken in total, these occurrences—the physical changes as well as the emotional weight of not being where you thought you'd be at this stage of life—is enough to make a man's world come crashing down around him. The convenient term for the collective problems hitting a man as he begins to gray? A midlife crisis.

Red Convertibles and Corvettes

"I worked as a university administrator for a number of years," says Joel, a retiree in Tempe, Arizona. "I was younger than my fellow administrators by a good ten years, so I thought it was funny that, over the course of the summer, most of the sensible family vans and station wagons in the administrator parking lot were replaced by red convertibles, Corvettes, and muscle cars. It's as if everyone suddenly wanted to recapture their youth. A few of my colleagues even began cheating on their wives, having affairs with students half their age. A few got divorced. I thought it was comical ... but I was reminded of all those weird signposts years later when I started to see that I wasn't where I thought I'd be at age forty. I really had a hard time coping with the fact that my tennis game slowed considerably ... and that in the bedroom things didn't always ... progress ... as I wanted. I was raised to believe that virility defined a man. So I began clutching at straws—getting into extreme sports like rock climbing—to try to prove myself. One day I was hanging from a rock face by my fingertips and I realized that I felt foolish ... as if I had tried to be a kid instead of take growing older ... growing up ... in stride. And I realized I was having a psychological problem ... a midlife crisis."

While Joel's tale is similar to that of countless men across the nation, there may be cause to rethink his conclusion that there's a psychological condition called a midlife crisis floating in the time stream, just waiting to strike your mind when you've put another candle on the birthday cake. In fact, a growing number of medical practitioners are beginning to attribute the so-called midlife crisis phenomenon to acute hormonal, physiological, and chemical changes that occur when a man reaches middle age. A male menopause, if you will.

> "... a growing number of medical practitioners are beginning to attribute the so-called midlife crisis phenomenon to acute hormonal, physiological, and chemical changes that occur when a man reaches middle age."

According to Theresa Crenshaw, M.D., the medical community is only now beginning to understand the biochemistry involved in male menopause (sometimes called viropause or andropause). In her book *The Alchemy of Love and Lust*, she describes three different testosterone phases in man. The first, as we've mentioned in chapter 2, occurs in a man's adolescence and postadolescence, when testosterone levels wildly fluctuate minute by minute. The second phase occurs when a man is "in his prime," from his twenties to his late thirties, when testosterone levels peak and remain consistent. The third phase, the andropausal phase, occurs as a man hits midlife. And that's the phase in which testosterone levels drop. In some men, the decreases are almost unnoticeable. But in some other men, the levels drop dramatically.

Since testosterone is what makes men men, some significant things take place when the levels drop. Sex drive diminishes. Psychologically, a diminished sex drive plays havoc with a man's emotions. And since testosterone acts as a natural antidepressant, a reduction of the hormone can actually cause more severe depression over the diminished sex drive.

Midlife also marks a decrease in dehydroepiandrosterone (DHEA) levels—DHEA impacts a man's sex drive, so a decrease also heralds a diminished sex drive. A significant drop in DHEA can lead to impotence in men.

A vicious cycle of sorts occurs during these downward swings in DHEA levels: Stress has been known to lower DHEA levels. A lower DHEA level means a diminished sex drive. A man begins to worry about his waning drive and gets stressed out. DHEA levels drop enough further. And so on.

Women aren't the only ones who complain of headaches. When men hit midlife, hormonal changes can cause their libidos to go limp. Experts recommend that partners keep open lines of communication. And don't hesitate to seek professional assistance.

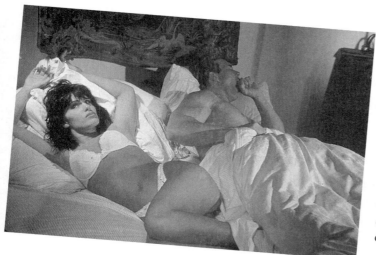

Decreases in testosterone and DHEA aren't the only things to worry about. According to psychotherapist Jed Diamond in his book *Male Menopause*, midlife is marked by decreased levels of dopamine, oxytocin, vasopressin, growth hormone, melatonin, and pregnenolone—a veritable stew of hormones that, at adequate levels, maintain a man's physical and emotional well-being. However, decreased levels can contribute to weight gain, decreased sex drive, depression, and general poor health.

"I knew something was happening to me," says Keith, a marketing consultant in New York City. "I felt sluggish, moody, bloated. My wife joked that I had PMS. I began reading up on midlife issues and found a lot of interesting stuff on male menopause. It made sense . . . the notion that my body was changing physically and hormonally. And that was affecting my behavior."

Medical Conflicts

Still, some in the medical community refuse to believe that a male menopause occurs, treating men suffering from a midlife crisis with antidepressants and therapy—just as medical practitioners did decades ago when treating menopausal women. At that time, some doctors thought menopause was "all in a woman's mind," just as some doctors today think male menopause is "all in a man's mind." Further, some women's groups decry the use of the term menopause in male menopause, thinking it takes away from an event that was, until now, exclusively a woman's rite of passage. Then there are those who think male menopause is just a convenient excuse for men to revel in childish behavior.

"When I identified what I was going through as male menopause," Keith says, "my wife's first impression was that I was making excuses . . . 'You men are always looking for a way out,' she said. But then I started comparing what I was going through with what she was . . . and but for the exception of her [menstrual] period stopping, every symptom matched between us. That's when we both realized a major change was happening in both of us . . . not just her."

According to Diamond, the symptoms of male menopause can include:

- taking longer to recover from injuries and illnesses
- less endurance for physical activities

- feeling fat or gaining weight
- difficulty reading small print
- forgetfulness or memory loss
- loss or thinning of hair
- irritability
- indecisiveness
- anxiety and fear
- depression
- loss of self-confidence and joy
- loss of purpose and direction in life
- feeling lonely, unattractive, and unloved
- reduced interest in sex
- increased anxiety and fear about sexual changes
- increased fantasies about having sex with others
- loss of erection during sexual activity
- the force of ejaculation isn't as strong as it once was
- erections take longer to occur.

"Then there are those who think male menopause is just a convenient excuse for men to revel in childish behavior."

A daunting list, but Diamond believes the move to midlife is positive, regardless of the problems. He writes:

"The purpose of male menopause is to signal the end of the first part of a man's life and prepare him for the second half. Male menopause is not the beginning of the end, as many fear, but the end of the beginning. It is the passage to the most passionate, powerful, productive and purposeful time of a man's life."

Given that the average American lifespan is in the mid-seventies, hitting 40 or 50 doesn't mean the end of life. It just means that a second adulthood has arrived, one in which a man can use all the knowledge and resources accumulated during his first adulthood (the twenties and thirties) and apply them for the rest of his days.

To accomplish this, Diamond recommends a 12-step program—no, not one of those. This one involves nutrition, self-exploration, and physical fitness to ease a man's passage to his "second adulthood." Here a summary:

1. **Eat right.** A traditional Asian diet, heavy on grains, vegetables, and fruits is best for your body. This type of diet limits meat and eliminates virtually all dairy products. Diamond points to the fact that Asian countries have lower incidence of heart disease, diabetes, and cancer, and that the life expectancy in Japan is the highest in the world. He attributes this to the traditional Asian diet.

2. Stay physically fit. Develop—and stick to—a program that combines aerobic conditioning, strength-building, and flexibility exercises. At any age, you can tweak your libido without hormones simply by working out. In a University of California study of 95 out-of-shape men, average age 47, 17 took strolls for an hour three days a week, while 78 did strenuous aerobic workouts. After nine months, the strollers reported no change in sexual desire or activity, and an increase in sexual problems. But the aerobic exercisers reported a jump in sexual desire, a 30-percent increase in frequency of intercourse, fewer sexual problems, and more pleasure from orgasm.

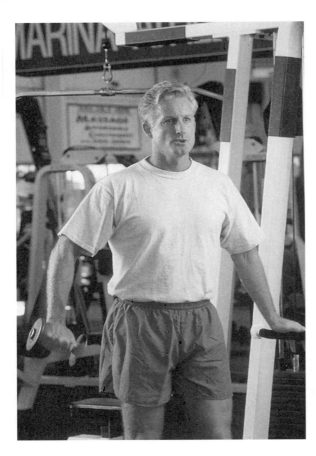

A Harvard study of male swimmers aged 40 to 69 came to the same conclusion. Those in their forties reported having sex about seven times a month; those in their sixties, only slightly less often. Eighty percent of the swimmers also said they considered themselves more attractive than most other men their age. Significantly, their wives and girlfriends rated them even more attractive than they rated themselves.

Weight loss can also bring about a jump in sexual vigor. When 44-year-old *Newsweek* correspondent Thomas M. DeFrank enrolled in the Duke University Diet and Fitness Center program, lost 47 pounds and saw his cholesterol drop from a hazardous 242 to an exemplary 166, he discovered an unexpected fringe benefit: "To my utter amazement—and the delight of my slightly shell-shocked girlfriend—I was suddenly imbued with the sexual energy of a 20-year-old lifeguard," he wrote.

Comments like DeFrank's prompted Duke University's Ronette Kolotkin, Ph.D., to survey the sexual effects of weight loss on 70 people, average age 42. "Moderate weight loss [8 to 30 pounds] significantly improved the men's sexual functioning and satisfaction," Kolotkin says. "At every age, participants said losing weight boosted libido, increased frequency of intercourse, and enhanced sexual enjoyment. Sexuality is one way the body celebrates its vitality. Renewed interest in sex is the body's way of saying thanks for losing weight."

3. Vitamin supplements. Diamond says the following daily formula will boost your energy levels:

- 10,000 international units (IU) of mixed carotenoids
- 800 IU of vitamin E
- 200 mcg. of selenium
- 2,000 mg. of vitamin C two or three times a day
- 30 mg. of zinc
- 80 mg. of coenzyme Q

4. **Herbal supplements.** Diamond feels herbs can "rebalance" a physiology that has been thrown for a loop because of hormonal changes. He cites:

- wild yam for hormone-building assistance
- black cohosh as a relaxant
- damiana as an antidepressant
- St. John's Wort to deal with depression and stress
- saw palmetto to aid in maintaining a healthy prostate.

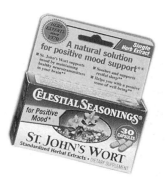

5. **Get regular checkups.** By getting an annual checkup, men can practice preventative medicine, instead of reacting to maladies.

6. **Check hormone levels.** Increasingly, medical practitioners are seeing the value of hormone replacement therapy for men. It's something that's been practiced for years in Europe . . . but then again, the medical community in Europe is uniform in its belief that there is such a thing as male menopause. Check with practitioners in your area regarding hormone checks and treatments.

7. **Reduce stress.** It's easier said than done, but stress can lead to other ailments. Meditation is a good stress reliever, as is physical activity (see number 2 above.)

   Perhaps the most important factor in retaining your sexuality long term is just to avoid getting anxious about it. Stress is a major desire killer for anyone, but it's especially pernicious for men over 40—guys who are not only preoccupied with work, bills, and family, but who also may believe the myth that after the Big Four-O, they're sexually over the hill. "Stop worrying that 40—or any age—signals the beginning of the end," San Francisco–based sex therapist Louanne Cole Weston, Ph.D., says. "You can have great sex at any age." In fact, women often prefer men who don't have rockets in their pockets but instead become aroused more slowly.

8. **Embrace a sexuality appropriate to the second half of life.** This is key. Instead of the "hot, fast" rules of sexual engagement practiced by twentysomethings, men in their forties and fifties need to

readjust their expectations—and themselves. Intimacy wins out over lust, and relationships win out over nameless, faceless sex.

9. **Become initiated into elderhood.** Diamond stresses that the word "elder" shouldn't be viewed as a negative—in most cultures (except ours, unfortunately) elders are the people in the community with the most wisdom and experience. Therefore, elders are revered. Diamond suggests getting in contact with the New Warrior Network (1-800-870-4611) for their program on elderhood.

10. **Join a men's group.** Talk to other men. Share. Support by other men lessens the stigma of male menopause.

11. **Explore your lifework.** According to Diamond, in the first half of their lives, men seek out careers that will provide the most security and financial support. In the second half of their lives, men should seek out that which fulfills them. At the start of this phase, you face one of two developmental choices: You can do nothing and stagnate. Or you can seek out new interests, ideas, and different horizons, generating a fuller life.

12. **Become a mentor to a young man.** In Diamond's view, men need to take responsibility for themselves—and for young males. By "acting out" in middle age—that is, trying to recapture youth with the red convertibles and young blondes—midlife crisis men send a clear message to our youth. That message: Growing older is something to fear. Seeing that, young people, in turn, will devolve into arrested adolescence, avoiding growing older—and growing up— because it's frightening.

Instead, Diamond suggests mentoring, imparting wisdom to young men, in order to show them that middle age is nothing to fear. That way, middle-aged men can help shape the impressions of youth and help young people grow to a new level of maturity.

#3   The Changes in Lovemaking Styles

Given the physical changes that can occur during male and female menopause, one of the most important challenges for couples as they get older is to understand that styles of lovemaking may change. So, it's important to keep the lines of communication open. Talk with your significant other about your feelings and any inadequacies you suspect may be cropping up in the bedroom. Chances are, your loved one will be compassionate and willing to work through any trouble spots. Above all, don't think that your sexual life stops at forty.

"Men don't stop having sex because they grow older," agrees Los Angeles urologist Dudley Seth Danoff, M.D., author of *Superpotency: How to Get It, Use It, and Maintain It for a Lifetime*. "They grow older because they stop having sex. Sex makes older men feel happier and younger. It can give as much joy at 70 as it did at 20. Some men say it's ever better."

Likewise, many women enjoy a heightened libido after menopause, because they no longer have to worry about birth control or fear an unwanted pregnancy.

Learn to Enjoy the Buildup

As you get older, you may not be able to get an erection in the blink of an eye, but look on the bright side: Long, leisurely lovemaking can be pretty awesome. In fact, many women claim to have their best sex ever after 40, primarily because the men in their lives have to take it slow. As long as you and your partner keep open lines of communication—and understand the changes that are occurring in each of your bodies—you can maintain a healthy sex life for the rest of your lives.

Another piece of advice: Don't be driven by orgasm. As a man gets older, he may not ejaculate as frequently as he did when he was young. And intercourse may be uncomfortable for her. Neither is a problem that can't be dealt with; they're just facts of aging. Accepting your changes will enable you to enjoy lovemaking for the intimacy and pleasure it brings to your relationship.

#4   Empty Nest Syndrome

You're in your fifties. The kids are off at college. You and your wife are alone in the house together for the first time in 18 years. But instead of taking the opportunity to swing naked from chandeliers, have sex on the kitchen floor, and talk all night long about absolutely nothing, you just stare at each other like strangers. Hello, empty nest syndrome—one of the leading reasons couples divorce later in life.

If you and your spouse find yourself in this position at any point in your later years, we suggest that you immediately flip to chapter 9, Hot for the Long Haul, to see if there are some ways in which you can rekindle your love. Sometimes it just takes a little work to get reacquainted and to remember what brought the two of you together in the first place. Something sparked the romance. And you may be surprised at how easily you can get that spark back.

> "... instead of taking the opportunity to swing naked from chandeliers, have sex on the kitchen floor, and talk all night long about absolutely nothing, you just stare at each other like strangers."

On the other hand, some things just can't be fixed, in which case you might want to flip to chapter 7 for our Troubleshooting advice about coping with a divorce.

#5 The Medical Milieu

Several medical conditions may impact your sexuality as you grow older. Here is a roundup of the most common:

Testicular Cancer

Youth is a disadvantage when it comes to testicular cancer, a disease that primarily strikes men between the ages of 20 and 34. Though thousands of cases are detected annually, Caucasian men are the most vulnerable. Very few Native Americans, Hispanics, or Asians experience it, and almost no African Americans.

Fortunately, testicular cancer can be detected early through self-exams, and when treated promptly, has a 93 percent cure rate, according to the National Cancer Institute. The key is to perform frequent self-exams. Just as women are advised to examine their breasts monthly, men need to give their testicles a good feel, preferably on a daily basis.

". . . testicular cancer can be detected early through self-exams, and when treated promptly, has a 93 percent cure rate, according to the National Cancer Institute."

Don't freak out if you discover a lump. It may just be a cyst. But be sure to schedule a doctor's appointment pronto. Your physician will probably be able to make a diagnosis with a physical exam; however, a sonogram may be required for confirmation.

If the lump turns out to be a tumor, a surgeon generally removes the testicle for a biopsy, a precaution that's also taken to prevent the cancer from spreading to the scrotum, lymph nodes, and other parts of the body. (Testicular cancer is highly curable when detected early, but spreads quickly when ignored.) Treatment usually includes radiation, chemotherapy, and surgery, depending upon the severity of the condition.

Please keep in mind that a single testicle can provide enough sperm and testosterone to father children and maintain a healthy sex life. And the chance of a reoccurrence of the disease can be as low as 1 percent. But again, the key is early detection.

Prostate Concerns

No matter how health-conscious you are, some prostate trouble is inevitable during your life span, says Rosenthal. But it's not as scary as you might think—and it doesn't have to interfere with your sex life. Here's a look at what might crop up.

Benign Prostatic Hypertrophy (BPH) By your fifties and sixties, you may begin to notice changes in your urinary and sexual function caused by enlargement of your prostate gland. Normally the size of a walnut, the prostate can increase to 15 times that and weigh as much as a half-pound if left unchecked. An oversized prostate can obstruct your urinary passage, or in the worst cases, totally block urine outflow.

This condition, called benign prostatic hypertrophy or BPH, tends to happen very gradually and is almost inevitable if you live to see your eighties. Studies show that 85 percent of all men who reach 85 will experience BPH. And you'll have the condition long before exhibiting any of the symptoms. Among them are an increased need to urinate during the night, difficulty getting the stream started, a stream that's more like a drippy faucet than a fire hose, painful or uncomfortable urination, an urge to urinate more often, dribbling after you think you're through, and blood in the urine. Fortunately, the only effect BPH may have on your sexual functioning is a decrease in the force of your ejaculation.

Treatment: If your doctor discovers the problem during a routine exam, chances are he'll just recommend waiting and watching. He'll also advise you to cut out caffeine and spicy food, which tend to irritate the bladder, drink lots of water, ejaculate as often as possible and de-stress. If you're exhibiting symptoms, he may prescribe the drug finasteride (Proscar), which shrinks the prostate by up to 30 percent.

Surgery becomes necessary if blood is detected in the urine. There are three procedures that have proven successful in alleviating BPH. With a transurethral resection of the prostate, a small tube is inserted through the urethra to the prostate. A lens in the tube has a loop of wire through which an electrical current is passed to cut the blocking tissue.

Another type of surgery involves carving away a chunk of the prostate and the sphincter muscle. (With BPH, the sphincter is unable to relax, thus making it difficult to urinate.) The downside of this procedure is retrograde ejaculation—a part of the semen goes into the bladder during orgasm.

A final operation known as transurethral incision of the prostate involves slicing the gland (rather than removing a portion of it) to minimize pressure on the urethra. Aside from being less invasive, it results in less retrograde ejaculation.

Prostatitis This is an inflammation of the prostate gland and can happen at any age. Acute prostatitis and chronic prostatitis are caused by a bacterial infection. Fever, chills, nausea, vomiting, inability to begin urinating, or painful, burning urination are evidence of acute prostatitis. Chronic prostatitis has similar symptoms except you may not have a fever. The most common prostatitis is a nonbacterial form, which also results in fever, chills, nausea, and vomiting, but fewer urination problems. And a final type, prostatodynia, is a painful condition that is believed to be caused by a muscle spasm or pinched nerve.

Treatment: Both acute and chronic prostatitis are treated with a course of antibiotics. Some doctors also recommend supplementing your medicine regimen with more frequent ejaculations to eliminate

Testicular Self-examination

The best time to examine your testicles is during or after a shower or warm bath, when your scrotal sac is relaxed. Check one at a time. Put your index and middle fingers of both hands under the testicle, and rest your thumbs on top. Gently roll the testicle between the thumbs and fingers and feel for any small lumps. Also feel for swelling or hardening of the entire testicle. Though it's common for one testicle to be larger than the other, take note if one is larger than it normally is.

Other signs you should watch for: a dull ache in the lower abdomen or the groin, pain or discomfort in the testicle or scrotum, or fluid in the scrotum. If any of these symptoms last as long as two weeks, call your doctor. For more info, call the National Cancer Institute at 800-422-6237 or the American Cancer Society at 800-227-2345.

the bacteria. The cause and cure for nonbacterial prostatitis are still unknown, so the best advice your doctor will give you to alleviate the symptoms of this condition is a dose of Ibuprofen every few hours and a warm bath. Warm baths help prostatodynia, too, as does an alpha-blocker prescription drug that calms the stressed muscle.

> **"Normally the size of a walnut, the prostate can increase to 15 times that and weigh as much as a half-pound if left unchecked."**

Prostate Cancer This is the disease elderly men dread—and rightfully so. Prostate cancer kills more than forty thousand American men each year. Though prostate cancer is rarely seen in men under 40, the American Cancer Society recommends yearly rectal exams beginning at that age and a prostate specific antigen (PSA) test starting at age 50—or age 40 for African American males or any man with a history of the disease.

> **"Prostate cancer kills more than forty thousand American men each year."**

Sure, the sound of your doc snapping on his rubber glove may be unnerving. But consider the consequences: The longer prostate cancer goes undetected, the more difficult it is to cure. Because the disease usually starts in a part of the gland that is farther from the urinary tract, it rarely cause the kinds of early warning symptoms that would get your attention. Therefore that rectal exam becomes an all-important means of early detection.

What will your doctor be feeling for? A cancerous prostate feels like a hard knuckle (compared to a soft muscle when healthy). For an even more precise diagnosis, your doctor may recommend a PSA test. This blood test has been available since 1994 and correctly detects nine out of ten cancers. The downside: It frequently gives false positive results, citing prostate cancer that is really BPH or a prostate infection.

If the rectal exam or PSA indicate cancer, the next step is a biopsy. Your doctor will perform this procedure in his office, inserting a gun-like instrument into your anus and removing tissue samples via tiny needles in the instrument. (Don't worry. It's not nearly as bad as it sounds.)

Treatment: Prostate cancer is one of the more mysterious forms of the disease, as it does not respond to typical forms of treatment, like chemotherapy. Hence there are three alternatives:

- **Watch and wait:** Prostate cancer can progress very slowly. If the patient is 70 when it is detected, his physician may not be inclined to put him through surgery. The risk in taking this course of action is that the disease will advance too far to be treated.

- **Radiation:** If performed correctly, radiation is relatively safe with only minor side effects (such as fatigue). The risk is that it won't zap all of the cancer.

Eating for a Healthier Prostate

One way to slow the growth of prostate cancer, if you've already been diagnosed with the disease, is to make some dietary changes.

- **Avoid alpha-linolenic acids.** Say, what? Okay, alpha-linolenic acid is a fancy term for the fatty acids found in animal fats, mayonnaise, creamy salad dressings, butter, and margarine. Research has shown that high alpha intakes are associated with increased prostate cancer. So avoid them or keep them to a minimum.

- **Just say no to saturated fats.** It's a consensus among health professionals: Maintaining a low fat diet is critical in staving off prostate cancer. A Harvard University study confirmed that men who eat a lot of fat—the equivalent of three quarter-pounds of juicy red meat per day—have more late-stage prostate cancer than their fish-and-poultry eating counterparts.

- **Do the Ds.** Skim milk and fish are excellent sources of vitamin D, which acts as a cell regulator in the prostate.

- **Get milk.** Another benefit of guzzling a glass or two of skim milk is calcium. Studies suggest that when the body does not receive enough of this mineral, tumor growth may accelerate. The theory is still speculative, but docs recommend 1,000 milligrams of calcium per day just in case. Leafy green vegetables are another great source of calcium. Or you could swallow a supplement.

- **Soy your wild oats.** Soybean products—a great source of protein—have proven to halt the growth of prostate cancer. Compounds in the soybean, called genistein and daidzein, are the keys. And soy meals can be tasty. We recently had soy cheese quesadillas that were as delicious as the traditional versions.

- **Antioxidants rule.** Vitamins C, E, and beta-carotene have proven effective in limiting the cell injuries caused by early phases of prostate cancer. You'll get your fair share by eating yellow, orange, and dark green fruits and vegetables, nuts, and vegetable oils.

- **Celebrate garlic breath.** Research proves that a diet high in garlic reduces your chances of getting cancer of any type. If you don't want to turn off your partner by consuming mass quantities of the real stuff, try garlic supplements. Otherwise, douse yourself in cologne and carry some breath mints.

- **Tea time.** Compounds in Green tea, an Asian staple, have shown an ability to prevent the growth of skin and esophageal tumors. Researchers are hopeful that the beverage will have the same impact on prostate tissue.

- **Spice it up.** Some researchers believe that cumin, a spice derived from turmeric, fights prostate cancer. It's used commonly in Asian and Mediterranean dishes. Note: spicy foods can irritate the prostate in some men. You'll need to see how you react to this one before making it a permanent part of your diet.

Wonder Substance

An ongoing study being conducted by Dr. Edward L. Giovannuci at Harvard University indicates that a substance called lycopene, a sibling of beta-carotene, could be the newest cancer preventer. Preliminary evidence presented at a national prostate cancer conference suggests that a weekly diet of five or more tomatoes (rich in lycopene) may reduce your risk of prostate cancer by as much as 40 percent. The best sources of lycopene in order:

- canned tomato juice
- canned tomato paste
- raw watermelon
- raw tomato
- raw pink grapefruit
- guava juice
- dried apricot
- canned rose hip puree

- **Radical prostatectomy:** This is the only way to make sure you get all of the cancer (if it's caught in time). Studies have shown 85 percent of the men who undergo this surgery to be cancer-free ten years later. According to the American Cancer Society, the five-year survival rate following this surgery is 92 percent, provided the cancer is detected before it spreads to other organs. Of course, this surgery may impair your sexual functioning. Weaker erections are practically a given, and many men who have the operation are rendered permanently impotent. There is also a temporary period of incontinence following the surgery (permanent for a few). You'll want to do a lot of research to find the best surgeon. The more successful a doc's record, the more likely you are to fall outside the aforementioned statistics.

If the cancer spreads beyond the gland, treatment typically involves radiation in conjunction with hormonal therapy that shuts down the production of testosterone (the hormone that fuels the growth of the prostate).

Arthritis

It doesn't take a rocket scientist to figure out that the side effects of arthritis—stiffness, pain, and fatigue—can directly affect your sexual life. The question is: what can you do about it?

You can pop some pain relievers for temporary relief. But for the long term, you need to give more thought to the positions you use, the time of day you make love (some forms of arthritis act up in the morning, others in the evening), and what causes pleasure versus pain. In *Sex Over 40,* Rosenthal sites "spoon," "standing rear-entry," and "woman on top" as a few of the more comfortable positions. He also recommends doing some stretching exercises before sex to loosen the muscles and joints.

A warm shower or bath before lovemaking also can be a sensual way to help ease the discomforts of arthritis, and if your partner suffers from arthritis, you may need to use a lubricant. Some forms of the disease are accompanied by a condition called Sjogrens syndrome, which causes a decrease in the secretions throughout your body, including vaginal lubrication. Also consider oral sex—it's a great way to free up aching hands. For more information, contact the Arthritis Foundation at 1-800-283-7800 and request its pamphlet *Living and Loving.*

Heart Disease

You've seen it in countless movies and TV shows: an older guy gets it on with a young, nubile sexpot and dies of a heart attack in the midst of doing the deed. Well, you can relax, guys. The incidences of a partner dying during sex is rare. Rest assured, your pulse rate does not go up significantly when you are making love. In a study conducted at Case Western Reserve School of Medicine, men were outfitted with cardiac monitors to record their pulse rate continuously throughout the day. The highest it got was an average rate of 120 beats per minute (bpm). (Sex clocked in at 117 bpm.)

Still, if you have a heart condition, or a history of heart disease, you still may worry. And worrying is your biggest hurdle when it comes to maintaining a healthy sex life. The best advice Rosenthal gives is to discuss your concerns with your doctor. Ask him what you can and can't handle. And if your partner is worried that she may overwork you (the little sex kitten!), bring her along to ask questions, too.

Keep in mind that sex is like any other form of exercise. You should know your limits and never overdo it. If you're not exercising, get your butt in gear. Start walking on a treadmill, lifting light weights. Many cardiac rehabilitation centers offer training programs created for heart attack patients. You've got to get back on the horse—albeit slowly—because the stronger and more fit you are, the easier it is for your heart to do its work.

If you have a heart attack, your doctor will probably make you wait several weeks before resuming sexual relations. Our recommendation, again, is to start slowly. Try positions that are less strenuous, enjoy caressing your partner and talk about ways to make the transition more relaxing for both of you. She'll be nearly as worried as you are.

Beta-blockers such as Inderal are often prescribed to reduce anginal pain during sexual relations. Unfortunately, when taken in large doses, they can diminish sex drive.

High Blood Pressure

The various medications for high blood pressure are truly lifesavers, but they can also put a serious cramp on your sex life. Side effects range from enlarged breasts and depression to loss of sex drive and impotence. If your doctor prescribes blood pressure medication, be sure to ask exactly what it may do to you. Also see if there are some lifestyle changes you can make as an alternative to drug therapy. Some options might be to cut back on salt intake, lose weight and exercise, according to Rosenthal.

Diabetes

Diabetes takes it toll on the body in many ways. In men, it can cause nerve and vascular damage that results in impotency. While some patients experience this side effect due to neglect—they simply don't take care of their condition—Rosenthal says some of his patients don't even realize they have diabetes until they seek treatment for their sexual problem.

The best way to prevent the disease from causing permanent damage is to lay off the alcohol and follow a medicinal regimen that keeps your blood sugar stable. A urologist who specializes in sexual dysfunctions will be of great assistance—particularly if the problem is advanced.

The Worst of the Bunch

High blood pressure medicines are notorious libido killers. Avoid them if you can. And if you can't, ask your doctor if you can have anything but these worst offenders:

- Ismelin
- Catapres
- Reserpine
- Aldactone
- Aldomet
- Inderal

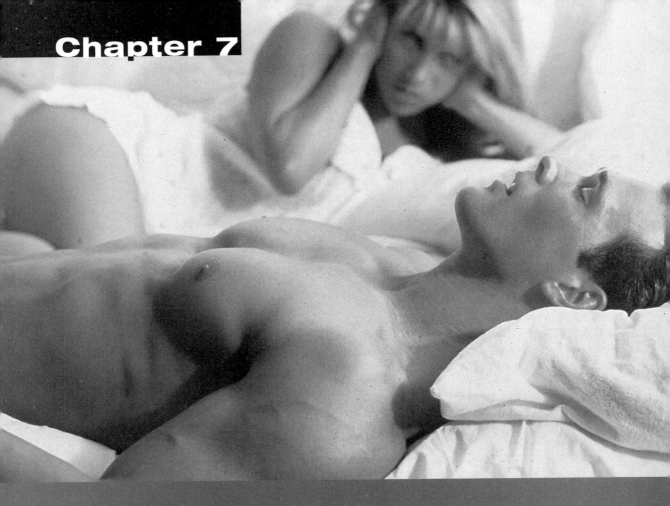

Chapter 7

Troubleshooting

We're in a computer-dominated age. We use them at work. We use them at home. We even surf the Internet. We've found a million different uses for the personal computer—from balancing checkbooks to printing customized greeting cards. And everything in between.

So, we, as a nation, are buying more PCs. We get them home, wrestle them out of their Styrofoam encasements, set them up, plug them in, turn them on and . . . nothing happens. That's when we consult the troubleshooting guide, to see if a common problem is the culprit. Oftentimes, the solution is simple—that's what troubleshooting guides are for, providing simple solutions to common problems.

Consider this chapter a sexual troubleshooting guide for the most complex of all computers—the human body. And, like computer troubleshooting guides, this one doesn't purport to solve every problem under the sun. For that you need special tech support in the form of your physician or therapist. However, this chapter does zero in on common problems—or, more aptly put, what's perceived as more common problems. The fact is, no one sexual malady afflicts a great percentage of men. If the problem you're experiencing isn't covered in these pages (all of them—and the various solutions—would take an entire book to cover!), consult with tech support. That is, check with your local health-care facility for a general practitioner or urologist regarding medical conditions, or a local sex therapist if you think the problem has behavioral or psychological roots.

Finding a physician is an easy deal, but finding a qualified sex therapist may be harder, depending on your geographic location. For starters, write to the American Academy of Clinical Sexology at 1929 18th Street NW, Suite 1166, Washington, DC 20009, or the American Association of Sex Educators, Counselors and Therapists at P.O. Box 238, Mt. Vernon, Iowa, 52314, and ask for a listing of therapists in your area. Typically, a qualified therapist can help you through your problem in a relatively short amount of time. If it takes a great deal of time (nine months to a year, for example), the problem may point to deeper psychological or emotional trouble and your therapist can direct you to a counselor, psychiatrist, or psychologist.

With that said, we present our troubleshooting guide—with nary a joke about your floppy disk or the performance of your hard drive.

The Quick Draw

Let's say you're getting romantic with your partner. The candles are flickering, she's clearly in the mood. Everything is just right. You're kissing, fondling, exploring, and just as things get exciting, bang, it's over. Suddenly you go from Superman to failure. This lack of ejaculatory restraint makes you feel as though your entire life is out of control.

We all know this is clearly not the case, though men have been conditioned to think that virility in the bedroom defines man as man.

The official name for coming too soon is premature ejaculation. Maturity has nothing to do with it, although the problem is associated with youth. "The habit is usually acquired during a man's teens," says San Francisco sex therapist Louanne Cole Weston, Ph.D. "He fears his partner may suddenly become unwilling, so he rushes through sex." Fear of getting caught in the act also causes many young couples to hurry up and finish. And often, adolescent boys engage in rapid masturbation to avoid getting caught, which causes a physiological and unconscious response. "As time passes, men—and especially women—decide that leisurely lovemaking is more enjoyable," Weston adds. "Unfortunately, by then many men are stuck with little ejaculatory control."

The key is gaining voluntary control over what has been involuntary. That's why many sex therapists prefer the term involuntary ejaculation, and it ranks as the top male sex problem. Among men questioned for the 1994 University of Chicago Sex in America survey, almost 30 percent said they'd climaxed too early during the previous year. (In comparison, only 10 percent reported erection problems.)

How early is too early? Toss your stopwatch. The temporal definition of premature ejaculation is highly subjective—Alfred Kinsey's report *Sexual Behavior in the Human Male* revealed that three-quarters of the twelve thousand men surveyed mentioned that the average duration of intercourse was from four to seven minutes. That being the case, a man who ejaculates three minutes into intercourse may not be a premature ejaculator. After all, he ejaculated halfway through the "average" session. However, he may be labeled a premature ejaculator if he wholly thinks he comes too soon. Ultimately, time is not the issue; control is. You're coming too soon if you ejaculate before you want to, whether that's three minutes or three hours into sex.

"Among men questioned for the 1994 University of Chicago Sex in America survey, almost 30 percent said they'd climaxed too early during the previous year."

Fortunately, involuntary ejaculation is one of the easiest sex problems to cure. Renowned New York sex therapist Helen Singer Kaplan, M.D., Ph.D., estimated that more than 90 percent of men can learn ejaculatory control within 14 weeks. "In fact," she noted, "results are so good that when I evaluate a man for involuntary ejaculation, I feel a jolt of pleasure because I know that, with rare exceptions, he will enjoy a much more gratifying sex life in just a few months." To learn ejaculatory control, you don't even need a steady lover.

Turn On, Tune In

Oftentimes, men think distracting themselves will help their involuntary ejaculation problems. Think of baseball. Balance the ol' checkbook. Remember Grandma's famous apple pie. Anything that would keep them from getting too aroused. That's what most men do, and it's a big mistake. "Distracting yourself is the worst thing you can do," Weston says. "Don't tune out your body. Tune into it. Become more familiar with your own sexual arousal pattern. Learn to recognize your 'point of no return.' Once you can, it's easy to make small adjustments that allow you to stay highly aroused without ejaculating."

With that in mind, here's how to last longer, based on ejaculatory-control techniques pioneered by sex researchers William Masters, M.D., and Virginia Johnson:

Sexbit 12

If your partner faints after a round of hearty sex, it may not be due to your prowess in bed. A study of 1,073 women at the University of Cincinnati found that as many as 12 percent of all women are allergic to semen. Symptoms include wheezing, facial swelling, and even loss of consciousness within 30 minutes of intercourse or oral sex. The cure: condoms or an allergy shot—made from your seed.

The Sexual Response Cycle

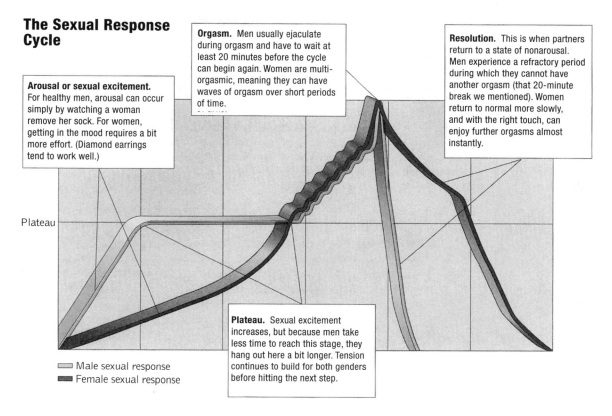

Arousal or sexual excitement. For healthy men, arousal can occur simply by watching a woman remove her sock. For women, getting in the mood requires a bit more effort. (Diamond earrings tend to work well.)

Orgasm. Men usually ejaculate during orgasm and have to wait at least 20 minutes before the cycle can begin again. Women are multi-orgasmic, meaning they can have waves of orgasm over short periods of time.

Resolution. This is when partners return to a state of nonarousal. Men experience a refractory period during which they cannot have another orgasm (that 20-minute break we mentioned). Women return to normal more slowly, and with the right touch, can enjoy further orgasms almost instantly.

Plateau

Plateau. Sexual excitement increases, but because men take less time to reach this stage, they hang out here a bit longer. Tension continues to build for both genders before hitting the next step.

Male sexual response
Female sexual response

Step 1: Learn how it works. Sexual arousal involves four phases:

- excitement
- plateau
- orgasm
- resolution

Excitement leads to erection and deeper breathing. The plateau phase involves intense arousal. When arousal passes the point of no return, orgasm occurs, followed by resolution, a return to pre-excitement. To last longer, you want to lengthen the time you spend in the plateau phase before going up and over the edge.

Step 2: Know thyself. Extending the plateau phase begins with masturbation. Focus on how you feel, not just on having an orgasm. Most guys quickly learn that

"Ultimately, time is not the issue [with premature ejaculation]; control is. You're coming too soon if you ejaculate before you want to, whether that's three minutes or three hours into sex."

they can keep themselves highly aroused without reaching climax by varying the tempo when they masturbate. Practice approaching your point of no return, then backing off from it. Repeat this until you feel confident that you can retreat from that point without ejaculating.

Step 3: Skip the potions. You need to become more aware of your arousal pattern. Drugs and alcohol interfere with this process. In addition, some drugs can cause involuntary ejaculation, notably phenylpropanolamine, an ingredient in over-the-counter weight-loss products (like Dexatrim) and many cold, cough, and allergy products. You should also forget about using anesthetic creams (like Sustain, Delay, Stud). They numb the penis, keeping you from tuning into your arousal pattern.

Step 4: Please your whole body. Guys often think they have one erogenous zone—the penis; that thinking is a one-way ticket to uncontrolled ejaculation. Full-body sex takes pressure off the penis, helping you last longer. Trading massagelike total-body caresses with one another will release tension, making you less likely to seek stress relief through a quick climax.

Or better yet, try the sensate focus technique. According to Robert W. Birch, Ph.D., in his book *Male Sexual Endurance,* sensate focus is a valuable tool in treating a number of male—and female—sexual disorders.

In his book, Birch refers to sensate focus as a couples' homework assignment; in essence, it's the creation of a situation in which couples focus on sensation. He recommends setting up parameters and ground rules for sensate focus sessions. For example, he believes the genitals and typical erogenous zones, such as breasts, should be off-limits during sessions—which means you and your partner should discuss your erogenous zones (what feels good, what gets you going . . . or gets you off) in advance. Then, those areas are strictly verboten during sensate focus.

Birch recommends a regular pattern of sensate sessions, for an hour at least twice a week. In the session, you and your partner lie in bed, preferably nude, cuddling. The goal at first is relaxation, not arousal.

Once you feel comfortable lying next to each other without touching—or with very light touching—you can move onto gentle caresses. Again, the goal is not immediate arousal, but more of an exploration of each other's bodies. Since sexual touching is a no-no, each of you has to explore different parts of your partner's body: the feet, back, arms, legs, stomach, and so on. That way, you discover new erogenous zones, which aid in pleasurable (i.e., more sexual) touching later on.

Birch suggests trying nonsexual touching sessions for at least two weeks before moving on to more sexual touch. By focusing on relaxation—and becoming more in tune with one another's bodies—you can then focus on relaxation during lovemaking, which greatly aids in prolonging orgasm.

Step 5: Take a deep breath. You will automatically breathe deeply during the massage sessions, but guys often tense up, fighting this natural response. Don't. You'll be amazed at how much it can improve your ejaculatory control. After all, deep breathing leads to better oxygen delivery, which means less stress, resulting in good wood.

Step 6: Stop. Then start. Once you develop good control during sensate sessions, start working on massage sessions that include genital touching. To begin, lie still while your partner strokes your penis with her hand. As you approach your point of no return, ask her to stop; she should quit stroking and simply hold your penis instead. Meanwhile, continue to breathe deeply and focus your sensations. When you no longer feel close to orgasm, she can resume the hand play. Once you develop good control while being fondled, practice the start-stop method with oral caresses and intercourse (with the woman on top, step 8).

A few times a week, work on accumulating a half-dozen starts and stops in each 20- to 30-minute session. (And remember: The focus of these practice sessions is on you and your sensations, but don't neglect your lover's needs.)

Step 7: Put on the squeeze. Masters and Johnson developed the squeeze technique to slow down overeager peters. It resembles the stop-start approach, except that during stops, the woman squeezes the head of the penis between her thumb and fingers to help the man retreat from orgasm. (Even a fairly intense squeeze won't hurt an erect penis.) These days, most sex therapists recommend the stop-start method instead because it feels more natural. But the squeeze does work. So if the stop-start doesn't work for you, try the squeeze.

Step 8: Roll over. Watch out for the missionary position. "For most men, control is easier with the woman on top," Weston says. "You don't have to support your weight. You just relax, which helps you gain control."

Step 9: Work your muscles. Even with the woman on top, some guys tense their leg and butt muscles during sex. Try not to; it hampers ejaculatory control. Concentrate on relaxing those muscles instead. Kegel exercises also help. They tone the pubococcygeus (PC) muscle, which runs between the legs and contracts during orgasm. (It's the muscle that allows you to stop urinating midflow.) Toning your PC won't just help you last longer, it will also intensify your orgasms. To do a Kegel, simply tense and relax the PC. It involves the same mechanics as stopping the flow of urination in midpee. Use that midpee stoppage as a test, and re-create that feeling by tensing your PC muscle. Do a half-dozen squeezes four times a day.

Step 10: Go pro. If these exercises don't lead to any improvement after a few months, try a sex therapist.

If sex therapy doesn't help, Prozac and similar antidepressants may, often within a month. Some men manage to maintain control after discontinuing their use, but it still requires a concerted effort. Moreover, these drugs have side effects—you may experience difficulty ejaculating or sometimes even a loss of sexual interest—so ask your doctor to discuss their pros and cons with you.

"Marathon sex isn't necessarily good sex, especially when you just want to impress, rather than pleasure, your partner."

Chances are you won't need Prozac or sex therapy. The vast majority of men can learn ejaculatory control on their own. As you do, be realistic: Marathon sex isn't necessarily good sex, especially when you just want to impress, rather than pleasure, your partner. But while lasting longer won't turn you into the object of every woman's desire, you will feel better about yourself and your lovemaking when you develop more control.

Impotence

While premature ejaculation is more prevalent overall among American males, impotence is more devastating. Simply put, an individual with premature ejaculation can have a semblance of a sex life and experience orgasm. With impotence, a sufferer cannot even achieve an erection, or loses an erection. And in a society where sexual prowess defines a man's virility, impotence can be an emotional world-ender.

". . . in a society where sexual prowess defines a man's virility, impotence can be an emotional world-ender."

Impotence and Age

Research indicates that impotence is not tied to age, but increases with it. According to *Reclaiming Male Sexuality*, studies by Alfred Kinsey confirm this. In Kinsey's 1948 study of twelve thousand males, he found that 1 percent of men aged 19 had impotence problems, while that number increased to 6.7 percent for men between the ages of 45 and 55. This number shot up to 25 percent for men between 55 and 75. The National Institutes of Health estimates that 20 to 30 million men have erectile difficulty.

It stands to reason that the passage of time increases the risks of impotence. For example, cardiac output decreases about 1 percent per year. That means that blood flow becomes more restricted, and because erections rely on blood flow to engorge the spongy tissues in the penis, less active blood flow means less rigidity in the penis. Or no rigidity at all. And our sense of touch also decreases with age. Electrical impulses through nerve endings slow down, causing delayed reactions to touch, such as that telltale surge and spring when the penis is stroked.

" . . . we must caution that there is no one cause—and no one cure—for impotence."

But even with these signposts, it is difficult to say that age *causes* impotence. Clearly, there are young men suffering from impotence. In fact, a Veteran's Administration study cited in *Reclaiming Male Sexuality* showed that the percent of impotence affecting young men and older men was essentially the same—it's just there were different reasons for the onset of impotence within the groups.

And there are countless cases of men suffering from impotence with no physiological problems—their impotence is tied to emotional duress or psychological issues. Ultimately, we must caution that there is no one cause—and no one cure—for impotence. In fact, for decades the medical community thought that up to 80 percent of erectile difficulties were psychological in origin. It was only until the seventies that Masters and Johnson postulated that the percentage was greatly exaggerated—citing that behavioral intervention treatments and psychological therapy didn't produce the results they should have. Today, the medical community estimates that perhaps as much as 80 percent of erectile difficulty cases are physiological in nature.

The single biggest culprit—aside from blows to the groin, sports fans—turns out to be lifestyle issues. Fatty diets, lack of exercise, and smoking can lead to erection problems. This makes sense. The arteries delivering blood to your nether region are some of the smallest in the body; they're generally the first to harden and fill with plaque from all those cheeseburgers. The result? Poorer erections . . . or few at all. Moreover, a growing number of doctors believe that erection difficulty may be an early warning sign of arterial disease.

Emotional or Physical?

According to Saul Rosenthal, M.D., author of *Sex Over 40,* there are telltale signs that will help men determine whether an erection problem is the beginning of impotence—and whether the problem is emotional (psychological) or physical in nature.

For example, if a man can achieve an erection but immediately loses it upon penetration, the problem is most likely emotional in nature. The same goes for a man who has had no difficulty getting an erection . . . until one day, with no warning, he cannot achieve one.

> "... if a man can achieve an erection but immediately loses it upon penetration, the problem is most likely emotional in nature."

However, if a man has, over time, had more difficulty achieving an erection, until he cannot get one, the problem is undoubtedly physical in nature. The same goes for a man who can achieve an erection with direct stimulation, only to find it subside once the stimulation stops. It may also be a physical problem if a man gradually loses his erection completely during intercourse. That points to a vascular concern—the valves in the penile veins are letting blood flow out of the penis and back into the general circulatory system.

Snap to It

In some instances, it's difficult to determine whether the problem is emotional or physical. That's where the snap gauge band comes in.

The snap gauge band is a Velcro device used to determine whether an individual can unconsciously achieve an erection. (The average number of erections per night is five; the average duration of nocturnal erections is 20 to 30 minutes.) If a man can achieve an erection while asleep, then a physician or therapist can determine that the causes are more emotional or psychological than physical.

The snap gauge band is snugly wrapped around the flaccid penis prior to bedtime. The band has three tiny plastic threads on it, and if a man achieves a nighttime erection, the band expands and the plastic threads break. That way, a man can wake up in the morning, look down and see if he unconsciously had an erection.

Sexbit 13

If a test of your testosterone level indicates that it's on the low side, your doctor may prescribe hormonal therapy (testosterone shots or patches) or he may recommend a more natural course of treatment—zinc supplements. This essential mineral is involved in the body's production of testosterone, and studies prove that zinc supplementation can increase levels of the hormone to normal amounts. Try 30 milligrams daily for several months, followed by another hormone-level check. Two other vitamins, A and D, are also involved in the production of testosterone. About 5,000 milligrams and 400 milligrams, respectively, should do the trick. And no, if your levels are normal, these regimes won't turn you into Super Stud.

A similar homespun test was widely used in the seventies; a ring of postage stamps was wetted and adhered to a flaccid penis at night. If the perforations between the stamps broke during the night, an erection had occurred.

Oftentimes, counseling and therapy can help men through their psychologically based impotence or erection problems. By getting to the root cause of anxiety—whether it be workplace stress, performance anxiety, emotional issues regarding the onset of male menopause, or the like—therapists can develop ways for men to address their fears and get back on track, sexually speaking.

Physical Afflictions

As mentioned in chapter 6, there are a number of illnesses that affect sexual performance—and a number that contribute to sexual dysfunction. According to the Massachusetts Male Aging Study conducted in 11 cities between 1987 and 1989, six medical conditions are most often associated with impotence: cardiovascular disease, high blood pressure, ulcers, allergies, arthritis, and diabetes. Please note that having one of these maladies doesn't automatically mean you'll become impotent. There are a number of intangibles involved. For example, reactions to medications may contribute to impotence. Or treatment methods. Or your physiological makeup, in combination with your illness.

Cardiovascular Disease

It seems logical. Cardiovascular disease occurs because of a hardening or blockage of the arteries. And the arterial system carries blood to the penis, causing an erection. So if there is general poor circulation, it stands to reason that there will be erectile dysfunction.

In *Reclaiming Male Sexuality*, George Ryan offers four home tests to determine whether you may have circulatory problems (which can later lead to impotence):

1. **Vigorous walk test.** Walk one mile. At a quick pace. If you feel pain in your calves, this may indicate insufficient blood flow.
2. **Cold penis test.** If your penis continually feels cold, you may have a circulation problem.
3. **Blue penis test.** And we don't mean sad. If your flaccid penis takes on a bluish tint, you may have insufficient blood flow.
4. **Penile hard areas test.** Feel along the base of your flaccid penis. There should be no uniformly hard areas. If there are, this may indicate vascular deposits, which can impede blood flow.

In any of these cases, consult your physician for further testing.

High Blood Pressure

Men treated for high blood pressure are more likely to experience impotence than other men. Refer back to chapter 6 for a list of high blood pressure medications that most often lead to impotence. And since many of these drugs also have a depression-causing side effect, the risks of impotence increase even more. Depression in and of itself can be a psychological cause of impotence and lowered sexual desire.

Ulcers

According to Rosenthal and Ryan, antiulcer drugs such as Tagamet and Zantac are the culprit here. When men switch medications, or stop taking them, the symptoms of impotence quite often disappear.

Allergies

The Massachusetts Male Aging Study showed that men with allergies were more likely to suffer from impotence problems. Frequently, it's the medications used to treat allergies that contribute to impotence. Among the most common culprits are:

- Ambenyl
- Antivert
- Benadryl
- Benylin
- Bonine
- Dramamine
- Dytuss
- Mepergan
- Nico-Vert
- Phenergan
- Remsed
- Stopayne
- Synalgog
- Vistaril
- Zipan

Arthritis

Arthritis can be a debilitating illness—with it comes stiffness, crippling pain, and a change in mobility. It may also create self-doubt and high levels of anxiety, since physical mobility is impaired. So, a physical problem leads to a psychological problem, which then leads to a physical problem—impotence.

Diabetes

According to the Massachusetts Male Aging Study, men with diabetes are three times more likely to be completely impotent than men without diabetes. Risk factors increase for men with diabetes, because sufferers are also likely to have vascular problems and high blood pressure. Additionally, diabetes causes nerve damage throughout the body, impairing the nerve responses to touch. The stress of coping with diabetes can also be a contributing factor to impotence.

Treatment for Physiological Impotence

There are five basic types of treatment for impotence: injectables, suppositories, vacuum pumps, surgery, and oral medication. Each has benefits and drawbacks; none help 100 percent of the men using the treatments. The following is a rundown of the various methods.

Injectables

Don't wince now. With this form of treatment, a drug is injected into the base of the penis, relaxing the smooth muscle tissue and opening up the veins near the penis to accommodate blood flow.

How did researchers come up with the, well, ghastly idea of sticking a needle into someone's John Thomas, you ask? Purely by accident, according to one health-care version of an urban legend. Seems a health-care professional dropped a syringe filled with the drug papaverine onto a male patient's torso. The needle made like a dart and hit the bull's-eye, landing directly on the man's penis, which became erect instantly.

Okay, so that's the tall tale. Here's the truth, according to *Newsweek* magazine. Surgeon Ronald Virag accidentally injected a smooth-muscle relaxer into the pelvic artery of a patient undergoing surgery. The result? The patient had a raging three-hour boner while anesthetized and under the knife. And so, another miracle of science was born.

These days, there are a variety of self-administered treatments available. The most common is called Caverject. Users typically inject the drug 20 minutes prior to sex; erections last sometimes no less than an hour.

Once you ejaculate, however, your erection doesn't necessarily subside—if the drug gives you an hour-long erection, you can't will it away. Therefore, users have to plan their lovemaking sessions. You can't wrestle your trouser snake into a pair of slacks to make the morning commute to work. Also, injectables take the spontaneity out of lovemaking. But then again, with serious erectile difficulties, spontaneity isn't even an option, so the injectables allow users a semblance of normalcy. And then there's the pain factor of injecting the same few spots again and again and again. But for most men, these are small prices to pay for the opportunity to make love again.

One other caution regarding injectables: Some men are so taken with the strong, unsinkable erections they get that they take injection treatments more than once a day. Some men who aren't suffering from impotence also try the injections for extra staying power. Big mistake. Abusing the drug (that is, using it beyond its intended prescription) can sometimes lead to priapism, a painful side effect in which a man's erection won't subside. Imagine pitching a tent. Now imagine that it won't go away . . . not when you sit down. Or stand. Or sleep. Or put on clothes. If the erection doesn't diminish, there's a very real possibility that irreparable damage to the penis will occur—leading to impotence that no treatment can cure.

Because of the dangers of priapism, some doctors also prescribe an injection of neo-synephrine (which causes a gradual reversal of the erection), for emergencies when a patient's erection won't subside. Interestingly, the Caverject literature defines a prolonged erection as lasting four to six hours; priapism in the drug's literature is defined as an erection lasting more than six hours and recommends seeking medical assistance after that six-hour time period.

Suppositories

Follow along. This treatment method involves inserting a gel form drug into your penis. But you don't use a syringe. Hmmmm . . . How do you do that? By inserting a small plastic pump tube into the tip of your penis to your urethra and squeezing the medication into your penis. There. We said it. You can stop squirming.

The suppository, called MUSE, must be applied five to ten minutes before sex; erections can last up to an hour. Like injectables, the erection doesn't necessarily subside after ejaculation, so planning is in order. MUSE is not known to be as effective as injectables, and its most common side effect is penile aching.

Vacuum Pumps

Ah, Austin Powers. Aside from his espionage skills and proclamations of "Do I make you horny, baby?," the International Man of Mystery is most known for his . . . Swedish sex pump?! Seems that even world-class jet-setting spies need a little help in the erection department.

Like its Swedish counterpart, the vacuum pump serves to create erections. With this treatment, a man places an elastic ring around the base of his flaccid penis. Then he slips the vacuum tube over it, creating a seal. (Or, the pump has a seal on it, which is rolled off the tube onto the penis shaft.) Air is then sucked out of the tube by a small ball pump or squeeze pedal. As the air is removed, a vacuum tight suction occurs, drawing blood into the penis, which then becomes erect. Since there is an elastic ring round the base of the penis, the blood can't escape. The tube is removed and . . . voila! The man can sustain an erection for up to 30 minutes.

The downside? Ejaculations may be difficult. And removing the elastic ring may be tough. Further, there is a potential for nerve or tissue damage if you don't remove the ring after 20 to 30 minutes. And talk about lack of spontaneity! Just imagine hauling this contraption out from under the bed just as your partner starts to murmur sweet nothings.

Surgery

There are two types of surgery: vascular surgery and penile implant surgery.

The former is used to correct vascular problems that may inhibit blood flow to the penis. It should be noted that it is typically quite expensive and isn't considered a "frontline" approach to solving erectile problems.

The latter typically involves inserting an inflatable rod into the shaft of the penis, which is inflated by way of a small saline-solution-filled pump located in one of the patient's testicles. After sex, the patient releases the fluid back into the pump by pressing a small internal release valve. Imagine a sex-oriented Reebok pump. That's the most common penile implant. The implant has problems, though: The saline fluid may leak and the hydraulics may not work. And the pump doesn't increase the user's length appreciably; it typically increases one's girth.

There's also a malleable version: a stiff bendable rod is surgically inserted into the shaft of the penis. With this method, the patient bends his penis upward when sex comes a-calling, and unbends it afterward.

Oral Medication

Oral medication is the road of greatest promise for most impotence suffers, particularly since the introduction of the revolutionary new drug Viagra. Viagra, commonly referred to as the Love Drug, works by allowing nitric oxide to relax the smooth muscle cells surrounding the penis, allowing stimulation to produce an erection. In clinical trials, the drug helped up to 81 percent of case subjects who had impotence problems. Unlike injections, suppositories, vacuum pumps, or surgery, oral doses of medication are viewed by men as neat and easy ways of treatment. And since Viagra is taken an hour prior to sex, a mood isn't broken by dashing off to the bathroom to "shoot up" . . . or pump up. The downstroke, so to speak? Viagra can cause headaches, diarrhea, and temporary eye problems.

According to the *Los Angeles Times,* within two weeks of its release, Viagra was became one of the "fastest-selling drugs in history." The demand "was unlike any other drug [doctors] had ever seen." Close to 20 thousand prescriptions had been written. Internet sites—many illegal—offered Viagra by phone. Studies to determine the effects of Viagra on women even commenced

"Viagra, commonly referred to as the Love Drug, works by allowing nitric oxide to relax the smooth muscle cells surrounding the penis, allowing stimulation to produce an erection."

within a month of the drug's release—the buzz was *that* good. Which speaks to the depth of our desire for sexual aids.

Another drug (for men), Vasomax, also shows promise (it's currently under FDA review). Like Viagra, this drug relaxes the smooth muscle tissue, and it also dilates arteries, so greater blood flow is achieved.

Medication and Impotence

Drugs—some of which you might not suspect—have libido-lowering side effects, at least for some users. According to Theresa L. Crenshaw, M.D., a San Diego sexual-medicine specialist, among the medications that might squelch your desire are:

- Many blood pressure medications, especially calcium channel-blockers

- Most tranquilizers: Librium, Valium, Xanax, etc.

- Any narcotic pain relievers: Demerol and anything with codeine

- Anti-epilepsy drugs, including Dilantin

- Most antidepressants (Wellbutrin is a notable exception)

Preventive Measures

In all cases, it's important to consult with your doctor on the most effective treatment for impotence. But as we mentioned in chapter 6, there are things you can do that may help prevent impotence from occurring.

- **Quit smoking.** Aside from the obvious risks of cancer, smoking constricts and hardens blood vessels. Constricted and hardened blood vessels means less blood flow to your penis. Nuff said.

- **Exercise.** Do it at least three times a week for 20 minutes to increase blood flow. You don't have to go nuts, sweating buckets on a stair machine. A brisk walk on the treadmill will suffice.

- **Cut out the hooch.** Even guys who easily bone up can become impaired by a few cocktails. The same goes for marijuana and other drugs.

- **Eat healthy.** According to Lynn Fischer, television chef and author of *The Better Sex Diet,* less fat on your plate is a key factor in preventing impotence, because you'll avoid hardening of your arteries. Fischer recommends getting about 10 percent of your calories from fat (5 percent from saturated fat) and limiting cholesterol and sodium to 100 milligrams and 3,000 milligrams per day, respectively.

- **Destress.** The benefits of adopting a laid-back lifestyle are immeasurable. For the purposes of this book, let's just say your sex life will improve tenfold if you take time to decompress.

- **Catch your zzzzzzs.** Fischer points out that "[lack of] sleep has become pandemic in our society. And it's affecting more than your performance at work . . ." Getting seven or eight hours of sleep a night is not a luxury, it's a necessity if you're running on empty. You'll be amazed at how vital you feel when you get up—and when you get it up.

A Bent Tale

Premature ejaculation and impotence may be the most notable sexual dysfunctions—probably because men consider them the absolute worst. But a third, lesser-known condition, called Peyronie's disease (after the physician to Louis XV of France) is equally harsh to the two out of every 100 men who suffer from it. Simply put, Peyronie's disease is an unnatural bending of the penis. But don't start sweating if your member slants a tad to the left or right. This is normal. What is considered abnormal is a penis that is crooked, possibly hard at the base and soft up top, and maybe even narrower around the middle as though someone put a rubber band around the shaft.

Researchers believe this penile abnormality is caused by an injury to the erectile chambers within the penis, which fill with blood to cause an erection. These chambers are encased in a sheath, the tunica albuginea, which stretches to accommodate an erection. But this sheath can only stretch to a point (10 to 13 times the normal erect state). If for some reason, you pop an ultra-mega rod the tunica albuginea will tear and scar, causing Peyronie's disease.

Yes, it can be painful. And yes, it can screw up your love life big time, putting you out of the game for months or even years. Though it is possible for the condition to correct itself over time, urologists are trying to be more proactive in treating patient's with Peyronie's. Some urologists attempt to soften the scar tissue via steroid injections, radiation, and vitamin E. More recent treatments include injecting the calcium channel-blocker verapamil (used to treat high blood pressure) into the scar tissue every two weeks for six months.

And finally, there are three surgeries. The first, called the Nesbit procedure, removes a patch on the normal side of the penis to straighten you out. The downside: you'll be a bit shorter—so to speak. Another procedure cuts directly into the scar tissue and requires skin grafting to straighten the penis. And the third, for men who also have erectile problems, involves implanting a prosthesis and possibly removing the scar tissue.

Most urologists also strongly recommend that Peyronie's patients stick to less acrobatic lovemaking. Certain positions make the penis more vulnerable to damage—namely the "woman on top, bending backwards." If things get wild, she could slip off, try to jump back on and . . . well, you get the picture.

Genital Compatibility

Sometimes the issue isn't about getting it up, but making it fit. Oftentimes, couples have difficulty in "meshing." That is, a couple perceives that there is a genital incompatibility between them.

The notion of a compatibility is definitely not new. Take, for example, the Kama Sutra. The 2,000-year-old Indian sex manual classified men and women according to the dimensions of their sex organs (the "stallion" male, the "gazelle" woman, and so on) and declared that some combinations would make for sexual fireworks, while others were potentially disastrous.

But sexual mythology aside (after all, the Kama Sutra also depicts sexual positions that could only be achieved without a backbone), so-called sex-organ incompatibility seems a bigger problem than it really is. And if a man and woman do experience some discrepancy

If you must take a certain drug, ask your physician if there is a substitute with fewer sex-depressing side effects. Or, in the case of antidepressants, consider a periodic "drug holiday."

The value of doing this was shown at McLean Hospital in Belmont, Massachusetts, where psychiatrist Anthony Rothschild, M.D., studied 30 people in stable, long-term relationships who complained that antidepressants had hurt their sex lives. Rothschild had them stop taking the drugs from Thursday morning until noon Sunday. Ten of the 20 people on Paxil and Zoloft reported increased libido and sexual satisfaction, while only two felt more depressed. (Only one of the ten Prozac users reported sexual improvement, apparently because Prozac takes longer to clear out of the bloodstream.)

If either you or your partner uses antidepressants, ask your doctor about taking weekends off; your love life might improve.

concerning, um, fit, there are plenty of things they can do to improve the situation.

Size Seldom Counts

Sex therapists and other experts agree that true instances of genital incompatibility, in which a couple is unable to have intercourse because of the size or shape of their genitals, are extremely rare. "Unless there is some abnormality of the male or female genitals, no size difference exists that would cause [total] sexual dysfunction," says Don Sloan, M.D., director of the human sexuality division at New York Medical College. If an abnormality does exist—such as an unbreakable hymen in a woman, or a penis that is two inches or shorter when erect (paging Howard Stern)—the person should consult a physician to see if the problem is correctable.

> ". . . the anatomy of a woman's vagina makes it compatible with virtually any size penis."

What's more, the anatomy of a woman's vagina makes it compatible with virtually any size penis. When a woman is sexually aroused, the outer third of her vagina narrows, gripping whatever penetrates. It's also extremely elastic. "[The vagina] is so accommodating that it molds itself to whatever is inside, whether it's a tampon or a ten-pound baby," Sloan says.

Sometimes, complaints about genital size have less to do with reality than with people's inaccurate ideas of what their genitals, or their partner's, are "supposed" to be like. A man who feels his penis is too small, for instance, is probably comparing himself to a false ideal. "Men worry that they are below average in size, but how do they know the average size of an erect penis?" asks Carolyn Libbey Livingston, Ph.D., a sex therapist and codirector of the Seattle Sexual Health Center. "Some men go by porn films, whose actors are cast on the basis of being exceptionally big."

Indeed, complaints about either partner's genital size may actually be a sign of anxiety about sex, or a smoke screen for some unspoken conflict in a couple's relationship. "If partners have an emotionally comfortable, loving connection, size isn't that great an issue," Livingston says. "Even if they're not each other's physical ideal, they can find ways to work with this and still have a good sexual relationship."

> "Sometimes, complaints about genital size have less to do with reality than with people's inaccurate ideas of what their genitals, or their partner's, are 'supposed' to be like."

Solutions to sexual problems can usually be found if a couple is willing to put in the effort, adds Lonnie Barbach, Ph.D., a San Francisco–based sex therapist and an editor of *Erotic Edge.* "You can either say, 'I need to be with someone who has a larger penis, a tighter vagina, whatever,' or if the relationship is worth it, you can stay together and improve your sex life."

Enhancing your lovemaking skills and improving sexual communication are desirable in any case. Meanwhile, if a couple does have some problem with sexual fit, the following techniques can make intercourse more pleasurable.

If the Fit Is Too Loose

The outer third of the vagina is the most sensitive part, and just about any size penis can stimulate this important area. But some men and women experience less sensation than they'd like if the fit of the penis in the vagina isn't sufficiently tight. If that's the case, you can:

Try positions that provide a tighter fit. Alex Comfort, M.D., author of *The New Joy of Sex,* suggests any position in which the woman's thighs are pressed together. Many couples find that "doggie-style" sex, with her on all fours and you kneeling behind, offers a tighter sensation as well as deeper penetration.

Another good bet is the coital alignment technique, or CAT. As you'll recall from chapter 4, in this position you rest your body against your partner, positioning yourself far forward between her legs, so that the base of your penis presses against her clitoral area. Then, instead of thrusting, the two of you move your pelvises in a gentle rocking motion.

"The technique provides ample stimulation for both partners, regardless of their genital dimen-

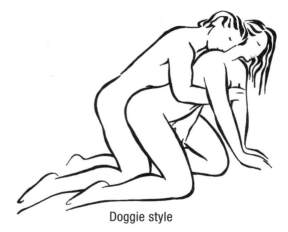
Doggie style

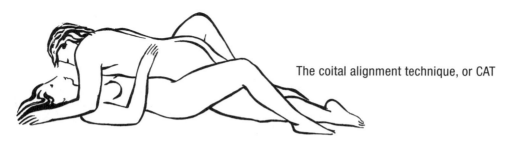
The coital alignment technique, or CAT

sions," says sex therapist Edward Eichel, who developed CAT and describes it in his book *The Perfect Fit.* For the woman, the base of the penis maintains steady contact with the clitoris throughout lovemaking, while the shaft presses her urethra against her pubic bone, stimulating a nerve-rich area inside the vaginal wall. And with CAT, many men experience a "soft, melting sensation that doesn't occur with ordinary thrusting," Eichel writes.

Ask her to practice "Kegels." Kegel exercises, which strengthen the pubococcygeal muscles of the pelvic floor, are often prescribed for women with postpartum incontinence and whose vaginas have stretched during childbirth. Practiced on a regular basis, Kegels not only tone the muscles around the vagina and increase its ability to grip during sex, but also enhance a woman's sexual sensations and even help her have more intense orgasms.

If the Fit Is Too Tight

Occasionally, a man with a very large penis will hurt his partner when he penetrates her. In these cases, Livingston counsels women to learn how to relax the vaginal walls.

Some more suggestions:

Be gentle. Though some women enjoy hard thrusting, others find it uncomfortable—especially if the man is bigger than average. "If your penis, whatever its length, hits an ovary and hurts her, don't go in so far," advises Comfort. A good option is to make love with your partner on top, which allows her to control the depth and angle of penetration.

Use a lubricant. Many vaginal lubricants can ease intercourse. Don't use household products such as cocoa butter or cooking oils. As always, if you're using a condom, avoid petroleum-based products such as Vaseline, which can turn latex into Swiss cheese.

Whatever your situation, it never hurts to experiment. A creative, energetic, mutually pleasurable sex life is what's important, even if the two of you are already a perfect fit.

Troubleshooting Relationships

And then there are those times when you're not a perfect fit . . . and no amount of accommodation will help. Take, for example, Brad and Alison.

At the end of a wild sunrise romp, Alison caressed Brad's chest and nervously broke the news. "'You're very special to me, but it's over,'" he recalls her saying. "'I've found somebody else.'" Brad was stunned. "After six months of great sex and great dates, I figured Alison had commitment on her mind," he says. "Instead, I got the big kiss-off."

Reading the Signs

Shocked as Brad was, chances are he could have seen it coming, says Harold H. Bloomfield, M.D., a Del Mar, California–based psychiatrist and coauthor of *How to Be Safe in an Unsafe World*. "Most men misread or ignore the red flags that signal trouble in a relationship," he adds. "They excuse or justify a woman's behavior and attitude because they want the relationship to succeed."

If you learn to spot the signals that she's itching to leave, however, you might prevent a breakup and build a more solid relationship. Keep an eye out for these clues:

She starts dressing down. Dramatically. Is there a deterioration of her grooming? "The first sign your woman is going to dump you is that she stops wearing good lingerie and quits shaving her legs," says E. Jean Carroll, advice columnist and author of *A Dog in Heat Is a Hot Dog.* "This often means she doesn't feel sexy and doesn't care if she pleases you."

Solution: You can find small ways to please her. Revitalize her sensual side and make her feel more desirable. Be free with compliments. Buy her a fun, meaningful gift. It doesn't have to be expensive, either. Carroll recommends a gift certificate for a spa treatment.

Her lovemaking fizzles. When a woman takes off her clothes, she removes her protective armor. When the armor returns, take note. "Watch out if passionate and uninhibited lovemaking suddenly becomes more rigid," Bloomfield says. "Making excuses or constantly saying 'Not now' is a signal that she doesn't feel safe feeling out of control with you."

Solution: You can ask yourself whether you've betrayed her trust. If you have, apologize and do your best to restore her faith in your relationship. Make intimate plans, even if you haven't breached her trust. "And that doesn't mean sex," says Kathleen Mojas, a clinical psychologist in Beverly Hills, California. "It means having fun again and connecting with each other." If you both enjoy tennis, play. If you like sailing—well, captain, sail. Fun, shared experiences breed intimacy and can shine up a lackluster love life.

She's always angry. When even your breathing sends her into fits, your days are numbered. "If her temper, attention span, and conversations suddenly become abrupt, she may be trying to sabotage the relationship," Carroll says.

Solution: You can let her vent. Go ahead, it'll clear the air. It may be she's mad at someone or something else—or she might just be angry with you. Try to resolve the issues together. If she continues to act like a snapping turtle, make a move. "Leave her alone and go date someone else," Carroll advises.

She's unavailable. She starts giving one-word answers, and usually the word isn't "yes." The cuddling and eye contact are gone, too. Maybe she insists on doing things by herself, spending weekends

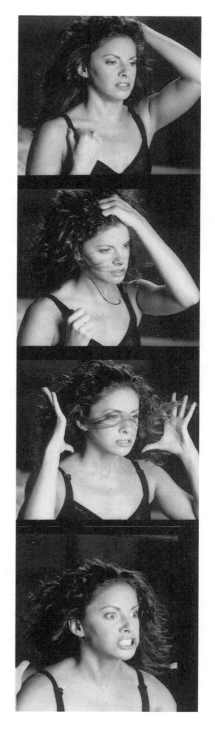

separately and so on. "This is an obvious giveaway that she's checked out emotionally or even physically," Mojas says. "She's creating distance."

Solution: You can talk about your feelings without accusing her of anything—she could just be swamped at work. Tell her you miss her companionship. Let her know how much she means to you and how much you value the relationship. As a last resort, Carroll says, "Encourage her to go and do what she has to do."

Suddenly, she's a critic. She used to love your closet full of Gap. She raved about your lime-zested shrimp risotto. Now she gripes about your wardrobe and ranks your kitchen skills below those of the McDonald's fry guy. Or worse, she gripes about your culinary skills and rates your wardrobe below the fry guy's. "She doesn't care what you think anymore, so she's letting her real feelings show," Carroll says. Since she's probably already planning an exit, what does she have to lose?

Solution: You can keep your pride. You can decide whether you want to stay or leave. But you shouldn't drag out the heartbreak unnecessarily. "Don't let women treat you badly," Carroll says. "If a woman is ready to dump you, let her go."

Your Cheatin' Heart

Richard arrived home early, hoping to surprise his wife after a long week working late at the office. Ann was surprised, all right—frozen in the hallway, white as a sheet. "Rich," she said, "I'm not alone."

Whether you're Traditional Macho or Nouveau Sensitive, discovering a lover's infidelity is always a crash course in Advanced Emotion. Twenty-five percent of husbands surveyed in the University of Chicago's landmark Sex in America study said they'd cheated on their wives. About 15 percent of wives admitted to cheating, and some research by Annette Lawson in the late eighties suggests that young married women actually cheat more than their male counterparts. (Another study found that unmarried women in steady relationships were more likely to cheat than married women.)

Many women, having grown up hearing about and sometimes seeing philandering fathers, almost expect—not necessarily tolerate—men's straying.

> **"Twenty-five percent of husbands surveyed in the University of Chicago's landmark Sex in America study said they'd cheated on their wives. About 15 percent of wives admitted to cheating, and some research by Annette Lawson in the late eighties suggests that young married women actually cheat more than their male counterparts."**

But you can bet most cuckolded husbands never see it coming. "Men don't expect crap like that the way women do," says Bonnie Eaker Weil, Ph.D., author of *Adultery, The Forgivable Sin.* "Men don't put up with cheating as readily. They're more devastated in many ways."

"Men fall apart when they're cheated on," agrees family therapist Frank Pittman III, author of *Private Lies* and *Man Enough.* "They've been raised to think that it's a sign of their failure as a man. Usually it centers on penis size or sexual technique, but sometimes it's even blamed on an inadequate car or income. It brings up all of a man's insecurities: The times he got bested by a bully as a child or asked a girl out on a date and she laughed at him."

Guys Get a Bum Rap

Completely irrational? Not quite. Guys are generally blamed by society, even mental-health professionals, for a partner's infidelity. "There are many, many advantages to being a man," Pittman says. "The lines in the men's room are much shorter than the lines in the women's room; men don't have periods—those sorts of things. One of the disadvantages of being a man is that if your wife screws around on you, you've got to focus your attention on figuring out what you did wrong. That's just the way it is."

Pittman sees it this way: Males minimize sleeping around. They convince themselves that it's meaningless, something purely physical to supplement their main relationship. Females, on the other hand, attach meaning to infidelity, including their own. "Women as a rule think about what they're displeased with in the marriage before they get into an affair," he says.

That leaves the cuckold with two choices: to write off the relationship and lick his wounds, or to try salvaging his marriage. Both paths lead through the five stages of grief—denial, bargaining, anger, depression, and acceptance.

However, for salvaging to succeed, you'll have to eat more humble pie, because angry as you may be, you won't get far pointing your finger. "Demanding that she take full responsibility for her actions will not improve the relationship," Pittman says. "That's one of the tricks I've learned through years of dealing with thousands of cases of infidelity." Eaker Weil agrees that while it would be unfair to place all the blame for a wife's behavior on the husband, the husband should realize he may have played a part in it. "Maybe he's been a workaholic, maybe he travels a lot, or hasn't been giving her emotional comfort and support," she says.

Damage Control

Old news, right? Men and women have always viewed emotional issues differently. The new variable is the working world. "Women today can support themselves and, often, can get sex anywhere," Eaker Weil says. So guys have to bring something new to the table: their softer, more supportive side.

To do this, think compromise instead of conversion: You're trying to meet your mate halfway. And as with any compromise, you'll do well to know as much about the other side as possible. For instance, Eaker Weil notes that sometimes women just need to vent. "They like to share and unload when they're overwhelmed," she says. So instead of lending a hand—after all, guys like fixing things—lend an ear.

Looking back, Richard realized he didn't do that nearly enough. "If only I hadn't been so critical and resentful, so focused on my own career," he says. In fact, he completely missed telltale signs that she'd gotten fed up and gone astray—lack of interest in sex, mysterious telephone hang-ups, the need for more "space."

Ann said she wanted to work things out. Richard agreed, on the conditions that she would stop seeing her lover and start seeing a therapist with him. He made a good call: Muddling through something as dire and draining as adultery without professional guidance can be an exercise in futility. In fact, whereas 35 percent of couples stay together after a spouse's infidelity has been revealed, Eaker Weil says that 98 percent of her patients stay together. Ann didn't make it into therapy with Richard. She did want to work it out, she said, but she needed space. He spent time at a friend's house in the suburbs, first just weekends, then three nights a week, then four, five . . .

To smother his rage, he drank 6 to 12 beers on a typical night, chasing them with tequila shots, pot, cocaine. Richard couldn't concentrate at work; he'd show up drunk and develop a splitting headache by noon. He became obsessed with fantasies of revenge focused on Ann's lover. Eventually, he discovered that Ann had been seeing him all along; once again, Richard missed the cues.

Through a variety of means, from therapy to keeping a journal to intense physical workouts and close friendships, Richard slowly pieced together facts about himself that helped him understand how he may have helped derail his relationship. Two years after that first night, Richard walked into an Alcoholics Anonymous meeting. For the first time in his life, he was tackling problems head-on, not skirting them.

"The key for me was finding out what I really felt, then letting myself feel it, then embracing those feelings," he says today, happily remarried and still sober. "Everybody has to go through those stages. By blocking them, you're just blocking your life."

Altered Mates

Is she cheating on you? Look over the telltale signs listed below. And while you do, bear in mind that guys often misread women's behavior, seeing infidelity where none exists. Remember Othello. If you suspect something might be amiss with your mate, don't go psycho on her. Instead, keep a rational eye on the situation, and try talking it out with her.

Change in sex life: Sudden loss of interest in sex or an abrupt, renewed interest in it, replete with new techniques, positions, behaviors, and so on.

A new look: Suddenly starts looking more sexy by losing weight, making an unexpected alteration to her hairstyle, significantly changing her mode of dress.

Repeat offender: Mentions the same person often—"He's so handsome, so funny"—then abruptly stops mentioning him.

Name calling: Stops using pet names or saying "I love you."

Multiple personalities: Becomes markedly more self-centered, selfish, arrogant, irritable, fault-finding, critical, emotionally distant.

Spaced out: Needs more "space" to find herself, be her own person.

No show: Attends school at night, gets a night job, or suddenly extends hours spent on the job but has little to show for it.

Missing person: Disappears for hours without clear explanations as to where.

Deeds undone: Stops doing the little things she used to do for you or, then again, starts doing good deeds for you with a vengeance (a typical way people deal with guilt).

Alone in a crowd: Where she used to enjoy doing things alone with you, she now needs to bring other people along.

Caller no-ID: You receive frequent hang-ups when you answer the phone, but your partner doesn't.

Coping with Divorce

While the stakes are high in any relationship, the stakes are even higher when the couple is married.

Say you met the perfect woman, you became a couple "until death do you part," you split. Now you feel like half a couple in a market already glutted with retreads. Friends disappear. You're sure you're a failure, alone in this world. Alone maybe,

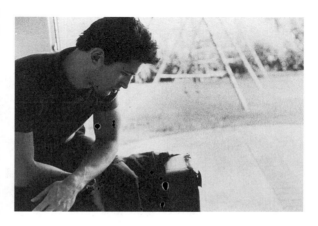

but not without company. About 50 percent of all marriages in the United States end in divorce. Still, regardless of how stranded or rotten you feel, remember this: Countless people have survived the ordeal. After weathering the storm, you can emerge better prepared for stronger, more lasting relationships.

Whether you sought the divorce or were blindsided when your once-loving wife breezily introduced her new boyfriend, a breakup hurts. "Just as you mourn the death of a person, you mourn the death of a relationship," says Mel Krantzler, a psychologist in San Rafael, California, and author of several books on divorce. "Next to the death of a loved one, divorce is the most traumatic experience in a person's life."

You probably feel alienated from the circle of friends you and your wife shared. Once you prided yourself on your independence, but now you feel shamed by desperate neediness. Your buddies don't understand. One moment you're morose and depressed, the next angry and vengeful. If you ended it or cheated on your wife, you may experience a curious mix of guilt and relief. If your wife dumped you or had an affair, you may seethe with anger.

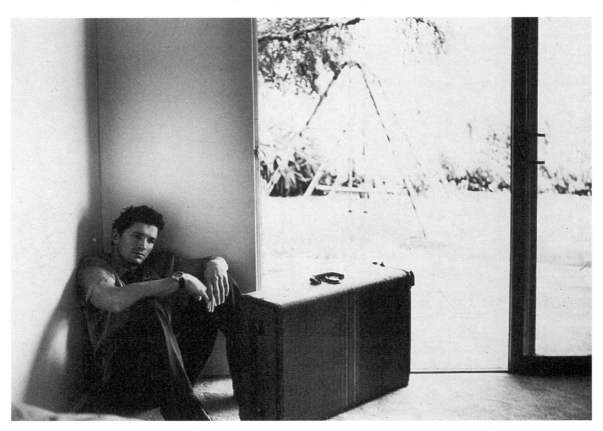

It's not unusual for the shock to last several months, and if you don't confront the feelings, you'll risk becoming emotionally stunted. You may even become clinically depressed and not know it. "Feelings are there to be understood, not condemned," Krantzler says. "Many men are so out of touch, they wouldn't understand their feelings if they hit them over the head with a baseball bat. Acknowledging how you feel is not a sign of weakness, but a sign of strength, and it allows you to find something good in something bad."

You also need to:

Take responsibility. No matter how nasty your ex was, you bear some blame for the breakup. A significant amount of the time, the breakup is the result of the interaction of both partners. It is rarely a singular flaw in only one of the partners.

"If you blame your partner and don't take responsibility yourself, that's a formula for reproducing the same kinds of problems," says counselor Ron Petit, who went through a divorce himself 17 years ago. "Those unconscious patterns are going to take over again."

> **"It's not unusual for the shock [of divorce] to last several months, and if you don't confront the feelings, you'll risk becoming emotionally stunted."**

Maintain balance. Take advantage of the chance to do all those things you put off while you were married. Go backpacking with your buddies. Learn to play the accordion. Whatever.

Reach out. Share feelings with friends and family. Consult a local hotline, social-service center, men's center, or church; many run good divorce workshops and do not necessarily push the religious angle. Or read one of these books: *Divorcing* by Mel Krantzler and Melvin Belli; *Learning to Love Again* by Mel Krantzler; or *The Good Divorce* by Constance Ahrons. Also, check out www.divorce-online.com, a virtual support group for divorced men and women.

The Wrong Way

Some coping mechanisms just don't work. "If you're just trying to avoid pain, you never get a chance to look at yourself," says psychologist Constance Ahrons, Ph.D., who directs the marriage and family therapy program at the University of Southern California. "You drown your sorrows in alcohol, women, running or working 20 hours a day." Consider a different approach if you feel yourself slipping into one of these all-too-common categories:

The super stud. The most misguided way to cope with a bad relationship is . . . another bad relationship. Some guys try to plug the breach in their emotional levee by quickly rebounding to another woman. Others become wildly promiscuous to compensate for years of monogamy or to reaffirm their attractiveness. Sure, the sex may seem fantastic at first, but many born-again rakes eventually find themselves unsatisfied. "Rather than making a commitment to one particular person, they try to screw them all. It's an act of transmitted vengeance against the ex-wife," Krantzler says. "After a while, it gets very boring."

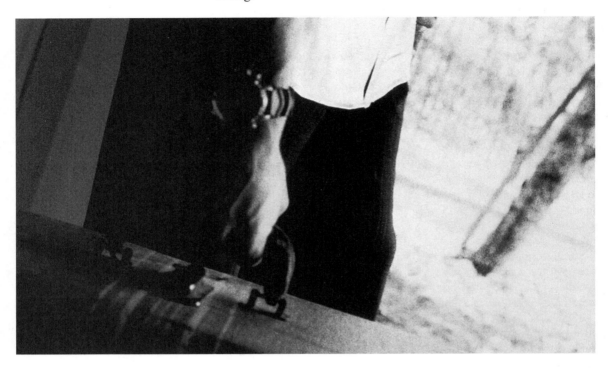

The escape artist. Some people move to a new city to avoid confronting their emotional demons. Workaholics bury themselves at the office. Computer users become online addicts. Substance abusers dull their pain with alcohol or drugs. Others try to reinvent themselves with new cars or clothes. These behaviors mask problems while inhibiting your ability to overcome them.

The obsessed. Beware when anger becomes a 24-hour obsession long after the split. In the most extreme cases, men stalk or even murder their estranged wives. Some turn divorce into a malignant extension of the failed marriage. "They live with that for months and years, and it really corrodes them," says William I. Doherty, Ph.D., director of the marriage and family therapy program at the University of Minnesota. "It hurts them physically and emotionally. Research indicates that chronic anger is bad for the heart and other organ systems, and it makes the individual inaccessible for other relationships."

The hermit. Again, it's not unusual to feel lonely after a divorce. But when isolation persists over many months, it's time to seek professional help with what may be a serious depression.

Courtroom Drama

As if the emotional toll weren't enough, divorcees often face legal wrangling. Not surprisingly, these *Kramer versus Kramer* battles can quickly turn into uncivil proceedings. Always consult a lawyer, even if your a split is amicable. You're still going to have to deal with assets, debts, or kids. Don't hide anything from your lawyer—embarrassing revelations of affairs or hidden assets may come back to haunt you. Also, make a list of all assets and debts. These include bank accounts, stocks, insurance policies, and all property worth at least $500. Remember to close all joint bank or credit-card accounts.

If the breakup is more venomous, beware of abuse allegations. Some women falsely allege physical or sexual abuse to nuke their husbands in court. "It's often used as leverage in bitter divorce cases," says Timothy J. Horgan, a New York divorce lawyer. "It immediately gets the father out of the house and keeps him away from the kids. The person making the accusation has a tremendous advantage at the outset of the case because the father is being investigated."

Other tips:

Stay put. Don't move out of the house without consulting your attorney. Your wife's lawyer may argue that you abandoned the family.

Back off. Quarrels and physical confrontations may give your wife the evidence she needs to slap you with a restraining order.

Remember your kids. They're hurting, too. Reassure them that you still love them—you just won't be living with Mom anymore. Don't turn children into pawns in the battle with your ex-wife, don't bad-mouth her in front of them, and don't compete for their loyalty. Let them know they're not responsible for the situation.

But don't overdo it. Spend as much time with your kids as possible, send cards, call them. But avoid becoming the stereotypical "Disneyland Dad" who showers them with expensive gifts, treats, and outings every time he sees them. Maintain an appropriate level of discipline.

Though it may be hard to believe at first, you can emerge from divorce a wiser, more mature person. "Divorce is as American an institution as apple pie," Krantzler says, "but you can join the ranks of millions who have been divorced and have renewed their lives by learning from the past rather than repeating past mistakes."

Sexual Compulsion

You'd think that after two decades of being inundated with information about every addiction imaginable, it would be a snap to figure out

To Date—or Not to Date?

Divorce doesn't mean you have to take a vow of chastity. But experts advise divorced men to be cautious about diving into new relationships too quickly. Wounds and unresolved tension may sabotage a second chance. Many men try to rebound too soon and watch new relationships go down in flames. Some experts suggest waiting a short while before starting to date, others up to a year. You will have to decide.

A few tips: Analyze the unresolved issues raised by your divorce. Were you too bossy? Too compliant? Once you get a better handle on how you contributed to the breakup, you will be more ready to try again. Don't use dating as an emotional crutch simply because you want a woman to keep you company, cook for you, or hang on your arm. That could be a recipe for another failure. Get other parts of your life in order first: Enjoy hobbies, exercise, spend time with friends. Once you restore balance in your life, you'll be ready to move on.

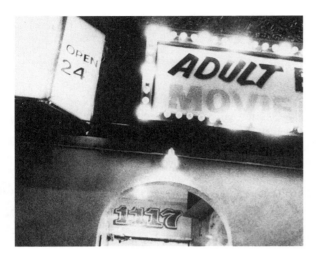

whether or not we're seemingly addicted to something. But most of us are as confused as ever about what constitutes an out-of-control craving, or compulsion, especially when it comes to sex.

Officially, there is no such thing as an "addictive personality." It isn't listed in the American Psychiatric Association's thick book of mental disorders. And most addiction experts will tell you that anyone has the potential to become addicted to something under the right circumstances. "If I told you to create a profile of the traits, the background, the sociological, environmental, ethnic, religious, and economic characteristics of the typical 'addict,' you couldn't do it," says Jokichi Takamine, M.D., an internist at St. Johns Hospital in Santa Monica, California. "That's because it's anyone."

Luckily, our understanding of why compulsive behavior happens is improving. And as it does, we're learning more and more about how to treat it.

Constant Craving

The old theories about what causes compulsive behavior—a rotten childhood, too much pressure, psychological trauma—are at best incomplete explanations. For one thing, they don't tell us why one man will obsessively seek out anonymous sex, while another with a similar background or upbringing will be content to pursue a monogamous relationship.

In *The Craving Brain*, Manhattan internist and researcher Ronald A. Ruden, M.D., presents an intriguing theory of compulsive behavior that focuses on brain chemistry. Some people have a "craving brain," Ruden says, because of either a genetic predisposition, hormonal imbalance, or because of environmental stress. "I don't even like using the word addiction anymore," he says. "I prefer the term 'craving response disorder,' because it really defines the problem and the process."

According to Ruden, a craving brain is low in serotonin, the natural chemical that helps us feel sated and content. And as we know from chapter 2, low serotonin levels signal an aggressive—almost wanton—sex drive.

Ruden surmises that if we don't have enough serotonin, we may go out looking for something that will create it. Then we discover—often accidentally—that certain activities or substances do the trick by first elevating another brain chemical, dopamine, which then triggers serotonin production. What's addicting, then, isn't the specific activity or substance, but the resulting dopamine rush. And we get hooked on whatever provides it.

Dopamine is the "gotta have it" chemical we crave when we don't have enough, Ruden says. Serotonin, on the other hand, is the "I got it" chemical. When we have enough serotonin, the sexual craving response stops—but only temporarily, since the serotonin levels in such a brain deplete quickly. Soon the whole process starts all over again.

This automatic response has been hard-wired into us for millions of years. Originally it had a noble survival purpose: Because sex felt good, we sought it, and the species survived. Because fat tasted good, we ate it, and it protected our bodies against the cold and nourished us during times of famine. Today, unfortunately, survival on such a primal level is not an issue and a lot of the things we seek can backfire and do us more harm than good.

> "Today, unfortunately, survival on such a primal level is not an issue and a lot of the things we seek can backfire and do us more harm than good."

Take, for example, pornography. Some sex compulsives actually start using porno films and magazines in an addictive fashion. Like Rich L.: On January 11, 1990, Rich L. masturbated while watching a pornographic video. He knows the date because he marks his sobriety from porn with it—Rich now considers himself a recovering porn addict.

"I was using porn frequently," he says. "I would go on binges, which meant I would rent a lot of videos and just spend all my time masturbating. Then I'd feel really demoralized and want to stop. But I'd do it again."

No good data exist yet to indicate how many men could be accurately described as porn "addicts," but John Sealy, M.D., medical director of the Sexual Disorders Unit at Del Amo Hospital in Torrance, California, believes the number of sex "addicts," about half of whom have porn problems, at least matches the number of gambling compulsives—about 5 percent of the population.

Still, casual viewing of pornography doesn't necessarily mean there's a problem. "Younger males who are not in serious relationships have very rich masturbatory fantasies when using these kinds of pictures," says psychiatrist and sex therapist Harvey Rosenstock, M.D., founder of the Rosenstock Clinic, a general psychiatric clinic in Houston. "It substitutes for what they don't have available at that time. There's no problem with that."

In fact, Rich L. says he feels viewing sexual images actually helped him at first. He had an inhibited upbringing, and his initial experimentation with sexual material showed him that sex was a healthy part of human nature, not something to be ashamed of.

But as he began to compulsively use more and more pornography, Rich L. found himself trapped in the classic belief system of the sexual addict. In *Out of the Shadows,* Patrick Carnes, a leading figure in the field of compulsive sexuality, lists the compulsive's core beliefs:

1. I am basically a bad, unworthy person.

2. No one would love me as I am.

3. My needs will never be met if I have to depend on others.

4. Sex is my most important need.

These are the four signposts of a lonesome road. "Sex addicts are very lonely, very detached people," Sealy says. "Their common core belief is: 'If anybody really knew me, they wouldn't want to be my friend.'"

For the compulsive, great amounts of energy go into keeping up a happy facade while wracked with feelings of detachment. "Feeling you have to take extraordinary precautions to conceal your behavior is a signal that it has gone beyond normality," Rosenstock says.

The Road to Recovery

"A craving brain takes away choice," Ruden says. "Addiction recovery is all about giving the craving brain its freedom of choice back again."

Unfortunately, "addiction" is a complicated problem, which is why artificially changing our brain chemistry with drugs isn't enough to take care of it. "It will be a long time before we can look to a simple pill or patch to cure all addiction in one fell swoop," Ruden says. "There are too many factors involved for that fantasy to come true anytime soon."

Takamine agrees. "You can't lay everything on one's personality or brain chemistry," he says. "There are stress factors. There are environmental factors. There's genetics. There are outside influences—family, how you were brought up, your character, your attitude." Until someone does develop that magic pill, we'll have to keep on diagnosing and treating compulsive behavior the old-fashioned way—from a multi-discipline perspective. Fortunately, for those who are willing to go through it, these methods work.

For example, 12-step groups have cropped up around the country to help sex "addicts." If you think you need help but don't want to attend a support group yet, you might try simply discussing your concerns with someone you can fully trust. "That automatically suggests you're open for some kind of dialog," Rosenstock says. "You've already taken the first step—realization of a problem."

A second step may be therapy, but that alone may not be enough, according to Sealy. "You need the power of the group experience to counter the shame," he says. "This is the only addiction with this much shame associated with it. But you don't have to live in isolation, despair, and shame."

Stopping the Compulsion

If you think you may have become addicted to sex or pornography, take the Sex Addicts Anonymous test we've included later. If the answer is yes, here's what you can do about it.

Educate yourself about your own compulsion. Read all you can, seek out experts and teachers.

Get help. As mentioned previously, 12-step groups can prove to be invaluable. In fact, Ruden asserts that 12-step groups—all of which use the same support-group model for abstinence, self-improvement, and helping others—are the best solution for many addicts. "Recovering people need to be able to identify with others of their own ilk." Ruden uses the metaphor of a herd of oxen: "If one ox gets separated from the rest, he becomes acutely anxious. When he finds his herd again, he'll plow right into the middle of it until he's surrounded by his own kind. Only then will he begin to relax. Many people work the same way." Also, seek out help in the form of therapists, psychiatrists, and psychologists. They can provide an interdisciplinary approach, involving medication, therapy, and behavior modification, to get you on the road to recovery.

If you fail, try again. "Keep seeking out treatments and people who have solutions until you solve your problem," Ruden advises. "It may be a lifelong quest, but so be it. Bear in mind that slipping once doesn't mean you can't succeed again; it just means you have to start over.

Find your aha! moment. This is what you're really looking for when you're trying to shake a compulsion: a moment of clarity when you finally "get it," when your obsession with what you've been doing or using suddenly drops away. Statistics show that the more active you are in seeking treatment, the greater your chances will be of having a moment like this. Ruden speculates that this moment may even be accompanied by permanent chemical changes in the brain, allowing the conditioned craving response to become undone. Obviously, much more investigation is needed here, but it's a fascinating idea.

"Addiction is so treatable," Takamine says. "If you're just willing to say, 'I've got an addiction; where can I get help?' you'll get it, and you'll put people like me out of business."

At age 44, Rich L. joined a 12-step program. Although he has yet to maintain a lasting love relationship, he describes himself as better off than he has ever been. He's had far more intimate contact with real people these past six years than ever before. "I think it's important for people to hear stories from other people who've had the addiction and are in the process of recovering," he said.

Are You a Sex "Addict"?

Sex Addicts Anonymous (SAA) provides a self-administered test to assess whether you may have a sexual addiction. SAA recommends seeking more information or counseling if you answer yes to two or more of these questions.

1. Do you keep secrets about your sexual or romantic activities from those important to you? Do you lead a double life?

2. Have your needs driven you to have sex in places or situations or with people you would not normally choose?

3. Do you find yourself looking for sexually arousing articles or scenes in newspapers, magazines, or other media?

4. Do you find that romantic or sexual fantasies interfere with your relationships or are preventing you from facing problems?

5. Do you frequently want to get away from a sex partner after having sex? Do you frequently feel remorse, shame, or guilt after a sexual encounter?

6. Do you feel shame about your body or your sexuality, such that you avoid touching your body or engaging in sexual relationships? Do you fear that you have no sexual feelings, that you are asexual?

7. Does each new relationship continue to have the same destructive patterns that prompted you to leave the last relationship?

8. Is it taking more variety and frequency of sexual and romantic activities than previously to bring the same levels of excitement and relief?

9. Have you been arrested or are you in danger of being arrested because of your practices of voyeurism, exhibitionism, prostitution, sex with minors, indecent phone calls, etc.?

10. Does your pursuit of sex or romantic relationships interfere with your spiritual beliefs or development?

11. Do your sexual activities include the risk, threat, or reality of disease, pregnancy, coercion, or violence?

12. Has your sexual or romantic behavior ever left you feeling hopeless, alienated from others, or suicidal?

Helping Hands

Contact these groups for more information on sexual addiction:

- Sex Addicts Anonymous 612-646-1970
- Sex and Love Addicts Anonymous 617-332-1845
- Sexaholics Anonymous 615-331-6230
- Sexual Compulsives Anonymous 212-439-1123
- Del Amo Hospital's Sexual Disorders Unit 800-533-5266
- American Associations of Sex Educators, Counselors and Therapists 319-895-6203 (fax requests only)

Chapter 8

Relationships

You've learned the difference between love and lust. Been schooled in the history of romance. Mastered foreplay and cunnilingus. Charted out a variety of sex positions. Now what? Where do you go to put all this knowledge—all these newfound skills—to use? Welcome to the wonderful world of relationships. The problem is, keeping a relationship isn't as easy as it seems. First, we'll show you where to begin—that is, finding the opposite sex, with commentary from single women. Then, we'll take you through the fine art of seduction. And, after you've met and seduced them, you'll need to follow the rules of dating, based on wisdom culled from a variety of relationships experts. Finally, it's on to the heavy-duty duties of relationships.

Meet Market

With the possible exception of money, nothing weighs more heavily on men's minds than where to find women. You could turn to your male friends for advice. But anyone who's spent time in locker rooms knows that when it comes to dating, men lie even more to other men than they lie to women.

So ditch the braggadocio and half-baked "strategies" of your friends. Instead, listen to this completely unscientific panel of women, all of them attractive and single. Their basic message about making the first connection? Be yourself. If you're out with friends, joke around, dance, play pool. "In a social setting, I'm not drawn to the loudest guy," says literary correspondent Dominique, "but I do tend to notice the ones who are animated, who look like they're having fun."

Some other things to consider as you move into the meet market:

Alpha Males Need Not Apply

Think you need to be tough—act tough—to get a woman to notice you, because it always seems like the really good girls like the really bad boys? Well quit your posturing, stow that new leather jacket, and put the Harley up for sale. According to writer Rosemary Daniell, tough isn't bought, it's earned. Witness her report on a life spent pursuing brooders brimming with machismo:

I've been through a lot of guys in my life, largely because my predilection for strong men called for a lot of trial and error. Like many Southern women, I had been brought up to choose the sensitive Ashley Wilkeses of the world rather than the tough Rhett Butlers.

"You are who you marry," my mother told me over and over. The kind of men she favored for me were the white-collar ones who went downtown to Atlanta each day, a briefcase under one arm, a

or . . . What to Do with All This Great Information

Brooks Brothers coat over the other. Oh, I had tried to escape her imperatives via a failed first marriage to the angry Sean Penn of our town, but I heeded her advice with husband number two, a young accountant type. In the suburbs, I cried as I watched him through the kitchen window, carefully laying out perfect squares of zoysia grass.

Then I tried for some white-collar, brainy toughness, marrying a Boston intellectual, Columbia- and Yale-educated. An aspiring writer, he liked to tell me what books to read and how to revise my poems, but my passion wavered as I realized that I had to be less in order for him to be more: His mastery of the cutting remark chipped away at my self-respect. When my first book was published, things fell apart at fast-forward, ending in a third divorce.

During the next few years, I dated, among other men, two famous tough-guy Southern poets who were as well known for their sexism, for giving drunken readings, and for arguing about which comma went where, as they were for their writing.

Fed up with trying to find someone who embodied both the edge I wanted and what Mother called "good husband material," I began my search for a bona fide tough guy. These men were usually great dancers and great in the sack but given to throwing my diaphragm across the room, muttering things like "I don't want anything to come between us, baby." Monogamy wasn't in their vocabulary, either.

Some of the men I took into my frilly Savannah apartment during that (pre-AIDS) period were downright dangerous, men who looked good but who turned out to be drug dealers or convicted felons. One, like a tomcat spraying his territory, threw damp towels around my bedroom and made deals over my telephone. Then, warning me not to sleep with anyone else while he was away, he left as abruptly as he had arrived.

I danced with a witch doctor in a Guatemalan jungle disco and lived in a hotel-cum-brothel in Costa Rica, then traveled with a Contra supporter to a refugee camp on the Nicaraguan border. Sitting in a village bar, I sipped rum-and-sodas, grateful that my friend, an Indiana Jones–type (who, true to form, was cheating on his wife), had decided that because of bad weather we would not, after all, go up in the single-engine plane parked out back with the bullet hole in its side.

Working as one of the first women aboard an offshore oil rig, I found myself surrounded by muscular men who routinely made comments like, "I'd marry yo dawg to git to you, honey." I soon had a boyfriend to protect me from the rest, a roughneck who, when visiting me in Savannah, would throw his bowie knife at the roses in my wallpaper. He drank so much one time that as I drove him to the airport the next day, I had to stop the car to let him throw up. "Ah always git this way when I have to leave somebody ah love," he said, grinning as though he expected me to go along with his delusion.

These were not real tough guys. These were cartoon characters.

I met Zane near the end of this tough-guy quest. He was still in the military, a paratrooper with steel-blue eyes and 14 fewer years on the planet than me, when I, a former war protester, met him. Albeit a reader of Albert Camus and Joseph Conrad, Zane had come from that delicious-looking blue-collar group, with biceps developed by actual work (and at which many middle-class women only allow themselves surreptitious glances).

Zane's genuine masculinity made me feel more feminine by comparison: I could be as gutsy and aggressive as I wanted, but he had the real cojones. And for the past eight years of our marriage, my choice of a true tough guy has been borne out.

Now a trucker, Zane has demonstrated time and again how true toughness compares to the pseudo kind. He's not, and never has been, afraid of expressing when he feels on the verge of tears, when he needs time alone,

> "Working as one of the first women aboard an off-shore oil rig, I found myself surrounded by muscular men who routinely made comments like, 'I'd marry yo dawg to git to you, honey.'"
> —writer Rosemary Daniell on her experience with tough guys

or about how he fears that time down the road when his parents will no longer be here. (I realized I was falling in love during my first visit to his parents' home when I saw Zane—unaware I was watching—tenderly kiss his white-haired mother on the head.)

The primary thing that this genuine tough guy is willing to do is to be honest about himself and make changes. Zane says that being a man means admitting when you made a mistake and shutting up and listening when the woman in your life is right.

I never considered Brad Pitt a heartthrob until I heard that he lets hundreds of little green lizards run wild in his house, and that a couple of his famous girlfriends had left him, complaining that he didn't bathe often enough. Most important, however, was that he was generous to down-and-out relatives. Guys who don't have a soft spot, guys who are unkind—they don't qualify. Nor do the self-labeled: According to one biography, author Norman Mailer, quintessential self-designated tough guy, feared Southern men when he was stationed at Fort Bragg, North Carolina, during World War II. He considered them the essence of machismo. Guys like Mike Tyson and O.J. may have been tough in the sports arena, but are they really willing to look at themselves? That takes real guts. True toughness is like true north. It may be found in a weight room or on the sports field, but it's also in the kitchen or living room. And it's the only kind of toughness I find worthwhile in a man.

Take Pride

You needn't have the build of an Olympic swimmer or spend hours primping—just take pride in how you look. Comb your hair. Brush your teeth. Wash your clothes. "It doesn't take a lot to impress a woman," says Deena. "Some color coordination and understanding of fabrics will go a long way."

Smooth Is Unsettling

Sure, that "shaken, not stirred" routine works in the movies. Then again, James Bond can also leap from a moving train into a car with an explosive suitcase in each hand and land with his cufflinks still in place. In real life, the ultra-suave approach tends to unsettle women. "Sorry," says Deena. "It's hard to take something that's so well-practiced seriously. I mean, how many women have heard the same line?"

> **"You needn't have the build of an Olympic swimmer or spend hours primping—just take pride in how you look."**

The Top Secret, Surefire, Magic, Guaranteed Hypnotic First Line

Here it is: "Hi, how are you doing?" or "Hi. I'm (your name here)." Too simple? Nope. If a woman is feeling outgoing and likes your bearing, she'll respond. If she doesn't, you're doomed anyway.

Walkin' the Dog

Entire social scenes revolve around canines. In fact, dog parks have become the singles bars at the turn of the millennium, with owners meeting, greeting, and comparing notes on breeds and breeding . . .

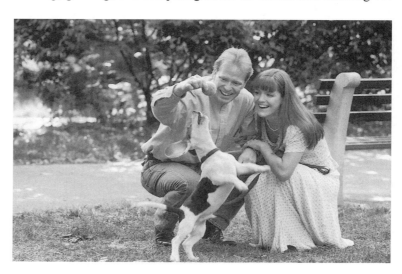

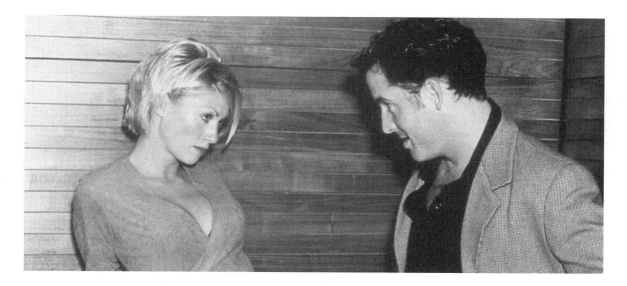

which eventually leads to talk of other kinds of breeding. Best yet, you won't need a first line; she'll ask your dog's name, and the door will be open.

The Eyes Have It

Yeah, you might feel shy. But for God's sake, look at a woman once you start talking to her. Averted eyes say you're pulling a snow job—and women hate few things more than a liar. Also, if you're looking downward, she'll assume you're just angling for a close-up of certain parts of her body—and that puts you in the I'm-a-closet-sexist-pig-out-on-the-town category, which is a no-no in these enlightened times.

It's just as bad to look around the room as you unfurl your rap. "Ugh," says painter Reiko. "When a guy's scanning the crowd as he's making small talk, I definitely feel insignificant. It's like he's just shopping, so it seems like there's a huge potential for being used."

Anguish Ain't Sexy

It's OK to be a sensitive guy; just don't start off baring your soul and sharing your innermost thoughts. Furrowed brows and a permanent sulk are flashing warning lights to most females. "What woman wants to date a man who acts like one of their girlfriends?" Sasha asks.

A Shoe-in

No woman will expect you to be a male Imelda Marcos, but well-chosen shoes will show attention to detail and score huge points. Ultimately, good shoes are a sign of a well-heeled man. A few suggestions from the panel: sandals (European style), boots, or well-made leather dress shoes.

If you insist on wearing athletic shoes, ditch your puffy cross trainers and invest in some kicks that look good with jeans or shorts, e.g., Puma Clydes, Adidas Stan Smiths, Converse Chuck Taylors, Nikes, anything by Simple.

Finding the Right Places

Show us a great place to "meet chicks," and we'll show you two dozen guys standing forlornly on the sidelines. Losers? Maybe. More likely they're just out of place; feeling like a fish out of water will make even the coolest man clammy.

"People can read discomfort a lot more easily than we'd like to think," Reiko says. "Women will pick up on it if a man feels uncomfortable." So play to your strengths. If you hate dancing, don't loiter in dance clubs. An awkward talker? Stay away from cocktail parties.

To find your home away from home, here's an annotated guide to myriad meeting places.

> **"Show us a great place to 'meet chicks,' and we'll show you two dozen guys standing forlornly on the sidelines."**

Bars. It's a safe bet most women feel open to meeting someone new here.

The upside:

- As we all learned in college, alcohol relaxes drinkers' inhibitions.
- Feeling ballsy? Send a drink as an opening gambit.
- Most people in bars are already feeling social.

The downside:

- Unless you're an extremely quick closer, it takes a high tolerance for booze and secondhand smoke to make good on the bar scene.
- Most women distrust men who spend a lot of time hanging out in bars. Men, however, often think too much with their penises to hold the same opinion of women.

Nightclubs. Emporiums filled with gyrating flesh and pulsating music, dance clubs serve as a prime venue for meeting strangers.

The upside:

- You don't even need to talk to a woman. Just go up and start dancing with her.

- Most women like men who can dance. It shows a certain self-confidence and easygoing sense of fun. And there's a belief that if you've got good moves on the dance floor, so will be the case when it comes time for the horizontal mambo.

- You can always act like you only want to dance.

The downside:

- Loud sound systems make real conversation difficult.
- Dancing makes you sweat, and it's hard to stay composed with a forehead Niagara flowing.
- She may, in fact, only want to dance.

Bookstores. Especially when accessorized with comfy couches and coffee bars, bookstores loom as the new hipster hunting grounds.

The upside:

- You can easily figure out someone's interests by seeing which aisles she's browsing. (You may want to avoid the parenting section.)
- It's free.
- Women will think you're well-read.

The downside:

- If you never actually buy (or even read) any books, the staff will peg you as a shameless pickup artist—or a cheapskate. And she'll figure it out pretty quickly, too.
- Higher than average bookworm-wallflower quotient.
- Many women are just there trying to buy a damn book. (Watch for repeated eye contact before you make a move.)

Friends. Many people meet this way, and friends love to orchestrate each other's amorous lives.

The upside:

- It's pretty easy to find out the basics: Is she dating anyone? How long has she been single? Why did her last relationship end? Has she ever done time?
- Introductions are a breeze, whether it's a blind date or just "accidentally" showing up when you know she'll be with your friends.
- Other people do your scouting.

The downside:

- She gets the scoop on you, too. (Got any skeletons in that closet?)
- If the date (or, worse yet, the relationship) goes south, you'll end up having to do some furious spin control.
- Your friends may set you up with people whom *they* would date—if they weren't married.

Laundromats. Ever since that infamous Levi's 501 jeans ad, people consider laundromats oddly sexy.

The upside:

- A woman's laundry can reveal her marital/parental status. Clues: jockeys, diapers.
- Washing and drying cycles hold women hostage for lengthy stretches.
- "Can I borrow some Tide?" is an acceptable first line.
- Women can see how tidy you are.

The downside:

- Most laundromats feature uncomfortable plastic chairs and TVs blaring worthless talk shows—hardly environs conducive to romance.
- If it's laundry day, you'll most likely be wearing the dregs of your threads.
- Women can see how tidy you are.
- You'll have to ditch your Spiderman underroos.

Supermarkets. Since everyone's got to eat, you'll see all sorts of potential dates.

The upside:

- You can do a quick personality profile and marital/parental status check by examining a woman's shopping cart contents. Clues: Hungry Man dinners, baby food.
- Store layout allows you to scope out prospects rapidly.
- Even if you strike out, you've still done your shopping.

The downside:

- She can do a quick personality profile by examining your shopping cart contents.

- People rarely talk to strangers in markets, so your opening line may signal a blatant pickup bid.

Weddings. Hands down, the premier spot for flirting.

The upside:

- You're decked out, and so are the women.
- Meeting someone is as easy as arching an eyebrow and saying, "So, whose side are you from?"
- Liquor.
- Most important, it's almost blasphemous—no matter what your real-life experience—not to believe in romance at a wedding, so the emotional pumps are primed.

The downside:

- The possibility of falling for a woman who:
  1. lives far away
  2. is related to you.

The One Other Place

Sure, there are the traditional places where the opposites attract. But what about the workplace? For a guy fresh out of college, this would seem to be tempting territory to meet interesting, intelligent women. Indeed, studies conducted to determine the most frequent places where people who eventually become a couple meet have found that work repeatedly ranks right up there with parties, and way ahead of singles bars and the street, as the likeliest place to form a long-lasting relationship.

Then there's the safety factor. You know she's employed, and there are people around who would probably tell you if she were, say, an ax murderer on work-release. You're spared the social anxiety of trying to strike up an acquaintance with a total stranger. And you start out knowing that the two of you have something in common—at best a consuming fascination with related careers, at worst a common frustration with a nightmare boss or a dysfunctional company.

But be cautious. The work waters can be shark-infested. Depending on the course of an office affair—and on your employer's view of passion on the payroll—you could find yourself blissfully married or unemployed or both. You could end up in a dream relationship, or spending eight hours a day under the gaze of somebody you loathe, who loathes you back, and whose loathing is based on intimate first-hand knowledge.

The downsides of office affairs have never been so apparent than in these litigious times. Just think about the Anita Hill–Clarence Thomas debacle, the charges against Robert Packwood, and headline-grabbing claims made against President Clinton by practically every woman in the country. Each case caused plenty of debate about what constitutes sexual harassment; and there are plenty of individuals—male and female—who feel it is an issue that should never be taken to court.

Still, the mere possibility of lawsuits or other work romance troubles have led many businesses to either regulate or absolutely outlaw employee romance. And the courts are supporting their right to do so. In 1993, Wal-Mart fired two workers at one of its New York stores for violating a company policy that forbade married employees from dating coworkers (one of the employees was separated from her husband). The state of New York sued Wal-Mart on the workers' behalf, but an appellate court ruled in favor of the company.

> "Depending on the course of an office affair—and on your employer's view of passion on the payroll—you could find yourself blissfully married or unemployed or both."

Still, motivated couples can be resourceful. Sally T. (not her real name, because her employer doesn't know she's dating a colleague) works for an advertising agency in New York City. "A lot of flirtation always goes on in an office, and most of it's insignificant," she observes. "But if someone's willing to risk following through and threatening the peace of the workplace, that's a sign they're serious."

Her coworker Oliver, who initiated their relationship, doesn't minimize the complications of love on company time. "Before we got together," he recalls, "I spent hours and hours—most of the day, in fact—flirting with her in the office, and it cut into my work. I'd rather we'd met through friends," Oliver concedes. "But friends just don't come through; I haven't met that many people socially that I'm interested in going out with." And though their company doesn't forbid employee dating, the two don't want to face the consequences of going public. Also, Oliver and Sally agree that the air of slight danger and mild conspiracy adds some spice. "It is kind of exciting," he admits. "It eroticizes all kinds of normally dull things, like E-mail, even meetings, have a certain frisson."

Despite the benefits, however, New York City–based therapist and couples counselor Carol Dougherty offers a different view. "There are too many problems," she says. "Competition with coworkers, for instance, or charges of favoritism. Do you keep it surreptitious or tell people? What if you break up? What about the situation where one person's already working there and hires somebody because he's attracted to her?"

The risks, in other words, are real. Although they may disagree on whether the pitfalls are worthwhile in the end, Dougherty and the veterans of office romance we spoke with are unanimous in their advice to anyone teetering on the brink:

- **Understand the risks.** Most companies don't actually forbid employee dating, but courts have upheld their right to fire you if you violate an explicit and uniformly applied policy. And even if your employer is tolerant in this respect, nobody should have to remind you that what passes as a routine come-on in a singles bar can, when delivered in the workplace, spark a sexual harassment charge. In these hypersensitive times, think before you flirt.

- **Beware the casual fling.** If even judicious workplace dating can lead to trouble, imagine what you can expect if you stumble into bed at random after a few cups of eggnog at the company Christmas party.

- **Remember that rank matters.** Mr. Maintenance Man can aspire to snare Mme. Treasurer, and secretaries do marry vice presidents, but the risk factor is proportionately higher when rank enters the picture. Coworkers won't like it. Charges of favoritism are inevitable. And mixing power with sex is like throwing gasoline onto the barbecue coals. Virtually all the most sordid (and most massively publicized) horror stories of workplace interactions gone awry involve bosses and subordinates. Beware.

- **Don't confuse your love life with your work life.** "It's weird when we're outside the job and find ourselves drifting into shop talk," Oliver says. "We have to stop each other." Especially in the first stages of a relationship, job gossip can help bridge the inevitable awkward silences. But sooner or later you're going to have to explore parts of yourselves that your work life doesn't touch. Love may bloom on the job, but it's not likely to thrive if you treat it as a mere extension of your wage-slave life.

- **Think ahead.** It may be depressing in the first flush of affection to anticipate the end of a relationship, but this is one context in which you can't afford not to. If your love affair with a friend or neighbor crashes and burns, you can always get an unlisted phone number, buy a wig, change your name, flee the country. But if your ex is a coworker, you're going to have to see her—and cooperate with her—day in and day out, possibly for the rest of your working life. So agree at the outset that if the worst happens, you're both going to be adults: distant, perhaps, but cordial, helpful, and professional.

None of these cautions should (and, of course, none of them will) stop you if you're determined to pursue a workplace relationship. Try to anticipate the dangers, by all means, but remember that love and work are like everything else: full of the uncertainties that make life interesting.

The Fine Art of Seduction

You know where to go to hook up with members of the opposite sex. So how do you make that critical transition from meeting to mating? It's called seduction. And before you start dating—and mating—you need to make that connection. Follow these guidelines, distilled from today's men and women who've found consistent success in the science of seduction.

Radiate. If you want women to see you as a sexual possibility, you've got to see yourself that way. Feel—and revel in—your own sexuality. Lose the "I'm-a-geek-and-you-probably-won't-like-me" attitude. "You have to radiate your sexual self the way some women do," says Zoe, a decorative painter in Santa Monica, California. "The only way to do that is to be comfortable in your own skin. If you don't, you're probably not going to feel comfortable around a woman."

Receive her signals. One could make the case that men don't seduce women; women tell them to come hither, sending messages both verbally and via body language. "If they're interested, women often try to make it easy for you to seduce them," says Bernie, a freelance writer from New York City. "The problem is that most men don't try to figure out what women are saying."

A few good signs, according to Jeanne Martinet, author of *Getting Beyond Hello*:

- eye contact and a smile
- hair twirls
- pointless fidgeting
- light touches—of her own body or yours.

"Flirting is the heart of the seduction; it's where you overcome the fact that you don't look like Tom Cruise and don't drive a Rolls-Royce."

Flirt. Of course, for better or for worse, it's still up to you to at least appear to make the first move, so flirt. He who flirts well and flirts often will not sleep alone every night. Flirting is the heart of the seduction; it's where you overcome the fact that you don't look like Tom Cruise and don't drive a Rolls-Royce. Flirting is a way of showing genuine interest in becoming better acquainted with someone. Flirting is banter, play; it's saying one thing while meaning another, and fully intending that both your meanings will be understood.

Judy Kuriansky, author of *The Complete Idiot's Guide to Dating*, offers these rules for flirts:

- Use flattery. It's the fastest way to a person's heart. If you're truly taken by the way a person looks or acts, feel free to compliment. A rule: Be sincere.

- Listen. "The most powerful aphrodisiac is your undivided attention," Kuriansky writes.

- If you discover a common interest, talk about it.

- Smile. Kuriansky cites a study concluding that people who smile more tend to make more money and have less stress. But for flirting purposes, she notes, a smile makes you look friendly, warm, and open. And that's attractive.

- Trust yourself. "Believe that you can do it, survive it, and come out feeling good about yourself," she writes.

- Be responsible. Be truthful, careful, and clear about your intentions.

I'm in the mood for love. Let's say she agrees to a date. Where to go? Dark and atmospheric restaurants are always great date sites, especially for the better-heeled. But there are other options for those with fewer dollars. Try this: Cook a meal. If you're insecure about your culinary capabilities, remember this most important point: If you're cooking for her, she's at your place.

Love shack. According to ancient tradition, the Bachelor Pad is a foul and sordid place, disheveled and faintly redolent of tossed-off sweatsocks and funkifying sheets, bathrooms that violate state health codes, and sinks full of dishes. Sounds great, doesn't it?

Don't forget that women have to tolerate being there. Clean your little love nest, and make sure there's lots of toilet paper in the bathroom. Be neat, but not sterile. A cool mess—clutter that reveals something about your life, like music or books—is OK. One of our love pundits even stores his motorcycle in his living room, deliberately parked against a white backdrop so it almost seems like a piece of furniture or sculpture. It's unexpected.

In the bedroom, start by getting rid of any photos of your ex. Then make the place inviting. Start with clean sheets and some decent blankets and comforters. You want the environment to be simultaneously safe yet exotic—a secret little chambre d'amour. Put simply: lots of pillows and some candles for the night table.

Musical truth. Music contains more romantic energy than any other force in the universe. Why? It doesn't matter. It just does. The question is: Which musicians and melodies will best contribute to the mood of the moment and make your date more amenable to your advances? Anything if you play an instrument that's not a tuba or a kazoo. Otherwise, try anything by Billie Holiday. Or Marvin Gaye. Or Barry White, Chris Isaak, Luther Vandross, or Al Green. If all else fails, get something, anything, with lots of saxophone.

The Dating Rules for Men . . . or the Postseduction Principles

You met her. And seduced her. Now you're dating. Except it seems like there's an awful lot of authorities steering the romance . . . especially from her end.

Witness: First there was *The Rules: Time-Tested Secrets for Capturing the Heart of Mr. Right*. That begat *The Rules II: More Rules to Live and Love By*, which begat *The Rules Dating Journal*. And *The Rules Note Cards*, which begat *The Real Rules: How to Find the Right Man for the Real You*. It even spawned *The Rules for Cats* and *The Rules for Dogs: The Secret to Getting Free Treats for Life*. It's a veritable cottage industry of Rules.

The *Rules* books have become a phenomenon because they revel in a specific set of edicts that a woman has to follow in order to be successful with men. And in these confusing times, women grasp at anything that seem to provide a sense of order and logic to what is typically illogical (affairs d'amour). In essence, the *Rules* woman follows not her heart but a list of directives suggested by the authors.

> "Which musicians and melodies will best contribute to the mood of the moment and make your date more amenable to your advances? Anything if you play an instrument that's not a tuba or a kazoo."

For instance, a *Rules* woman will not call you and will rarely return your calls (Rule No. 5). She will always end a phone call first (Rule No. 6). If you hear a "ding" while you're on the phone with her, it might be a timer going off to let her know it's hang-up time. She will dump you if you don't buy a romantic gift for her birthday or Valentine's Day (Rule No. 12). She will not go Dutch (Rule No. 4), and she will always end a date first (Rule No. 11).

The book's authors believe that men respond to challenges, and if pursuing a woman isn't a challenge, a man will lose interest. Accordingly, the *Rules* woman litters her trail with obstacles. Judging from the popularity of the book and its spin-offs, the mindset has taken hold. If a manufactured challenge is what you want, a *Rules* woman could be for you. But if you're looking for a more honest relationship in which a woman reacts to you, not Mr. Preconceived Typical Male, we're with you.

So, we queried some prominent love experts to compile our own set of dating and relationship "rules" that should get us all through the day—no contrivances, no timers, and no manufactured, prefab romance.

Rule No. 1: Listen. "Many women want a man who listens and empathizes," says Deborah Tannen, a reigning guru on communication differences between men and women and the author of *You Just Don't Understand: Women and Men in Conversation*. Listen, she says, but don't necessarily advise. If you're a good listener, your attentiveness will be appreciated, and you'll also pick up on what makes her really purr.

Rule No. 2: Laugh, and make her laugh. Life's tough. "A sense of humor makes the going endurable," says San Francisco Bay Area psychotherapist John Amodeo, Ph.D., author of *Love & Betrayal*. You don't have to be Bill Murray; just maintain a sense of humor about the world and, more important, about yourself.

Rule No. 3: Give freely. Psychologist David Buss, Ph.D., says all females look for a man who is generous with his resources. "In a study across nearly 40 different cultures, females valued the financial capacity of potential mates more than males did," Buss says. But that doesn't mean she only wants your money. If you offer other precious resources, like your time, energy, and affection, she'll notice.

Rule No. 4: Expand your sensuality. "The human male has more sensual common ground with a male ape than he does with a female of his own species," quips Stephen Johnson, head of The Men's Center of Los Angeles, a nonprofit counseling agency. Beyond basic vision and taste, men may not be as aware of their senses as women. But we can develop them. Use all your senses to praise her: Compliment the color of her clothes, the sound of her voice, the smell of her perfume and skin.

Rule No. 5: Be on time. Nothing erodes a relationship like rudeness—and few things are ruder than being late. And while spontaneity is often appreciated over the course of a relationship, you shouldn't always wait until the last minute every time you invite her out. *The Rules* trains a woman to turn you down if you call on Wednesday for a Saturday date. That's fair. Plan ahead, especially for those first encounters.

Rule No. 6: Romance her. For *The Rules* authors, failure to be romantic is a capital offense. They explain to their readers: "If you end up marrying a man who gives you a briefcase instead of a bracelet on your birthday, you may be doomed to a life of practical, loveless gifts and gestures from him such as food processors, and you may spend thousands of dollars in therapy trying to figure out why there's no romance in your marriage."

We agree, though we're not too sure about the therapy part. Romantic gestures show that you act from the heart—and that you're interested in capturing hers.

Rule No. 7: Tell the truth. This rule trumps all the others. Weave a web of deceit and it will soon entangle you. Don't pretend that you like the ballet and the theater when you really prefer college football. Still, that doesn't mean you can't learn to like the erotic footwork and the melodies. "A lot of the much-touted differences between men and women are overblown," says Patricia Arroyo, a counselor at Dartmouth College in New Hampshire. "If both sexes would deal with each other more honestly, gender differences wouldn't go away, but it would be much easier to negotiate around that which naturally divides us."

> "We may get some heat from the feminists for saying this, but most women are like the TV character Ally McBeal: They want to have it all— but just get married first."

Taking the Plunge

You've done the Meet Market routine. You've seduced her . . . and maybe even played by The Rules. You know she's The One. She's 26, you're 28, and the two of you have been shacking up blissfully for more than a year when she starts to look disappointed by your lavish gifts—a leather jacket for Christmas, a sterling silver charm bracelet for Valentine's Day, a trip to Cancun for her birthday. Sheeeeesh! You put a lot of thought into those tokens of affection. What does she want?

Frankly, you on bended knee holding The Rock. We may get some

Sexbit 14

If you tend to ignore the romantic advice of parents and friends, you may want to rethink things. Research conducted at the Universities of Lethbridge and Waterloo in Canada indicates that Mom, Pop, and the buddies can assess the long-term success of your relationship better than you can.

heat from the feminists for saying this, but most women are like the TV character Ally McBeal: They want to have it all—but just get married first. And guys are the same way; they're just a bit more patient because they're not working against a clock.

With that observation on the table, our advice to any man who finds the right woman is to hold on as though your life depends on it. If she wants to get married, and you know that you want to spend your life with her, talk through your concerns (if there are any) and make a decision together about when the blessed event will occur. The longer you've been together, the harder it will be for you to procrastinate—unless your significant other is a gullible sap. And even gullible saps have their limits. Take too much time to pop the question, and the gullible sap may be the one you're forever wishing did not get away.

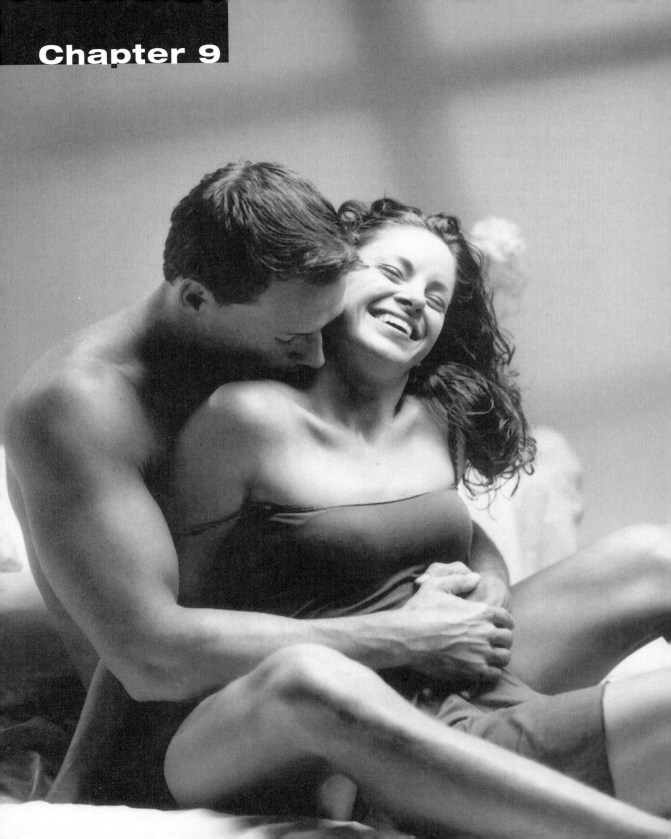

Chapter 9

You've been together for 5 years, or 10, or 20. For your last anniversary, you made a reservation at a special restaurant. You had champagne. You gave each other nice gifts. And afterward, you jumped into bed and . . . fell asleep?

Congratulations on extending your relationship past the initial passionate stage. It feels good, as comfortable as an old pair of jeans, doesn't it? But while not too long ago bedtime would have been just the start of the evening's celebration, lately you don't have as much desire as you used to, and the feeling seems mutual. It could be for a lot of reasons . . . you're tired, distracted, a little bit older, or maybe you're just plain bored with each other.

Are the two of you doomed to spend your nights watching Jay Leno when you could be tearing up the sheets? Hardly. Although your libido may have become a little rundown, it just takes a bit of effort to jump-start the passion again.

So think of this chapter as your ticket to sexual rejuvenation. In addition to highlighting creative ways to get through a rut, we asked both sex experts and real-life couples to share ways to get that spark back into a long-term relationship. You had it once. With a little innovation in the bedroom, kitchen, bathroom, etc., you can have it again—in spades.

Talk—and Chuckle—About It

We can't stress it enough: "Communication and laughter are the keys to keeping sizzle in relationships," says Roger Libby, an Atlanta-based sex therapist and host of a radio show called *The Pleasure Dome*. "You can be as sexually creative as you like, as long as you discuss your desires with your partner before you plunge in," he says. "Express your interests over time. That way you can both get a feel for each other's comfort levels. And realize, too, that things may not go exactly right the first time out, so laugh about it. Sex is supposed to be fun."

Sandra and Robert, a twentysomething couple from Madison, Wisconsin, are proof that dialogue—and a little friendly advice—work. "It took me three years to bring up the subject of cunnilingus with Robert," Sandra says. "I couldn't orgasm from vaginal intercourse, so I wasn't being satisfied sexually. I started to think we were sexually incompatible and that I had made a huge mistake marrying him. My friends told me oral sex would do it for me, but I figured it would be unpleasant for Robert, especially since he never attempted it on his own."

As it turns out, Robert was afraid Sandra would be against it, so he never asked. "We didn't have sex until we were together almost a year, so I figured she was really conservative."

Hot for the Long Haul

Sexbit 15
Optimism Reigns

It's very possible to maintain sexual desire and excitement in a long-term relationship.

Agree . . . . .83.0%   Disagree . . . . .5.9%   Not Sure 11.1%

(Source: Source: *Men's Fitness* Sex Survey of readers, 1998)

"Hell, no," says Sandra. "I finally got the guts up to ask for a little '69' and wow! I've gone from nonorgasmic to multiorgasmic; my only regret is that it took three years to happen."

Word Play

The moral of Sandra and Robert's story: If there's a sexual favor you'd like from your lover, don't wait three years to ask for it. And if you can't just ask outright, try this game: Get a couple of pens and some paper, and independently of each other, write down everything you wish your partner would do for you in the sex-and-affection department. Be specific. For instance, write: "I wish you would initiate sex once a week," or "I wish we would have sex in the shower."

Rank your requests from the easiest to the most difficult. Then set a time to make your requests, one each, once a month. Two rules apply:

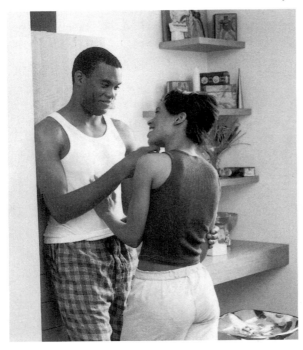

You each commit to give the other's request serious consideration, but neither of you is obliged to grant it. Even if you don't agree to everything on each other's list, chances are you'll get most of what you want and feel much closer as a result.

By the Books

Not everyone entering a relationship is as sexually experienced as the characters on *Melrose Place*. For these individuals, Joan Elizabeth Lloyd, author of erotic and self-help books such as *Nice Couples Do*, suggests an experiment she calls bookmarking. "Go to a bookstore, buy an erotic magazine, novel, or sex how-to. Take turns reading it, each time marking a section that you find intriguing. Pass it back and forth, until you can both agree on something that excites you. Then go for it."

At this point, you might want to flip back to chapters 4 (The Whole Shebang: Love, Lust, and Sex) and 5 (The Wilder Ride) for some great bookmarking opportunities.

Phone Home

As you get more comfortable expressing your desires, sex therapist Bernie Zilbergeld, Ph.D., suggests "simmering." When you feel any sexual charge, hold onto it. Call your lover and mention your momentary turn-on. Let her know you're filled with anticipation for your next meeting. No need to have elaborate phone sex; just let her know that your juices are flowing. Arousal is contagious, and anticipation adds zing to any rendezvous.

Sex First

Putting sex on the back burner is an easy choice to make for couples caught up in the daily pressures of work and family. But it's not smart. "If you want to maintain an active love life, you have to make it a priority," says San Francisco–based sex therapist Louanne Cole Weston, Ph.D. "Make sex dates for times when you both have energy, not late at night when you're both exhausted."

If there are children in the house, think naptime . . . think playgroups . . . think strongly about working out a deal with a neighbor. Arrange to have your kids play at their house on, say Saturday afternoons, while their kids hang out at your place on Sundays. That way you each get a couple of hours alone with your respective partners.

With a luxury like that, Libby recommends thinking of the entire house as a sexual playpen. We may be conditioned to view the bedroom as the "appropriate" place, he says, but consider the monotony of making love over and over and over in the same room for 50 years. Rather than compartmentalize sex, do it in the kitchen, in the bathroom, on the Persian rug. Test out every new piece

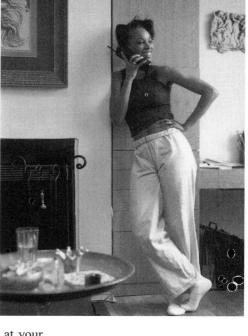

> **"I finally got the guts up to ask for a little '69' and wow! I've gone from nonorgasmic to multiorgasmic; my only regret is that it took three years to happen."**
>
> **—Sandra, on oral sex**

of furniture. "In other words, be adventuresome," Libby says, "It's the best way to keep love and lust going strong."

Work on the individual settings as well: Candlelight is more arousing than darkness. Music is more erotic than silence. Sexual lubricants enhance the pleasure of touch. Erotic videos can be a turn-on for both of you, which brings us to our next suggestion . . .

Get Creative

Let's say you've perfected the sex positions listed in chapter 4. Now what? Well . . . you could avoid monotony the easy way by merely mixing up the sequence of acrobatics—missionary today, rear entry tomorrow, woman on top the next day . . . blah, blah, blah. Or you can use your imagination.

> "If there are children in the house, think naptime . . . think playgroups . . . think strongly about working out a deal with a neighbor."

To many couples creative lovemaking means playing games. John and Donna, for example, figured out a way to turn their respective pet peeves into passion plays. John says he was bothered by his wife Donna's habit of not putting the caps back on their household supply of pens. Donna hated that John left change lying around, "on the kitchen table, the bathroom vanity, the night stand." Instead of nagging each other, and turning minor irritations into major differences, they've nipped the problem in the bud rather wisely. Each time John catches Donna in the act of leaving a cap behind, he doesn't complain. He just picks it up and puts in a dish on his nightstand. Likewise, Donna collects John's change in a dish on her nightstand. When either partner is feeling randy, he/she presents the other with a cap . . . or a quarter . . . for a sure thing. "When I hand over a cap, Donna can't say no," John says, "I've become vigilant about collecting those pen caps. I'm actually starting to like her habit."

> "Candlelight is more arousing than darkness. Music is more erotic than silence. Sexual lubricants enhance the pleasure of touch. Erotic videos can be a turn-on for both of you."

In author Ellen Kreidman's latest book, *How Can We Light a Fire When the Kids Are Driving Us Crazy?,* Earl and Marie recommend their version of erotic Monopoly. "Instead of paying rent when we land on the each other's property, we remove an article of clothing. Just in case the game lasts too long, the first one to Pass Go ten times, collects."

Debbie figured out a way to make her husband's obsession with

Monday Night Football work to her advantage. "We both bet on which team will win the game, and by what point spread. The loser has to do whatever the winner says. Recently, my husband made me cook and serve dinner totally nude. It was so much fun, I'm going to turn the table on him next time I win."

Creative Assistance

Granted, not everyone has the capacity to turn Monopoly or *Monday Night Football* into a sex game. Which is A-OK, because there are plenty of companies willing help you spice things up. For a price, you can buy books, games, and videos designed to spark your libido. There are classes you can take to become more sensitive lovers. Here's a look.

Read On

Anyone who loves surprises will dig Laura Corn's clever trio of books—*101 Nights of Grrreat Sex, 101 Nights of Grrreat Romance,* and *101 Grrreat Quickies*. Each offers . . . well, 101 seduction options, sealed shut until you and your lover tear them free. There are some for pleasing him and some for pleasing her. Here's a sample (for him), randomly pulled from our favorite Corn compendium—*101 Grrreat Quickies:* "#37. Passion Fruit: The bearer—who is bare—will present you with a sweet, delicious and incredibly juicy piece of fruit. As soon as he sits down, you must kneel and place the fruit in his lap. Now devour it. And do it slowly and sensually, while getting as wet and messy as possible. Don't be afraid to make a big, wet mess—because before this meal is over, you're going to lick your plate clean." Now excuse us for a few moments while we take a break for #40: Naughty Kitty.

If getting away for a romantic weekend isn't an option, sex authors Pepper Schwartz, Ph.D., and Janet Lever, Ph.D., provide an hour-by-hour game plan for having one at home in their book, *The Great Sex Weekend*. Tips can be obvious (unplug the phone and take the dog to the kennel) and schmaltzy (kiss each other as if it were the first time), but it's the underlying theme of the book that's important—make your love life a priority, even if it's just the occasional weekend.

Toss of the Dice

There are two dice, but instead of having numbers on all sides, they have suggestive words or phrases. Throw them, and whatever lands up, you do. That's the premise of Dirty Dice: Fooling Around By Chance, a game from Holiday Products that you can take with you just about anywhere. The upside? With rolls like "kiss" and "above the waist," Dirty Dice leaves lots of options open. The downside? Your partner may end up rolling "squeeze" and "ear," over and over and over again.

Board to Tears—of Ecstasy

There are at least a half a dozen board games with romantic or sexual themes. On the tame side, An Enchanting Evening provides an opportunity to reflect on the richness of your relationship. The game begins with you and your partner writing down a secret wish that can be shared later that evening. As you move around the board, you draw cards that direct your actions. You may have to respond to questions about your relationship, for example, or do some gentle, playful touching. There's nothing sexually overt about this game; you could give it to your parents for a fiftieth wedding anniversary gift.

> "... there are erogenous zones all over the body that can benefit from a sensual rub."

If you'd prefer something spicier, try Romantic Sensations. This game encourages you to explore your sense of touch and comes complete with sensuous massage lotion and bath gel. Sexsational is a board game with a fantasy spin. It begins with you and your partner writing down a "secret" fantasy you'd want fulfilled by the end of the game. Each of you takes turns picking "opportunity" cards, which require you to correctly guess how your partner would answer provocative questions. In theory, you'll be so hot after a round of Sexsational you'll fulfill your personal fantasies.

Titillating Tapes

After 20 years of marriage, you should know how to have sex. It just may not be earth-shattering—or even quivering—anymore. To shake things up, order a copy of *The Sexuality Library*. From the folks at Good Vibrations (800-289-8423), this collection of erotic books and videos includes a solid array of sex education tapes. Pop in *Sexual Ecstasy for Couples,* which offers tips on sharing fantasies and light bondage. Or *Accupressure for Lovers,* a video that teaches you how to "release ecstatic sexual energy" via 12 lovemaking points on the body.

We've already cited foot massage as a great method of foreplay. But

Sexbit 17

Mood lighting, anyone? According to the *Playboy Advisor,* using blue lightbulbs in the boudoir creates "a mysterious and sensual atmosphere" ideal for sex. Pink bulbs "provide light that is soft, romantic and flattering—it makes most people look much younger." And for those occasions when you want your bedroom to look like a brothel, screw in a few red lightbulbs. A well-stocked hardware store should have a wide selection of bulbs in each of these sexy hues.

there are erogenous zones all over the body that can benefit from a sensual rub. Yes, massage is a great way to relax stiff muscles and ease tension. But it's also fantastic for gaining a better understanding of your mate.

Creative Touch

"I totally recommend massage for people who are in some kind of significant relationship, whether it's explicitly sexual or not," says Sylvia Hacker, Ph.D., who taught human sexuality for 20 years at the University of Michigan's public health and nursing school. "It's the best nonverbal form of communication; it allows you to slow down and find out from each other what pleasures you."

For couples who, for whatever reason, aren't able to have intercourse, massage is a terrific alternative for expressing love and getting close physically. "The term massage is an overall umbrella for getting in touch with the body's potential for pleasure," Hacker says. "You can merely allow your skin to be touched for its own luxurious excitement, or you can choose to let it lead to orgasm."

From shiatsu to Rolfing to foot reflexology, many different massage techniques have been developed over the years, but sensual massage doesn't require mastery of any of them. In fact, a good erotic massage can borrow from several disciplines. It may involve the full body, or it can focus on specific parts, such as the neck, back, abdomen, legs, or breasts. All that's required for a good massage session is the willingness to find out what feels good to your partner, and to let her know what you like. And practice, practice, practice.

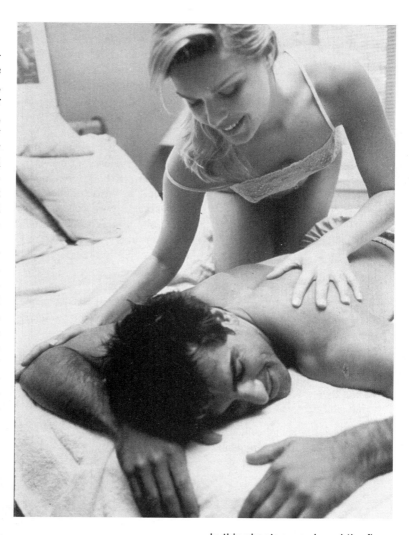

In this chapter, we shared the finer points of giving her an erotic massage, but one thing we didn't mention is the bonus: If you rub her the right way, she'll probably reciprocate.

▼ideo Primers

Turned off by XXX flicks? Perhaps the steamy R-rated entertainment on this list will get you and yours going.

- *Body Heat:* Kathleen Turner looked hotter than ever in this noirish take on the prototypical forties femme fatale film.

- *9½ Weeks:* For the most part this fetish flick flopped, but we loved the tasty refrigerator scene.

- *Last Tango in Paris:* This account of one man's descent into depravity is more psychological than sexual, but it's worthwhile for the butter scene alone.

- *Risky Business:* A high schooler and a hooker have hot train sex in this scathing indictment of materialism.

Love Shack

First, set the mood: Nitya Lacroix's *Massage for Lovers* (Harper-Collins, 1994) suggests creating an "altar of love." Choose a time when you both can relax for a long time without interruption. In a warm, uncluttered room, work on a firm, comfortable surface—a mattress may be too soft for certain strokes. If so, try placing a sleeping bag or folded blanket on the floor and working there. "Keep some warm towels nearby to cover her if she starts to feel cold," Lacroix advises. (You'll also need plenty of towels to absorb the massage oil.) Soft lighting—aromatic candles are a good source—adds to the erotic aura, as do some favorite tunes played quietly.

Oil Slick

Like a sports-car engine, the friction of a high-performance massage requires plenty of oil. Baby oil will work, but it doesn't have a sexy scent. In her book *Erotic Partner Massage* (Sterling, 1990), Christine Unseld-Baumanns suggests thinking with your nose: "Partner massage is part aromatherapy," she says. "A massage oil containing orange blossom, lavender, or balm oil is perfect for releasing tension." Whatever oil you choose, warm it in your hands first; you don't want to massage goose pimples.

Different Strokes

Your hands can apply a pleasuring touch in a variety of ways. Anne Hooper, a former *Penthouse Forum* editor, recommends these basic

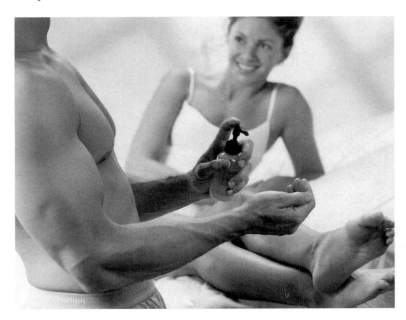

strokes in her book *Ultimate Sexual Touch: The Lovers' Guide to Sensual Massage* (Dorling Kindersley, 1995):

- **Sweeping strokes.** Best for massaging large body parts, such as the back. With open hands, use long, sensuous, sweeping strokes.

- **Detailed strokes.** For smaller, more complicated parts, such as the shoulders, hands, and feet. Movements should be firm and short. Avoid massaging areas where the bone is close to the skin.

- **Kneading.** A smooth move for the hips and buttocks or other fleshy parts. Use the thumbs and forefingers of both hands to rhythmically squeeze and release the skin.

- **Circling.** A great basic stroke for areas such as the back and shoulders. Place both hands palms down and move them in opposing circles. Lean onto your hands when you want to add pressure.

Get Her Back

Because most people are comfortable with back rubs, this is often the best place to start. Slather on oil, then start by using circling movements on the shoulder area. As you move toward the midback, apply some sweeping strokes, letting the flats of your thumbs gently massage the spine. Finish off with a good kneading of the buttocks.

Neck Romancer

To massage your partner's neck, suggests Susan Mumford in *The Complete Guide to Massage* (Penguin, 1995), put a little oil on your hands, then place them so that your fingers are pointing downward at the top of her chest and the flats of your thumbs are touching the back of her lower neck. Keeping your hands in full contact with her body, draw them outward over the shoulders and slide them around underneath the neck. For added invigoration, move up and "shampoo" the scalp with your fingers. (Be sure to wipe any oil off your hands before you touch her hair.)

Treasure Her Chest

You'll both miss out if you don't throw in a very intimate chest massage. Hooper's book describes how to do it: Slide the palm of your right hand diagonally across her right breast toward her left shoulder, then do the same on the left side. Repeat six times on each side. Next, splash on some oil and use the tip of your index finger to trace a spiral on her breast. Start on the outer edge and slowly spiral in until you reach the nipple.

- *The Postman Always Rings Twice:* This remake of classic film noir starring Jack Nicholson and Jessica Lange led to a generation of table-clearing sexcapades.

- *Crimes of Passion:* It's twisted. And gritty. And blue. As in China Blue, the alter ego of the architect portrayed by Kathleen Turner in this examination of fetish culture.

- *Fatal Attraction:* There's nothing sexy about boiling bunnies. But ya gotta admit, the sex after the attraction—and before the fatal—was sizzling hot. Kitchen countertops never looked so good.

- *Witness:* Okay, Amish amore isn't steamy, but the dance scene was electric.

The Ab Rub

The abdomen picks up stress quickly, so any soothing strokes will help, Mumford says. Ab massage has another benefit that's somewhat geographical: From the stomach it's easy to move on to other nearby, ah, parts. Kneel at your partner's side and spread oil on her abdomen using soft, circling, palms-open strokes. Add force to your movements as she becomes more comfortable.

Creative Cleansing

There is something totally erotic about slipping and sliding through postmassage sex. But if you'd prefer to proceed in a tidier manner, another great way to build arousal is to prepare a romantic bath for two. In author Mary Muryn's book *Water Magic* (Simon & Schuster, 1995), she devotes an entire chapter to "Pleasure and Sexuality Baths." By combining essential oils that are reputed aphrodisiacs, Muryn claims that a bath can do everything from strengthen an erection and heighten arousal to enhance fertility.

Certainly you'll want to set the stage. In other words, put the rubber duckies and tub toys away, and break out the candles, soft music, chocolates, and champagne. And don't worry if your bath is on the small side; cozier means closer. Instead of having to swim across one of those trendy monster Jacuzzis, you just reach out and touch each other.

You can go the bubble route, but those soap suds have a tendency to get in the way. That's why stores such as The Body Shop, H₂0 Plus, and Aveda sell nonfoaming bath products specifically oriented toward couples. You can also purchase some of the essential oils listed in chapter 2, and mix up one of Muryn's concoctions. Our favorite for couples who need to jump-start their libido is the "Wake-Up-Your-Sex-Life Bath." Make sure the water is mutually comfortable before adding the essential oils, as they tend to evaporate quickly. And consider mixing them in advance with vegetable oil, honey, or cream. Any of these added ingredients will ensure that the essential oils are properly dissolved in water and absorbed by the skin, says Muryn.

Wake-Up-Your-Sex-Life Bath

3 drops magnolia oil

5 drops nutmeg oil

5 drops Arabian musk oil

Creative Taste

They say the way to a man's heart is through his stomach. Well, the same may hold true for his libido, as well as hers. Oysters, celery, onions, asparagus, mushrooms, truffles, chocolate, figs, honey, caviar, bird's nest soup, and wine are a partial list of foods long reputed to be aphrodisiacs, substances that rev up desire and improve sexual performance.

Until recently, scientists dismissed the true potency of aphrodisiacs as quaintly fraudulent and insisted that the power of suggestion was all that fueled any reported benefits. "It's very difficult to separate effects on the mind from those on the body," says Varro Tyler, Ph.D., professor of pharmacognosy (natural products pharmacy) at Purdue University School of Pharmacy. "Sexual enjoyment involves both mind and body equally, so anything people consider arousing becomes arousing."

But they've been learning that some old reputed sexual enhancers, and some surprising new ones, actually work. Get your shopping list ready. The following are among the latest foods and herbs that'll put you in the mood.

Caffeine (in coffee, tea, cocoa, chocolate, and colas). Arab caliphs sipped coffee before visiting their harems, and Montezuma and Casanova ate chocolate to fortify themselves for lovin'. But caffeine may do more than simply keep you and your partner awake until the end of the ten o'clock news. University of Michigan urologist Ananias Diokno, M.D., found that coffee drinkers were considerably more active sexually than nondrinkers. No wonder business is booming at Starbucks.

Carrots. Phoebe Cates did an excellent job of highlighting the phallic qualities of this veggie in *Fast Times at Ridgemont High*. But Bugs's favorite treat also happens to be an excellent source of beta-carotene, a form of Vitamin A that helps keep the sex hormones in check.

Figs and avocados. Both contain niacin, also know as vitamin B_3, which lowers cholesterol and increases blood flow by dilating blood vessels. John Morgenthaler, coauthor of *Better Sex Through Chemistry* (Smart Publications, 1995), says that niacin triggers a pivotal histamine necessary for quality orgasms.

Ginseng. Asians insist that ginseng boosts productivity, the immune system, athletic ability, and prowess of a more intimate nature. American scientists remain skeptical. But James Duke, Ph.D., a botanist with the U.S. Department of Agriculture's Research Station in Beltsville, Maryland, and author of *Ginseng: A Concise Handbook* (Reference Publications, 1990), cites several Asian and Russian studies showing that the herb may indeed promote sexual function. Herbalists say ginseng preparations, which are available at health-food stores,

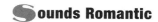

Sounds Romantic

Whether you're warming up with an erotic massage, or enjoying a long night of leisurely lovemaking, these tunes will put you in the mood—and keep you there.

Al Green, *Greatest Hits*

Anything by Barry White, Frank Sinatra, Enigma, and Nat King Cole

Chopin's piano waltzes

Debussy's *La Mer*

Deep Forest, *Deep Forest*

Donna Summer, *Four Seasons of Love*

Harry Connick, Jr., *When Harry Met Sally*

Peter Gabriel, *So*

must be used for several months before producing any noticeable stimulant effect.

Oysters. Scientists scoffed at their reputation until nutritionists discovered that they are, indeed, exceptionally rich in the trace mineral zinc, which is crucial for male reproductive health. Whole grains and fresh fruits and vegetables also contain zinc, while processed foods are often low in the nutrient. Deficiencies are associated with infertility and prostate problems. In fact, University of Rochester researchers have restored sperm counts of infertile men using zinc.

> "Oysters, celery, onions, asparagus, mushrooms, truffles, chocolate, figs, honey, caviar, bird's nest soup, and wine are a partial list of foods long reputed to be aphrodisiacs, substances that rev up desire and improve sexual performance."

Saw palmetto. This small palm tree native to the southeastern United States was recommended by early American folk healers as a breast enlarger, diuretic, and treatment for benign prostate enlargement. Recent research shows some support for the latter two benefits.

Tropical fruits. In *Sexual Nutrition,* Morton and Joan Walker write that certain fruits such as bananas, kiwi, mangoes, and papaya have a high content of chelating (binding) minerals and an enzyme called bromelain that act like pipe cleaners for blood vessels, including those in the penis. As you know from previous chapters, the more freely blood flows to your equipment, the more likely it is to perform when you need it to.

Wild yam. This tuber's sexual reputation springs from its age-old use as a remedy for gynecological ailments. It turns out that wild yam is a potent source of diosgenin, a chemical that resembles the female sex hormones used in birth control pills.

Yohimbine. For centuries, the bark of the African yohimbe tree has been reputed to restore potency. Studies conducted in the 1980s showed that it does raise erections in some impotent men by increasing blood flow to the penis. A few years ago, the Food and Drug Administration approved yohimbine as an impotence treatment. It's available in three prescription drugs: Aphrodyne (Star Pharmaceuticals), Yocon (Palisades Pharmaceuticals), and Yohimex (Kramer Laboratories). Yohimbine extract is also available in health-food stores.

Creative Travel

Whether it's long hours at the office or young children that are interfering with your love life, getting away for a week—or even a weekend—can go a long way toward getting back on track romantically. Of course, we're talking about traveling together—without work and without kids. And with a little forethought and planning you can choose a destination that guarantees romance. All-inclusive resorts such as Sandals' Couples in Jamaica, St. Lucia, and Antigua make it easy. In addition to a partners-only policy—no kids allowed—a Couples getaway includes unlimited food and drink, a wide range of sports and water activities for the adventuresome, and lush surroundings for mates who prefer to kick back with a fruity drink and a good book. Married couples who are feeling ultra romantic can even renew their wedding vows. The Sandals' resorts perform about 20 weddings per week—for free.

Interested in a more free-form trip? Here are our picks for the most romantic cities in North America, with a few suggestions on what to do when you get there.

Florida Keys

About 28 miles from Key West is Little Palm Island, rated by *Conde Nast Traveler* as one of the best hotels in the world. Here, you can stay in one of 30 thatched roof villas with in-room whirlpools, recline beside a free-form pool with a waterfall, and enjoy gourmet cuisine prepared by an award-winning French chef.

Even closer to Key West is Sunset Key, a small island 500 yards, or about ten minutes away. Operated by Key West Hilton, it offers one-, two-, and three-bedroom guest cottages reminiscent of the old, traditional Key West architecture. Call 888-477-7SUN for details and reservations.

Prefer the funky flavor of Key West itself? Pier House (800-327-8340) is a sophisticated hotel located in the historic heart of the city. It's decor is Old Florida with porches and shutters, and topless sunbathing is permitted on its tiny but pleasant private beach.

Chicago

Okay, so most people don't think of the Midwest as a romance Mecca. But we live in Chicago, and when it blooms in spring after a long cold winter, the city is breathtaking. In fact, there's nothing Second about it. Chicago has one of the best urban beaches in the country. On a warm summer night, you can walk for miles, enjoying the lake breeze and spectacular skyline. The newly renovated Navy Pier, though a bit touristy, has a five-story ferris wheel that screams romance—especially at night. The city's restaurant and theater scenes are top-notch; the shopping along North Michigan

> "Chicago has one of the best urban beaches in the country. On a warm summer night, you can walk for miles, enjoying the lake breeze and spectacular skyline."

Avenue and Oak Street is world class; and there are lots of fun neighborhoods—Lincoln Park, Old Town, and Bucktown, to name a few, which perfectly reflect the city's laid-back nature.

We recommend staying in a hotel around North Michigan Avenue. The Four Seasons (800-332-3442) is a luxurious, modern option, while the equally posh Drake Hotel (800-553-7253) exudes stately charm. Both are within walking distance to Oak Street beach and primo restaurants and shopping.

Montreal

If you like the romance of a French city, but don't relish the endless flight to Paris, consider a trip to Montreal. This charming city—with its cobblestone streets, friendly atmosphere, and French heritage—is, in some circles, actually preferable to Paris. And the exchange rate is much better. As we went to press, the U.S. dollar was worth about $1.50 in Canada, which means everything you buy is about 33 percent off. For a truly chi-chi escape, stay at the Ritz-Carlton Kempinski (514-842-4212). Aside from being the first Ritz in the chain and the oldest hotel in Montreal, it's the place where Liz Taylor and Richard Burton were wed.

If that feels like a bad omen, check out the Westin Mont-Royal (800-226-3000), a lux hotel whose guest list has included Madonna, Cher, and Pavarotti. Or if you want romance on a smaller scale, there are slews of bed-and-breakfasts in the area, some in old mansions. Call 800-267-5188 for more info.

New Orleans

For some of the best food in America, and a truly decadent time, head to New Orleans. Reserve a room on Bourbon Street if you're *really* up for a party. We stayed at the Royal Sonesta (800-766-3782) and booked a room with a balcony. Though we arrived after midnight, there were hundreds of people dancing in the street. During our four-day stay (the perfect amount of time to experience this funky Creole city), the crowd remained thick and lively.

If you'd prefer something less boisterous, the Hotel Maison de Ville (504-561-5858) is filled with antiques and four-poster beds. According to the Zagat Survey, an annual nationwide review of restaurants, the hotel's bistro is the best in town. And if you tire of Hurricanes—the city's signature fruity (and potent) drink—Hotel Maison de Ville serves complimentary port and sherry each evening.

Because New Orleans gets mega-muggy during the summer months, you'd be wise to visit in the early spring or fall. Be sure to walk along the lovely waterfront, take a riverboat ride, and get up early at least one morning to for a round or two of coffee and beignets at

Cafe DuMont. And if you're open-minded, check out some of the burlesque shows on Bourbon Street. They can be a definite turn-on.

New York

Theater, restaurants, carriage rides through Central Park. New York oozes romance—so long as you don't trip over the garbage that tends to accumulate in the streets. Seriously, though. New York is considered the U.S.'s most sophisticated city, and hotels such as the St. Regis (800-759-7550), The Pierre (800-743-7734), and The Carlyle (800-227-5737) cater to lovebirds. (Bobby Short sings in the nightclub of the latter.) Whether you're seeking romance in the winter (ice-skating at Rockefeller Center) or the warmer months, it's a wonderful place for couples to reconnect and, of course, it's the city that never sleeps . . . so why should you?

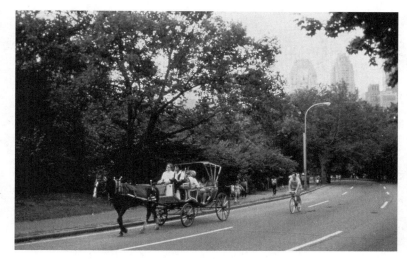

Okay, so the carriage ride through New York's Central Park is a bit clichéd. But it works when romance is in order.

San Francisco

San Francisco is postcard pretty and offers plenty of opportunities to revive that spark. You can do the tourist thing and explore Pier 39, the Japanese Tea gardens, and hippie-heaven on Haight-Asbury streets. A trolley ride is a must, as is trip to Chinatown. And prepare to eat. San Francisco has an excellent restaurant scene. But, as far as we're concerned, the most romantic adventures require a car and a drive along twisty, turning Highway 1. Stop at the Muir Woods, a redwood forest with trees predating Columbus's arrival, and then keep driving until you reach Point Reyes. The drive and the scenery will take your breath away.

If you have time during your trip, visit Napa wine country for tasty samplings. After all, wine is the liquid of love.

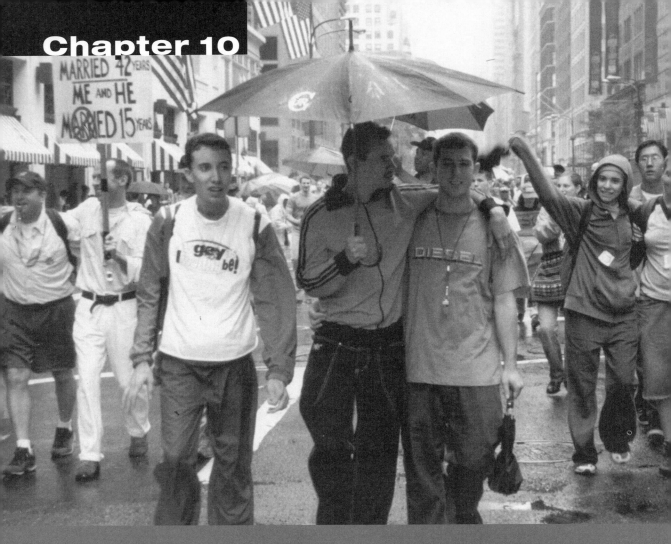

Chapter 10

Alternative

The Problem with Labels

Heterosexual. Homosexual. Bisexual. Each of these terms is used to classify a person's sexual orientation. If you're attracted to—and prefer to get intimate with—the opposite sex, you're heterosexual. If you'd rather get frisky with a member of the same sex, you're homosexual. And if you swing both ways, you're bisexual. The problem with these labels, like the myriad others in our society, is that they create stereotypes. And stereotypes create misunderstandings, prejudices, and oftentimes hatred.

Our objective in this chapter is not to share the details of a homosexual or bisexual lifestyle, but to create a better understanding of the complicated issue of sexual orientation. On the surface, it may seem rather easy to differentiate among the three labels. Either you like guys, girls, or both. But studies have shown that it's not nearly that clear-cut.

Much of what we know about sexual orientation and homosexual behavior, for example, was gleaned from two research studies by the Kinsey Institute— *Sexual Behavior in the Human Male* (1948) *and Sexual Behavior in the Human Female* (1953). Though other more recent research projects have delved into the subject of sexual preferences, including one that set out to debunk Kinsey's findings, none have been as extensive.

The Gist

Kinsey's study involved sixteen thousand individuals from a wide sampling of the general population who were asked to describe human sexual orientation more precisely. Respondents answered questions about their personal sexual preferences and experiences using a scale of zero to six, with zero representing people who considered their behavior exclusively heterosexual, three representing people who said they were equally attracted to men and women, and six applying to people who felt they were exclusively homosexual. Responses one through five dealt with ranges of preferences, and took into account such areas as dreams, fantasies, and changes in preferences throughout a individual's lifetime.

Interestingly, few people rated themselves either a zero or a six. If you apply that to society as whole, it means the majority of people wouldn't label themselves exclusively heterosexual or homosexual. In other words, sexual behavior isn't black or white. Most of us have experienced some gray, whether it be a physical attraction to a member of the same sex, a homoerotic dream or fantasy, or an adolescent exploration (you know, one of those "let's play doctor" games). And though Kinsey's statistics suggest that about 37 percent of males and 13 percent of females

Nation

had some overt homosexual experience in the course of their adult lives (that is, one that results in orgasm), it is estimated that only 10 percent of the population exclusively prefers same-gender sex.

Nature Versus Nurture

For those individuals who fall into that 10 percent category, the question society tends to ask is: What causes homosexuality? This is where major prejudices come into play. Because homosexuality in many circles—particularly religious ones—is considered abnormal, or "against God's will," there are plenty of people who feel the need to blame someone—a domineering mother, a depraved adult who takes advantage of a vulnerable kid, an abusive father, etc.

> ". . . sexual behavior isn't black or white. Most of us have experienced some gray, whether it be a physical attraction to a member of the same sex, a homoerotic dream or fantasy, or an adolescent exploration (you know, one of those "let's play doctor" games)."

However, research has shown that homosexuality has both genetic and environmental bases. For example, we know:

- that background and skin color have little bearing on sexual orientation. The proportions of various types of sexuality seem to be about the same in all cultural and racial groups.

- it's not a contemporary issue. Evidence of homosexual activity dates back centuries and has been found in a wide variety of cultures.

- humans aren't the only animals with same-gender desires. Just ask a farmer.

- baby brothers have a higher tendency toward homosexuality. Male homosexuality has been linked to the number of male siblings: a study has shown that the greater the number of elder brothers a man has, the more likely he is to be homosexual. The reasons could be

Sexbit 18

The Kinsey Institute's research into sexual identity may have been completed decades ago, but a more recent study at the University of Georgia seems to confirm the results—most people aren't solely hetero- or homosexual. Sixty-four "straight" men were first questioned to determine their anxieties regarding homosexuality. The researchers then attached monitors to the participant's penises and showed them clips of straight and gay XXX movies. It turns out, the men who expressed the greatest homophobia showed the most arousal while watching men having sex with other men. Interesting, indeed.

biological or simply an effect of the treatment of younger siblings within the family, according to *The Lovers' Guide Encyclopedia*.

- it could be determined at conception. Several research studies point to a genetic basis for sexuality. One conducted on identical twins (who have the same genetic makeup) and fraternal twins (who do not share the same DNA) showed that if one twin is homosexual, an identical brother is much more likely to be homosexual than a non-identical brother. More recent research claims to have identified the relevant gene and has noted differences in brain structure among heterosexual and homosexual men.

- the sex-is-dirty upbringing can contribute. "Puritanical attitudes toward sex, if they lead to a deeply rooted fear of the opposite sex, may also encourage homosexual behavior," reports *The Lovers' Guide Encyclopedia*.

Social Stigmas

Despite these historical observations, and research findings which indicate that homosexuality is *not* a choice, the lifestyle across most cultures remains unacceptable. Being "gay," a term used to describe homosexual men, or a "lesbian," a homosexual female, still carries many social stigmas, primarily due to misunderstandings and stereotypes.

Plenty of straight and homosexual men claim to have a "gaydar," but the truth is, gay men and lesbians do not stand out in the ways some heterosexuals think they do. Just because a guy dresses nicely and likes to decorate his home, for example, doesn't mean he's gay. Two men living together may just be friends. Homosexual men and women aren't obsessed with sex and they don't like to always "do it" one way. Their relationships and sexual practices are just as varied as those of heterosexuals. However, because of the taboos and social intolerance still associated with the lifestyle, homosexuals have banned together to form what has become (at least in the States) a highly politicized, and increasingly powerful, subculture.

> "Because homosexuality in many circles—particularly religious ones—is considered abnormal, or 'against God's will,' there are plenty of people who feel the need to blame someone—a domineering mother, a depraved adult who takes advantage of a vulnerable kid, an abusive father, etc."

We're Here. We're Queer. Get Used to It.

It began with the Stonewall riot in the late sixties, a time when New York City police routinely rousted gay clubs simply because there were gays inside. One night, however, the gays fought back. And that marked the beginning of "out" activism. Still, it was small-scale compared to the ground swell of activism that commenced in the early eighties with the discovery of HIV and AIDS. Because AIDS was initially considered a homosexual disease—it was initially labeled "gay cancer"—finding a cure was a low priority of the Reagan administration.

"Homosexual men and women aren't obsessed with sex and they don't like to always 'do it' one way."

This led to grassroots efforts ranging from Act Up sit-ins on Wall Street to candlelight vigils to nationwide fund-raising efforts and ultimately the banding together of an alternative nation. It pushed safe sex to the forefront of our social consciousness and led to medical efforts and research, which proved AIDS is not just a disease exclusive to homosexuals but one that impacts everyone—everywhere.

The Closet Door

It also prompted a desire among homosexuals to stand up and be proud, to reveal one's sexual identity. But "coming out" isn't always easy given the attitudes that still exist regarding homosexuality. Even though homosexuality is more openly discussed, America's religious Right, and the family values platform of many of our most prominent politicians, tend to encourage fear and "homophobia." Ellen DeGeneres may have been given the opportunity to openly dig chicks on prime-time TV, but not for long. Her sitcom's gay theme

"Ellen DeGeneres may have been given the opportunity to openly dig chicks on prime-time TV, but not for long. Her sitcom's gay theme survived one season."

survived one season. To think that anyone can admit their homosexuality and not be subjected to biases is naive.

Advocates of the coming-out process say that telling the truth is a relief. That's probably true. The cost of subterfuge—the constant camouflaging and editing of conversations—runs high. And we don't deny some of the other benefits of "coming out":

- You can share more of yourself and your life with others.
- You'll eliminate a lot of the confusion in your life, allowing you to gain a greater understanding of who you really are. Studies indicate that 30 percent of all suicides among young people stem from questions of sexual identity.
- You won't feel so isolated and alone. Sharing your lifestyle helps validate it.

- You will give the important people in your life an opportunity to support you.

- You can love—and be loved—easier because there are no barriers or secrets.

But that's the sunny side. The dark side of "coming out" involves risks—sometimes big ones. You may experience discrimination, job loss, and alienation from friends and family. You might find yourself on the receiving end of verbal harassment. Or worse, you could be physically harmed by a total stranger merely for admitting you're gay. So our advice is to avoid pressure. Think it through. And do what's right for you.

The Issues

Although homosexual men and women can be considerably more open about their lifestyle these days, there are still numerous issues that weigh heavy on their minds. To present a clear picture of the challenges gays and lesbians face, we spoke to John Gallagher, national correspondent for *The Advocate*. Here, in order of discussion, are the topics he deems most pressing.

1. **Marriage.** A controversial subject in and out of the gay community, same-sex unions are currently not recognized legally in any part of the U.S., and, in fact, have been officially deemed illegal in 28 states. What's more, President Clinton signed the Defense of Marriage Act in 1996, which withholds federal tax pensions and other benefits to partners of homosexuals.

   Despite this lack of government support, many members of the gay community continue to fight for the right to make a legally binding commitment. As we went to press, lawsuits filed by gay couples seeking marriage licenses have reached the Supreme Court in three states—Hawaii, Alaska, and Vermont.

   "Gays and lesbians have the same desire as heterosexuals to make lifelong commitments," Gallagher says. "They want the same things—a relationship, a home, a family." Right now, they're having commitment ceremonies, often conducted by more progressive members of the clergy. "But not allowing gay couples to make the commitment legal denies them many

> "... not allowing gay couples to make the [marriage] commitment legal denies them many of the benefits of that union, including tax incentives, adoption privileges, and insurance."
> —John Gallagher, national correspondent for *The Advocate*

of the benefits of that union, including tax incentives, adoption privileges, and insurance."

Interestingly, not all homosexuals are in favor of legal marriages. According to Gallagher, there is a portion of the gay community that feels "marriage" is historically a heterosexual model for a relationship. "Buying into a standard construct is not what gay liberation is all about."

We have no doubt that this issue will remain at the forefront of gay activism and political discussion over the next decade. In fact, we wouldn't be surprised if some of the country's more liberal states had loosened up their policies by the time you read this.

2. **Insurance.** Another critical issue is the ability to secure comprehensive medical and life insurance. According to Gallagher, most entertainment companies, as well as a growing number of large corporations (like American Express and Levi-Strauss), offer "domestic partnership" insurance—health and life insurance to same-sex couples in long-term relationships. Though Gallagher expects domestic partnership insurance to become more commonplace, he acknowledges that legalizing gay marriages would make it a requirement.

3. **HIV.** "It is now possible, thanks to the use of protease inhibitors, for a person with HIV to live a long life," says Gallagher. But while contracting HIV no longer seems like a death sentence, he points out that "it's still serious, people are still dying, and the treatment is extremely expensive."

Gallagher also notes that while mortality rates among gays with HIV has declined, rates of infection are beginning to creep up again. "People—especially young gay men—are tired of the 'safe sex' message and the constant reminder to wear a condom," he says. "That condom, while providing protection, is also considered a barrier to intimacy. It's a rubber wall."

". . . while mortality rates among gays with HIV has declined, rates of infection are beginning to creep up again."

Consequently, it's a very difficult time for AIDS prevention, Gallagher says. The condom problem, coupled with the feeling that AIDS "is a chronic disease that you can live with," is making it hard to communicate the need for protection.

4. **Alcohol and substance abuse.** "It's not that gays are getting drunk or stoned and having spontaneous sex. They're using the substance in order to have an excuse for having unprotected sex."

That's Gallagher's explanation for the growing problem of alcohol and substance abuse among homosexuals. "The pressure to conform to societal norms has many gay men and lesbians feeling ashamed of who they are and the sex they prefer." So they drink and do drugs—namely ecstasy and crystal meth—so they have something to blame for giving in to their desires.

Gallagher admits that drug and alcohol use aren't unique to the gay community, but "the ramifications of indulging and then having unsafe sex are far scarier."

5. **Family relationships.** Having a family is as important to many gay couples as it is to straight ones. "That many of us are adopting children and giving them loving homes is beginning to influence the way society looks at gays," says Gallagher. "When you see a gay couple raising a family, it's hard to buy into the rhetoric that all gays are hedonistic," he says.

The trend among homosexuals to adopt has been dubbed the "Gay-by Boom" from within the community.

> "When you see a gay couple raising a family, it's hard to buy into the rhetoric that all gays are hedonistic . . . "

"Ten years ago, we didn't think it was possible," says Gallagher. "But again, it boils down to gay couples wanting to have the lives that everyone else has."

Gallagher points out that there are two states that ban gays from adopting—New Hampshire and Florida—and some states only allow one partner to officially adopt a child. Because of these roadblocks, many couples are also exploring methods of assisted reproduction, such as using surrogate mothers.

Whatever the path to becoming parents, Gallagher says studies have shown that children reared in gay households suffer no psychological harm. "If you're loved, you're loved. That's what counts."

6. **Discrimination.** Conservative Americans and the religious Right have coined the phrase "special rights" to refer to the antidiscrimination efforts being taken on behalf of homosexuals. "It's a brilliant sound bite," says Gallagher. "It plays really well because there is no counter. No group should receive 'special' rights."

But in truth, he explains, a person can be fired from a job because he is gay. And it's not actionable in many states. It's also difficult to prove and it requires a person to get up in court and discuss his private life—something that's often difficult for gay men and lesbians to do.

Consequently, Gallagher claims there are fewer than 20 gay-based discrimination cases filed each year. "Most people just fold up their tents and slip away.

"But it's not just about being fired," he says. "Just as women still face a glass ceiling, gays do too. Companies have a we're-glad-to-have-you-but-don't-count-on-being-CEO attitude."

7. **Housing.** In many ways, this issue is also about discrimination, says Gallagher, and it's not just a problem in small-town America. A gay couple bidding on a co-op in New York, for example, can have perfect credentials and financial means, but if someone on the board has a problem with homosexuality, the couple can be voted out. Sketchy laws in most states offer little recourse, and even if an individual or couple were to challenge a decision, the courts haven't been very supportive, says Gallagher.

> "A gay couple bidding on a co-op in New York, for example, can have perfect credentials and financial means, but if someone on the board has a problem with homosexuality, the couple can be voted out."

8. **Military service.** During President Clinton's first term in office, the subject of gays in the armed services was big news. The "Don't ask, don't tell policy" he offered as a compromise to an outright ban was deemed a cop out by the homosexual community. Though the issue has quieted lately, it's still a major point of contention among homosexuals, "primarily for what it represents and the message the current administration is sending," says Gallagher.

"By not allowing openly gay men and women in the military, it's saying that we're not good enough to fight for our country. It's saying that only straights can be warriors," says Gallagher. "There's an attitude that no heterosexual would be safe in a military that admits homosexuals. This relies on the worst stereotypes and sends an offensive and destructive message—especially in a country in which patriotism is so important."

9. **Pressure to remain in the closet.** Though admitting one's homosexuality can be difficult, Gallagher feels that gay men and lesbians feel more strained by a need to keep their lifestyle preference a secret. "The fear of losing friends, a job, and family support are all reasons why many homosexuals refuse to 'come out'," says Gallagher. "But if all homosexuals were 'out' it would show strength in numbers. People would realize that a lot of individuals—their friends, their relatives, their coworkers—are gay. That

it's very commonplace. Knowing someone gay would make society less likely to discriminate."

But getting over that hurdle is tough, admits Gallagher. Because most of society is still judgmental when it comes to homosexuality, "coming out" means taking all of those risks. "And coming out is not just a one-time thing. You can tell your family you're gay and they can be totally cool with it. But to truly affirm who you are, it's something that you have to repeat every time you meet someone new. You come out over and over again. It's tough, which is why many homosexuals don't do it."

10. **Spirituality.** Though many organized religions openly reject homosexuality as "heresy . . . against God's will," many members of the gay community understandably want religion in their lives—in whatever form it might take. Many are willing to do battle to return to their faith of choice, says Gallagher, and they're beginning to make inroads. "We're seeing the ordaining of gay clergy and a greater willingness among some clergy to perform commitment ceremonies."

Bibliography

Bechtel, Stefan, and Laurence Roy Stains. *Sex: A Man's Guide*. Pennsylvania: Rodale Press, 1996.

Birch, Robert W. *Male Sexual Endurance*. Ohio: PEC Publishing, 1997.

Block, Joel D. *The Secrets of Better Sex*. New York: Parker Publishing Co., 1996.

Chia, Mantak, and Douglas Abrams Arava. *The Multi-Orgasmic Man*. California: Harper SanFrancisco, 1996.

Chichester, Brian, and Kenton Robinson. *Sex Secrets*. Pennsylvania: Rodale Press, 1996.

Corn, Laura. *101 Grrreat Quickies*. Arizona: Park Avenue Publishers, Inc., 1996.

Corn, Laura. *101 Nights of Grrreat Romance*. Arizona: Park Avenue Publishers, Inc., 1996.

Corn, Laura. *101 Nights of Grrreat Sex*. Arizona: Park Avenue Publishers, Inc., 1995.

Crenshaw, Theresa L. *The Alchemy of Love and Lust*. New York: Pocket Books, 1996.

Diamond, Jed. *Male Menopause*. New York: Sourcebooks, 1998.

Eisenberg, Arlene, Heidi E. Murkoff, and Sandee E. Hathaway. *What to Expect When You're Expecting*. New York: Workman Publishing, 1984.

Fischer, Lynn. *The Better Sex Diet*. Washington, D.C.: Living Planet Press, 1996.

Frumkin, Lyn R., and John M. Leonard. *Questions and Answers on AIDS*. California: Health Information Press, 1997.

Gach, Michael Reed. *Accupressure for Lovers*. New York: Bantam Books, 1997.

Hicks, Roger W. and Victoria Day. *A Lover's Guide to Massage*. New York: Sterling Publishing Co., 1996.

Jacobowitz, Ruth S. *150 Most-Asked Questions about Midlife Sex, Love & Intimacy*. New York: Hearst Books, 1995.

Joannides, Paul. *The Guide to Getting It On*. California: Goofy Foot Press, 1996.

Love, Brenda. *Encyclopedia of Unusual Sex Practices*. New York: Barricade Books, 1992.

Massey, Doreen. *The Lovers' Guide Encyclopedia*. New York: Thunder's Mouth Press, 1996.

Milonas, Rolf. *Fantasex*. New York: Perigree Books, 1975.

Morgenthaler, John, and Dan Joy. *Better Sex Through Chemistry*. California: Smart Publication, 1994.

Neporent, Liz. *Crunch: A Complete Guide to Health and Fitness*. New York: Doubleday, 1997.

Odzer, Cleo. *Virtual Spaces*. New York: Berkley Books, 1997.

Rosenthal, Saul H. *Sex Over 40*. New York: Tarcher/Putnam, 1987.

Ryan, George. *Reclaiming Male Sexuality*. New York: M. Evans & Co., 1997.

Skriloff, Lisa, and Jodie Gould. *Men Are from Cyberspace*. New York: St. Martin's Griffin, 1997.

Silber, Sherman J. *How to Get Pregnant with the New Technology*. New York: Warner Books, 1991.

Taormino, Tristan. *The Ultimate Guide to Anal Sex for Women*. California: Cleis Press, 1998.

Westheimer, Ruth K. *Sex for Dummies*. California: IDG Books Worldwide, Inc., 1995.

White, James, R. *The Best Sex of Your Life*. New York: Barricade Books, 1996.

Winks, Cathy, and Anne Semans. *The New Good Vibrations Guide to Sex*. California: Cleis Press, 1997.

Zilbergeld, Bernie. *The New Male Sexuality*. New York: Bantam Books, 1992.

Illustration Credits

Photos pages ii, xiii, 2, 23, 24, 67, 97, 100, 102, 136, 137, 153, 154, 174, 182, 199, 200, 202, 212, 217, 235, 236, 238, 246, 251, 255, 258, 259, 261, 269, 271: Courtesy of *Men's Fitness* magazine, photography by Katrina Dickson, Roni Ramos, Robert Reiff, Cory Sorensen, Laura Wagner.

Photos pages 5, 8, 27, 31, 44, 45, 46, 47, 48, 49, 50, 51, 52, 53, 54, 112, 113, 114, 115, 132, 141, 157, 180, 231, 253, 264, 272, 274: Photography by Robert Reif, courtesy of MagicLight Productions.

Video tape boxes pictured page 141 courtesy of Candida Royalle, Femme Productions/Adam and Eve.

Author photo: Courtesy of John and Beth Tomkiw.

Line art pages 10, 11, 20, 22, 28: By Michael Brown and Cassio Lynm.

Photos and line art pages 21, 74, 77, 80, 81, 85, 87, 90, 91, 108–109, 184, 186, 194, 215, 250, 266, 267: Courtesy of The Philip Lief Group. Photography by David Kelly Crow.

Line art pages 29, 121, 122, 123, 124, 125, 126, 229: By Richard Stodart.

Photos pages 70, 144–145: Photography by Tom Keller

Photo page 71, 72: Courtesy of Sagami, Inc.

Photo page 120: Courtesy of the Greater Miami Convention and Visitors' Bureau

Photo page 165, 168: Courtesy of House of Whacks, Paul Natkin

Photo page 203: Courtesy of Celestial Seasonings, Inc., Boulder, CO

Photo page 225: Courtesy of Pfizer

Photo page 240: Photography by Katrina Dickson

Photo page 279: © 1982 NYSDED, all right reserved

Photo page 280, 285, 289: Courtesy of the Lesbian and Gay Community Services Center, New York City, Archives (Photo page 285 photographed by David Morgan)

Index

Abdomen
  exercises, *51–52*
  size, 40
  touching/massage, 25, 274
Abortion, 98–99
Acrophilia, 170
Acrotomophilia, 170
Adoption, 98
Adultery, The Forgivable Sin, 233
Acquired immunodeficiency syndrome. *See* AIDS
Acyclovir, 61
Adrenaline, 42
Africa, AIDS cases in, 64
Age of first sexual experience, 5
Aging
  children and, 191. *See also* Childbirth
  empty nest syndrome, 205–6
  female response to, 40
  fifties decade, 188–90
  forties decade, 186–88
  frequency of sexual activity and, 187
  lovemaking style changes, 204–5
  male health, 201–4, 206–11
    arthritis, 210
    career and, 204
    check-ups, 203
    diabetes, 211
    elderhood initiation, 204
    fitness, 202
    heart disease, 210–11

herbal supplements, 203
high blood pressure, 211
hormones, 203
men's groups and, 204
mentoring, 204
nutrition, 201
prostate concerns, 206–10
sexuality, 203–4
stress reduction, 203
testicular cancer, 206
vitamin supplements, 202–3
menopause
  female, 188–90
  male, 198–204
premenopause, 187
sixties decade and beyond, 190
thirties decade, 184–85
twenties decade, 181–84
Ahrons, Constance, 237
AIDS, 4, 55, 61–67, 284, 286
  control of, 65, 67
  HIV and, 62–63, 66
  reducing risk of, 64–65, 67–70
  statistics, 63–64
Alchemy of Love and Lust, The, 32, 199
Alcohol, 252
  abuse, 226, 286–87
Allergies, 222
Alman, Isadora, 103
American Academy of Clinical Sexology, 106, 213
American Academy of Pediatrics, 14

Report of the Task Force on Circumcision, 16
American Association of Sex Educators, Counselors and Therapists, 213
American attitudes, 3–4
American Baby, 16
Amodeo, John, 261
Anal sex, 127–29
Anal stimulation, 27–28, 135, 146–47
Anasteemaphilia, 170
Anginal pain, 211
Anguish, 251
Animal sexual behavior, 120
Antibiotics, 57, 58–59, 61, 207
Antidepressants
  phenylethylamine (PEA), 33
  sexual dysfunction and, 226, 227
  testosterone, 34
Antioxidants, 209
Anxiety, 185
Aphrodisiacs, 32, 275–76
Aphrodyne, 276
Appearance
  importance of, to relationship, 7
  pride in, 250
Applied Research-West, Inc., 4
Arachnephilia, 170
Arava, Douglas Abrams, 28
Arm(s)
  exercises, 44–46
  touching, 25–26

About the Authors

John and Beth Tomkiw have been married for twelve blissful years. He is a freelance writer; she is an editor at *Playboy* magazine. Prolific writers, their work has appeared in a variety of consumer magazines, including *Men's Fitness, Playboy, Self,* and *Maxim.* They reside in Chicago with their daughter, Claire Elizabeth, and their Labradors, Betty and Veronica. This is their first book about fornication.

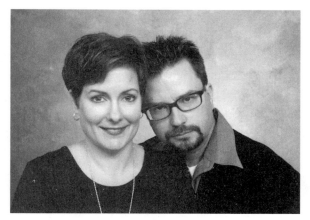

Beth and John